Frontiers in Arthritis

(*Volume 3*)

(Rheumatoid Arthritis: A systematic approach)

Edited by

Syuichi Koarada

Division of Rheumatology, Faculty of Medicine, Saga University, Saga, Japan

Frontiers in Arthritis

Volume # 3

Rheumatoid Arthritis: A systematic approach

Editor: Syuichi Koarada

ISSN (Online): 2468-6670

ISSN (Print): 2468-6662

ISBN (Online): 978-1-68108-661-3

ISBN (Print): 978-1-68108-662-0

General:

1. Any dispute or claim arising out of or in connection with this License Agreement or the Work (including non-contractual disputes or claims) will be governed by and construed in accordance with the laws of the U.A.E. as applied in the Emirate of Dubai. Each party agrees that the courts of the Emirate of Dubai shall have exclusive jurisdiction to settle any dispute or claim arising out of or in connection with this License Agreement or the Work (including non-contractual disputes or claims).

2. Your rights under this License Agreement will automatically terminate without notice and without the need for a court order if at any point you breach any terms of this License Agreement. In no event will any delay or failure by Bentham Science Publishers in enforcing your compliance with this License Agreement constitute a waiver of any of its rights.

3. You acknowledge that you have read this License Agreement, and agree to be bound by its terms and conditions. To the extent that any other terms and conditions presented on any website of Bentham Science Publishers conflict with, or are inconsistent with, the terms and conditions set out in this License Agreement, you acknowledge that the terms and conditions set out in this License Agreement shall prevail.

Bentham Science Publishers Ltd.
Executive Suite Y - 2
PO Box 7917, Saif Zone
Sharjah, U.A.E.
Email: subscriptions@benthamscience.org

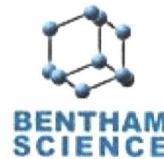

**BENTHAM
SCIENCE**

CONTENTS

PREFACE

Arthritis is a common condition, which affects joints and tissues surrounding the joints. It affects the patients widely and is one of the most common causes of disability. The eBook volume entitled "Rheumatoid Arthritis: A systematic approach," will provide a simplified but high-quality diagnostic interpretation of various radiographic images, including magnetic resonance imaging (MRI) and ultrasound. We hope to illustrate each disease by each volume, one by one. The contents of the series are based on my lectures that have been approved by our students and residents in Saga University, Japan. The diagnostic approach to make decision by conventional radiography is originated based on my experience of research and education in the division of the Rheumatology at the University of Pittsburgh, the U.S. However, arthritis images in the book are not only conventional radiographs but also images by multiple modalities. To make accurate diagnosis from radiographs, the methodology has been uniquely developed, through ABCDEGFGH (A; alignment, B; bone, C; cartilage, and D; distribution may be common, but E: extra-bone, F: further examination and G: goal and H; healing will be much more important) and improved by the experience of more than thousands of cases with rheumatic diseases in our institute.

In our various experienced cases, there are many interesting and rare cases. For example, there are a number of patients with Behçet's disease with arthritis. Our cohort also includes cases of adult onset at Still's disease (AOSD) with severe arthritis and are treated with various biologics and immunosuppressive drugs. Because we have established the diagnostic criteria of AOSD that has been approved world-widely, our hospital is one of the central institutes of AOSD in Japan and in the world. We have first proposed the method to prevent aseptic osteonecrosis of femoral head (AONF) induced by corticosteroid therapy in SLE patients. We found the novel marker of plasmablasts in IgG4-related disease (IgG4-RD). We also found that plasmablasts should be the targets for systemic lupus erythematosus (SLE) and various autoimmune diseases. We investigated new therapy for SLE and B cell targeting therapies. We performed ultrasound of the joints including hydro-US routinely (more than 1000 cases/year) and published reports of ultrasound. These original findings will be included in our series of arthritis which may be interesting for rheumatologists, orthopedists, physiatrists, pediatricians and general physicians. The series of "Frontier in Arthritis" will broadly cover osteoarthritis, rheumatoid arthritis (RA), SLE, juvenile arthritis, gout, systemic sclerosis, AOSD, Behçet's disease and so on. We present a systemic approach to understand the frontier of arthritis and diseases.

Syuichi Koarada
Division of Rheumatology
Faculty of Medicine, Saga University
Saga
Japan

List of Contributors

Akihito Maruyama Division of Rheumatology, Faculty of Medicine, Saga University, Saga, Japan

Mariko Sakai Division of Rheumatology, Faculty of Medicine, Saga University, Saga, Japan

Nobuyuki Ono Division of Rheumatology, Faculty of Medicine, Saga University, Saga, Japan

Syuichi Koarada Division of Rheumatology, Faculty of Medicine, Saga University, Saga, Japan

Yoshifumi Tada Division of Rheumatology, Faculty of Medicine, Saga University, Saga, Japan

Yuri Sadanaga Division of Rheumatology, Faculty of Medicine, Saga University, Saga, Japan

Yukiko Takeyama Division of Rheumatology, Faculty of Medicine, Saga University, Saga, Japan

CHAPTER 1

Basic Knowledge of Rheumatoid Arthritis

Syuichi Koarada[*], **Nobuyuki Ono** and **Yoshifumi Tada**

Division of Rheumatology, Faculty of Medicine, Saga University, Saga, Japan

Abstract: Rheumatoid arthritis (RA) is a systemic autoimmune disease characterized by proliferative synovitis and inflammatory arthritis with erosions. RA targets multiple peripheral joints including the metacarpophalangeal (MCP) and proximal interphalangeal (PIP) joints. Conventional radiography is still important, but recently, imaging of RA has been dramatically changed by magnetic resonance imaging (MRI) and ultrasonography (US). In this book, we aim to provide comprehensive understanding of RA by ABCDEFGH's new approach. A: alignment, B: bone, C: capsula articularis, intra-articular, D: distribution, E: extra-articular, F: further information, G: goal, and H: healing.

Keywords: ABCDEFGH's approach, Conventional radiography, Rheumatoid arthritis, Magnetic resonance imaging, Ultrasonography, Prevalence.

Rheumatoid arthritis (RA) is a chronic systemic autoimmune disease, which is primarily characterized by proliferative synovitis and inflammatory arthritis with erosions. The arthritis of RA affects symmetrically multiple peripheral joints and radiographs of a patient show erosive changes in the metacarpophalangeal (MCP) and proximal interphalangeal (PIP) joints. Although the conventional radiography is still important, recently, imaging of RA has been dramatically changed by the new modalities including magnetic resonance imaging (MRI) and ultrasonography (US). Sensitive imaging technology is necessary for the implementation of early diagnosis and preparation of individualized treatment protocols for RA.

An understanding of the clinical, pathophysiological and radiological characteristics of RA may be useful for the diagnosis of rheumatic diseases. In this volume, we present typical and distinctive X-ray findings of RA.

[*] **Corresponding author Syuichi Koarada:** Division of Rheumatology, Faculty of Medicine, Saga University, Saga, Japan; Tel: 81-952-31-6511; E-mail: koarada@cc.saga-u.ac.jp

The prevalence of RA is estimated to be about 0.5-1% of the adult population [1 - 2]. The ratio of women to men in the RA patients is 2-3 to 1 [1 - 2]. Although there is a possibility that RA will occur at any age, the peak age of onset is 45 to 65 years old [1 - 2]. The incidence of RA described in the literature is not racial or geographically different.

The pathogenesis of RA has not been elucidated but it is multifactorial. Genetics, environmental and immunological factors may affect this disease. RA has a specific genetic predisposition and approximately 70% of RA patients express human leukocyte antigen (HLA)-DR4 [3]. The concordance rate of twins is about 15-20% in RA [4]. There are other genes related to RA including STAT4 (signal transducer and activator of transcription 4), TRAF1/C5 (tumor necrosis factor-receptor associated factor 1/complement component 5), and PTPN22 (protein tyrosine phosphatase, non-receptor type 22).

It has been suggested that tobacco smoke, air pollution, occupational exposure to mineral oil and silica, infectious agents, and female hormones are involved in the disease. Autoimmunity, including antibodies such as anti-citrullinated peptide antibodies (ACPAs) and rheumatoid factors (RFs), is associated with RA. Immune dysregulation, antibody responses to modified peptides and increased production of cytokines and chemokines may contribute to pathophysiology of RA.

Because RA is a common disorder, most physicians are very familiar with clinical and radiologic features. For decades, rheumatologists have been evaluating the disease with conventional radiographs of joints using the ABCDs' approach. A; Alignment: deformities and fractures, B; Bone: mineralization, periarticular osteopenia, new bone formation, osteophytes, syndesmophytes, erosions, bone cysts, C; Cartilage: joint space and calcification, D; Distribution of the changes: pattern of joint involvement (regional, intra-articular, systemic, and time), S; Soft Tissues: swelling, and subcutaneous calcification. However, the latest information of advanced modalities including MRI and US also needs to be included in the approach. Furthermore, the state of the intra-articular and extra-articular structures can be clearly distinguished by the new modalities.

Therefore, the category of "S" should be reconsidered since the soft tissues consists of various structures. In this volume, "S" is divided into two categories " C" and "E". The category of "C" consists of components of the intra-articular structures, articular synovitis, joint effusion, intra-articular calcification, cartilage, and joint space. Also, the category of "E" consists of extra-articular structures including tendons, ligaments, skin, bursae, enthesis, subcutaneous soft tissues, nerves, arteries, and veins.

The following approach is helpful for the diagnosis of RA.

A: alignment
B: bone
C: capsula articularis, intra-articular
D: distribution
E: extra-articular
F: further information
G: goal
H: healing

This book is intended to provide a comprehensive understanding of RA by ABCDEFGH's new approach. However, the pathology of RA is very broad and it is difficult to cover all aspects of RA in this Book. We hope to further improve this book with criticism and suggestion from precious readers.

CONSENT FOR PUBLICATION

Not applicable.

CONFLICT OF INTEREST

The author (editor) declares no conflict of interest, financial or otherwise.

ACKNOWLEDGEMENTS

The authors thank Ms. K. Eguchi and A. Ibe for secretarial assistance.

REFERENCES

[1]   Gabriel SE. The epidemiology of rheumatoid arthritis. Rheum Dis Clin North Am 2001; 27: 269-82.

[2]   Dugowson CE, Koepsell TD, Voigt LF, Bley L, Nelson JL, Daling JR. Rheumatoid arthritis in women: incidence rates in group health cooperative, Seattle, Washington, 1987–9. Arthritis Rheum 1991; 34: 1502-7.

[3]   Deighton CM, Cavanagh G, Rigby AS, Lloyd HL, Walker DJ. Both inherited HLA-haplotypes are important in the predisposition to rheumatoid arthritis. Br J Rheumatol 1993; 32: 893-8.

[4]   Deighton CM, Walker DJ. The familial nature of rheumatoid arthritis. Ann Rheum Dis 1991; 50: 62-5.

CHAPTER 2

A: Alignment

Syuichi Koarada[*] and **Mariko Sakai**

Division of Rheumatology, Faculty of Medicine, Saga University, Saga, Japan

Abstract: Category A is alignment. Alignment includes mal-alignment, deformities and fractures, axis, subluxation, luxation, height of carpals, abnormal outline of bones. Mal-alignments and deformities of the joints are common in rheumatoid arthritis (RA). There are various deformities including swan-neck deformities, Button-hole deformities, ulnar deviation of the MCP joints, palamarsubluxation at the MCP joints, Zigzag deformities, splaying laterally of the digits, and so on. In the spine, atlantoaxial subluxation is important in RA.

Keywords: Deformities, Luxation, Mal-alignment, Rheumatoid arthritis.

INTRODUCTION

Category A: Alignment is the positioning of the bones in the joints.

Mal-alignments and deformities of the joints (Fig. **1**) are frequent in RA due to laxity and disruption of the capsules, ligaments, and tendons.

Findings of mal-alignment include abnormal axis, loss of height of carpals, deformity, (sub)-luxation, fracture, and abnormal outline of bones.

Plain radiographs of the hands include the posteroanterior view (PA view) (Fig. **2**), oblique view (Fig. **3**), lateral view (Fig. **4**), ball-catch view (Nørgaard view) (Figs. **5** and **6**), and so on.

DEFORMITIES

Deformities of the joints of patients with RA can occur in any joints, although they are frequently found in the hand, wrist, foot, and neck.

[*] **Corresponding author Syuichi Koarada:** Division of Rheumatology, Faculty of Medicine, Saga University, Saga, Japan; Tel: 81-952-31-6511; E-mail: koarada@cc.saga-u.ac.jp

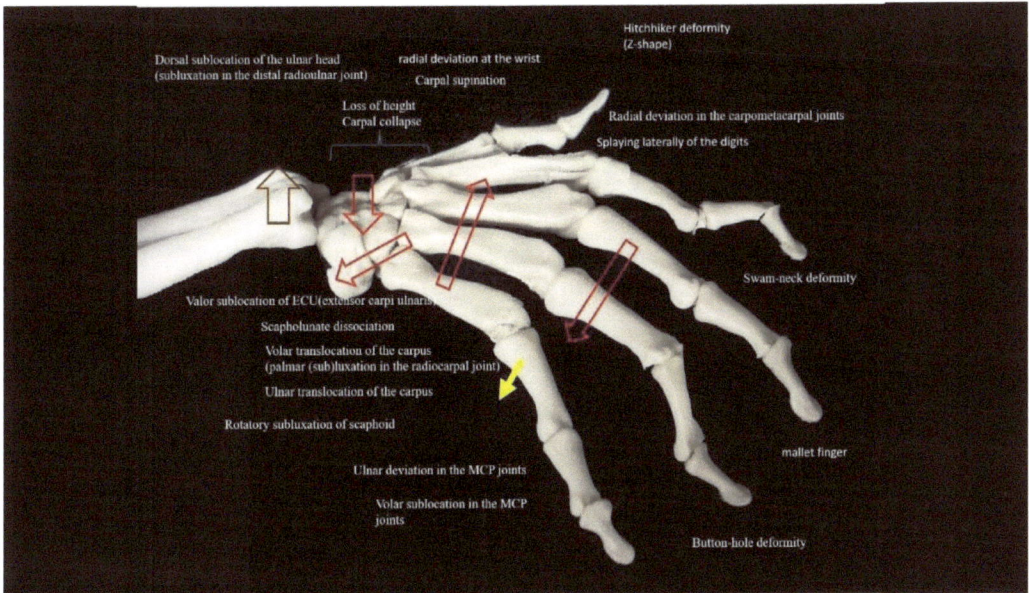

Fig. (1). Mal-alighments and deformities of joints of the hand and wrist in patients with RA.

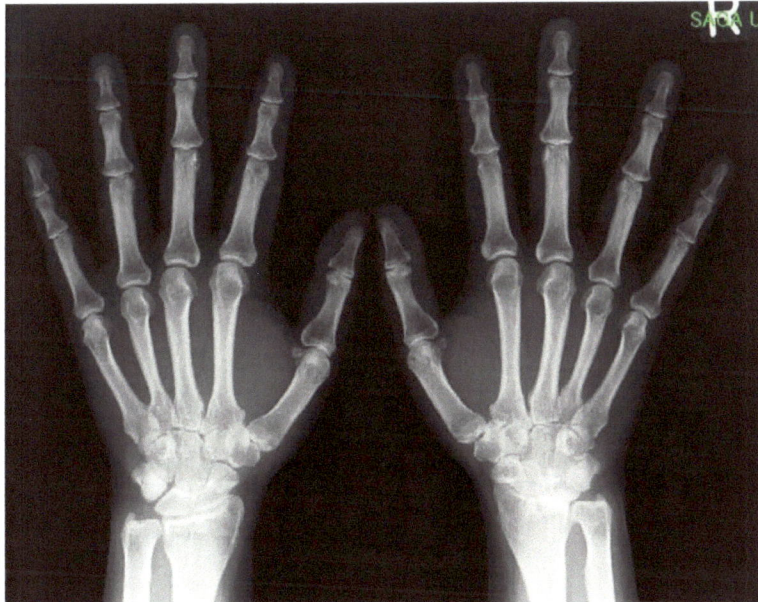

Fig. (2). PA view of the hands of a patient with RA.

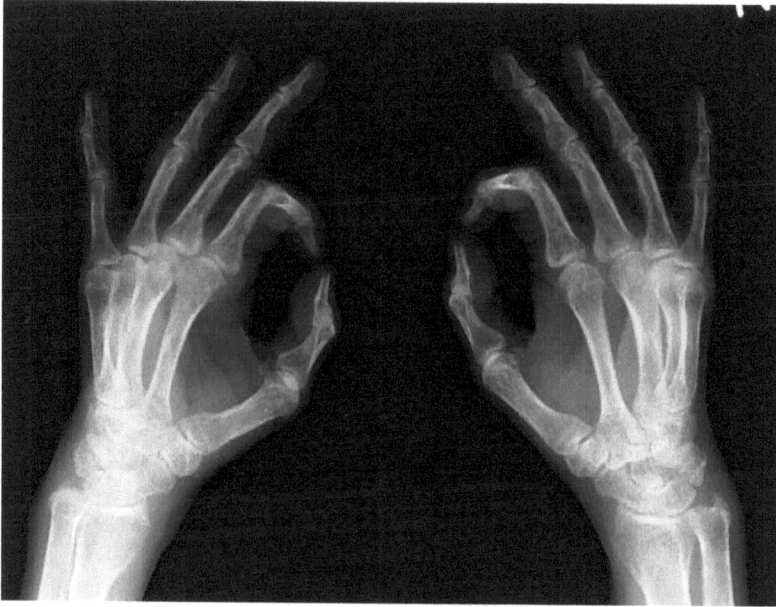

Fig. (3). Oblique view of the hands of a patient with RA.

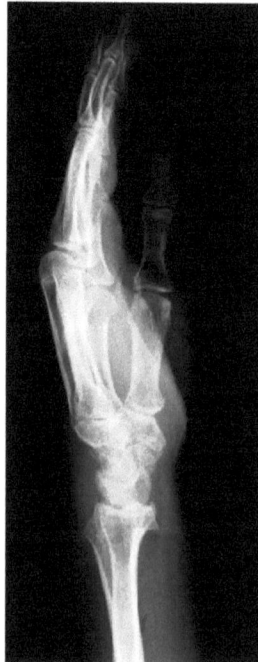

Fig. (4). Lateral view of the hand of a patient with RA.

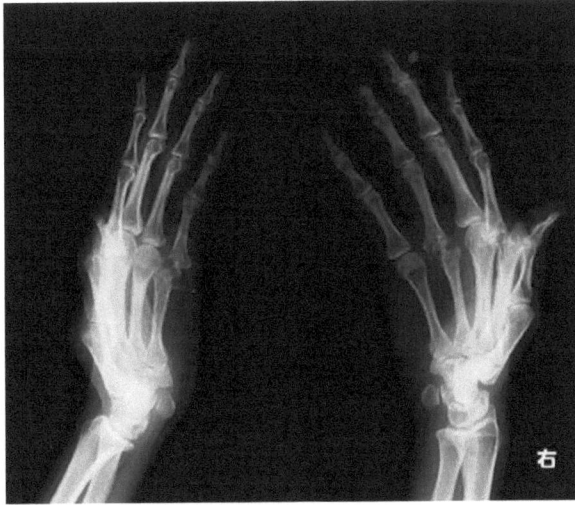

Fig. (5). Ball-catch view (Nørgaard view) of the hands of a patient with RA.

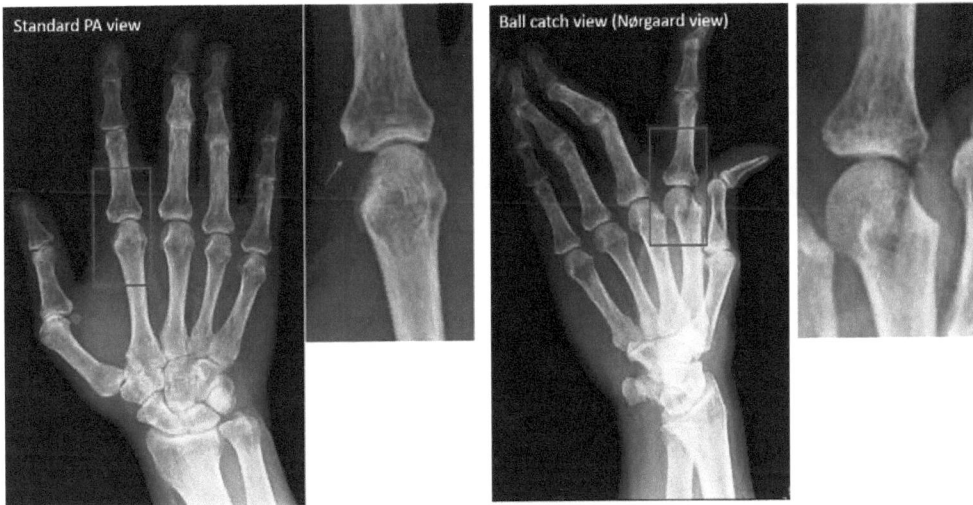

Fig. (6). To detect an erosion at the 2nd MCP joint of a patient with RA is difficult in plain PA view of the right hand. However, ball-catch view (Nørgaard view) clearly shows an erosion in the patient with RA.

Fingers and Thumbs

Deformities of the fingers and thumbs are very common features of RA because the balanced tendon mechanism is compromised by the arthritis. A schema of the hands and the wrists resembling ancient army (Figs. **7** and **8**). Radiographic anatomy of the skeleton of the hands and wrists is shown (Figs. **9 - 18**).

In RA, deformities of the fingers include swan-neck deformity, button-hole deformity (boutonniere deformities), and mallet finger, and hitchhiker's deformity

(Z-shaped deformity) of the thumb can also occur.

Structure of 1-5 lines, 3+3lines and larger I in upper limb

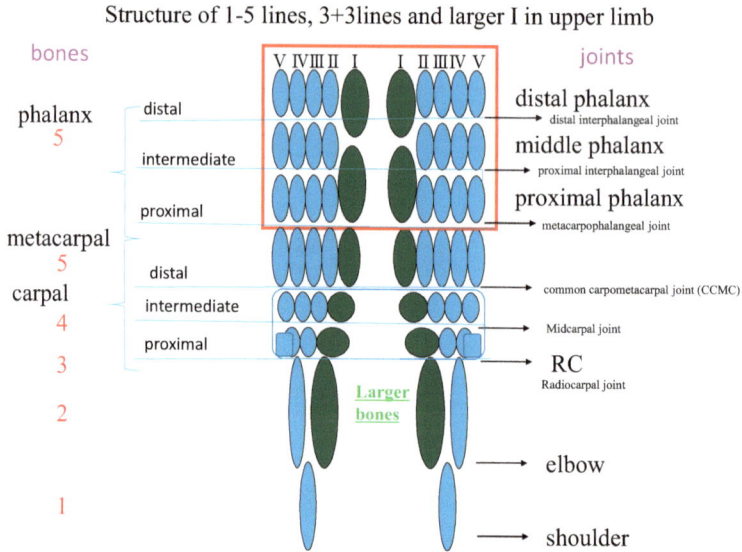

Fig. (7). A schema of the hands and the wrists resembling ancient army.

φάλαγξ, phalanx⇒phalangeal

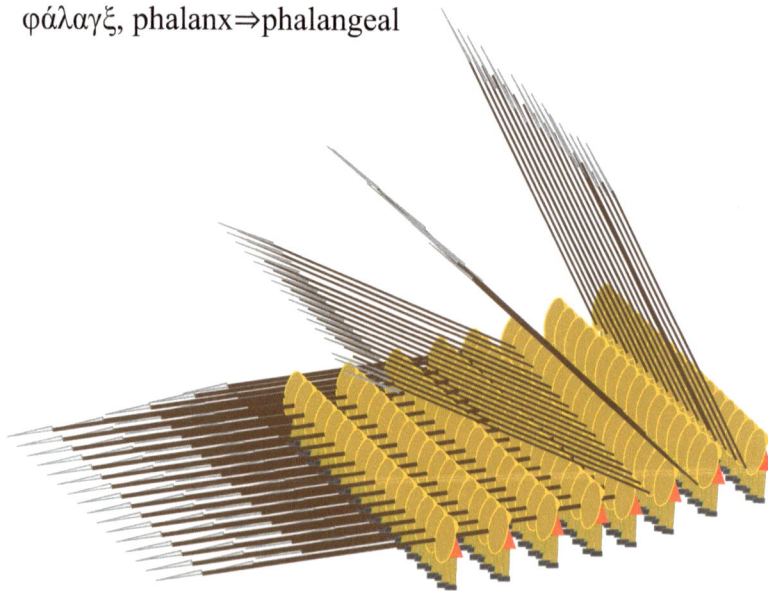

Fig. (8). Phalanx: an ancient Greek and Macedonian military unit resembles the structure of the hand bones. The phanx consists of several lines of soldiers in close array with joined shields and long spears (muscles and ligaments).

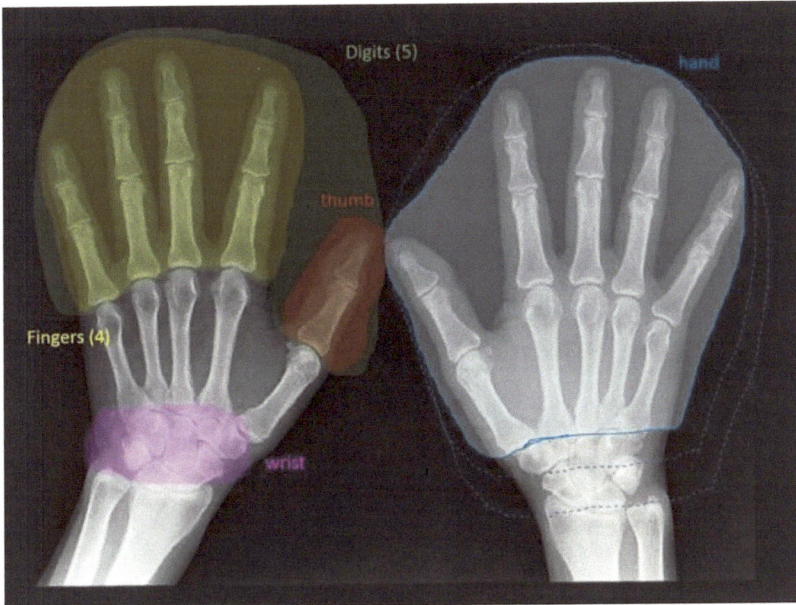

Fig. (9). Radiographic anatomy of the skeleton of the hands and wrists: PA view.

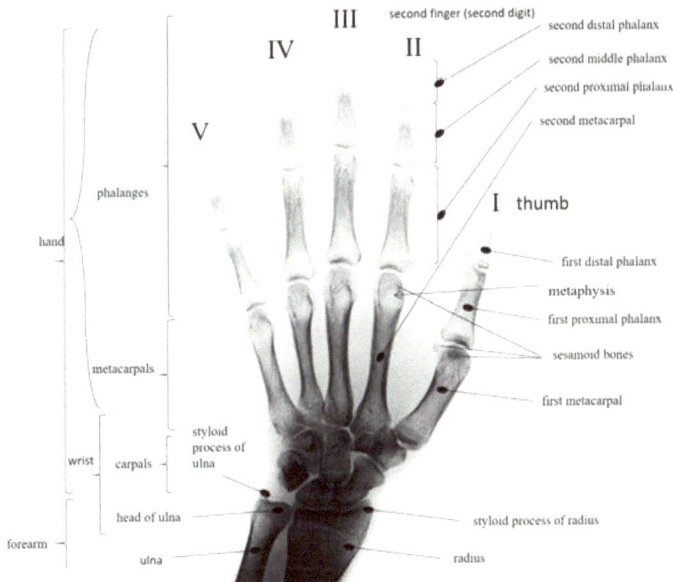

Fig. (10). Radiographic anatomy of the skeleton of the hand and the wrist: PA view.

Tuberosity of distal phalanx

Head of phalanx

Shaft(body) of phalanx

Base of phalanx

Head of metacarpal

Shaft of metacarpal

Base of metacarpal

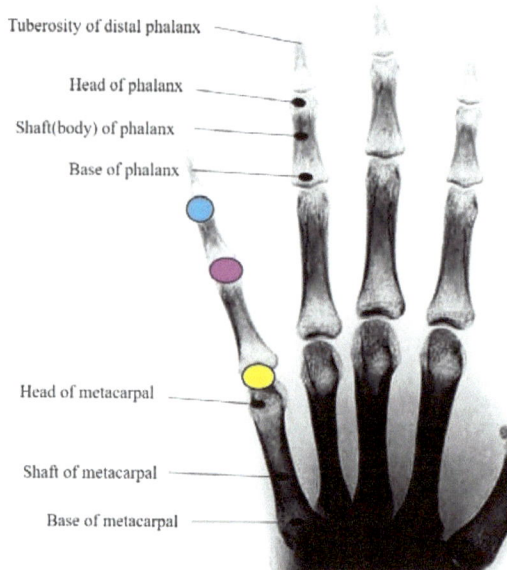

Fig. (11). The bones of the phalanges and metacarpals.

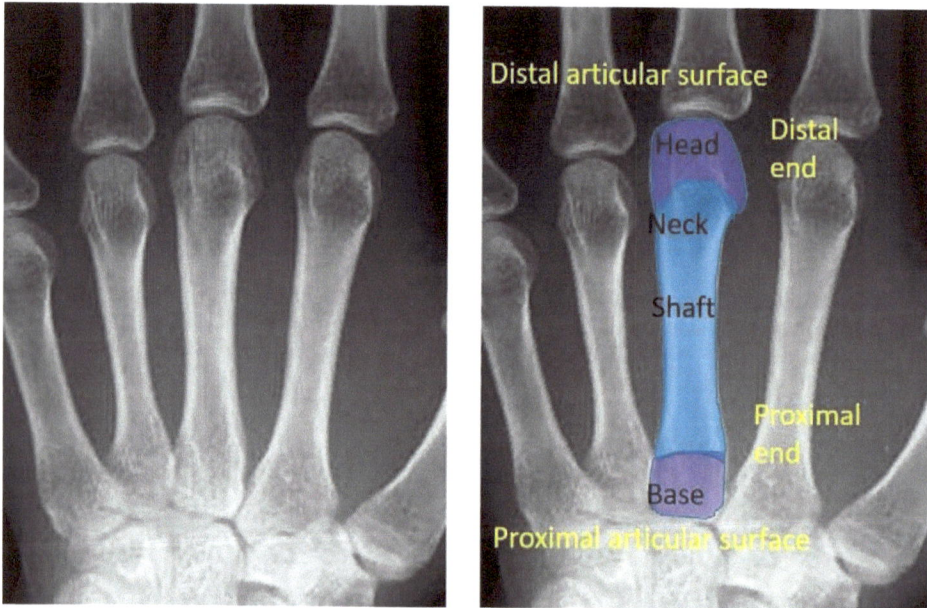

Distal articular surface

Distal end

Head

Neck

Shaft

Proximal end

Base

Proximal articular surface

Fig. (12). Radiographic anatomy of the skeleton of the finger: PA view.

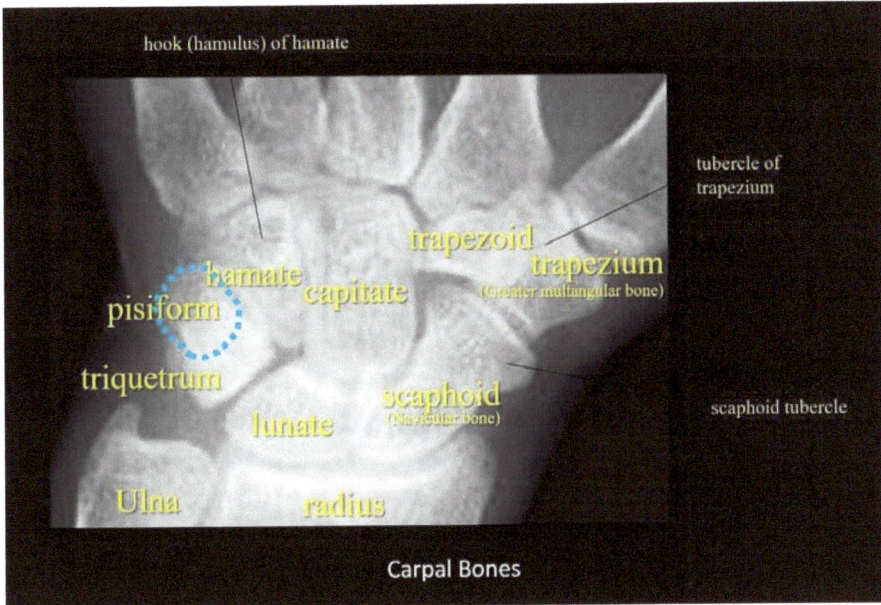

Fig. (13). Radiographic anatomy of the skeleton of carpal bones.

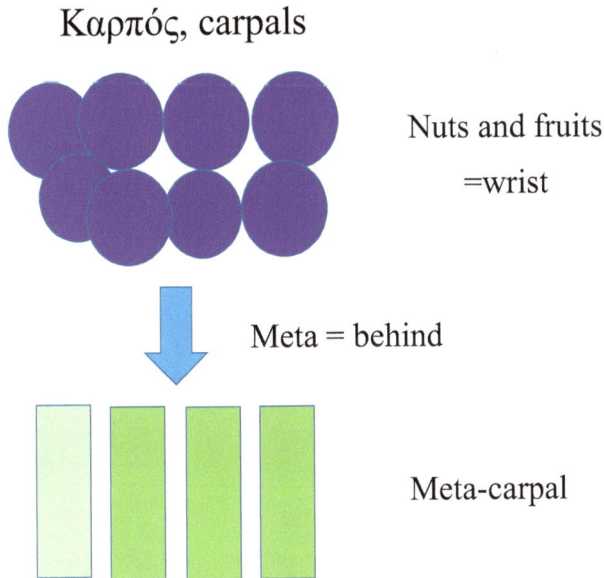

Fig. (14). A schema of the carpals resembling nuts and fruits.

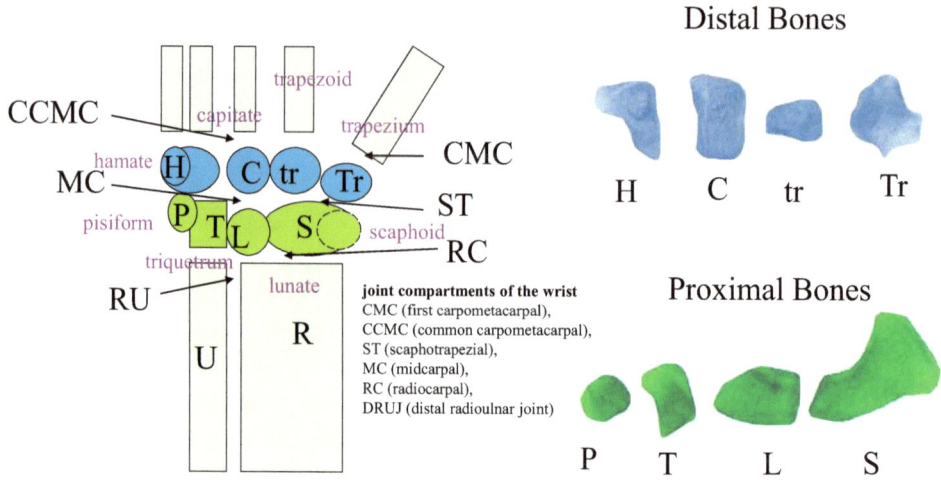

Fig. (15). Joint compartments of the wrist.

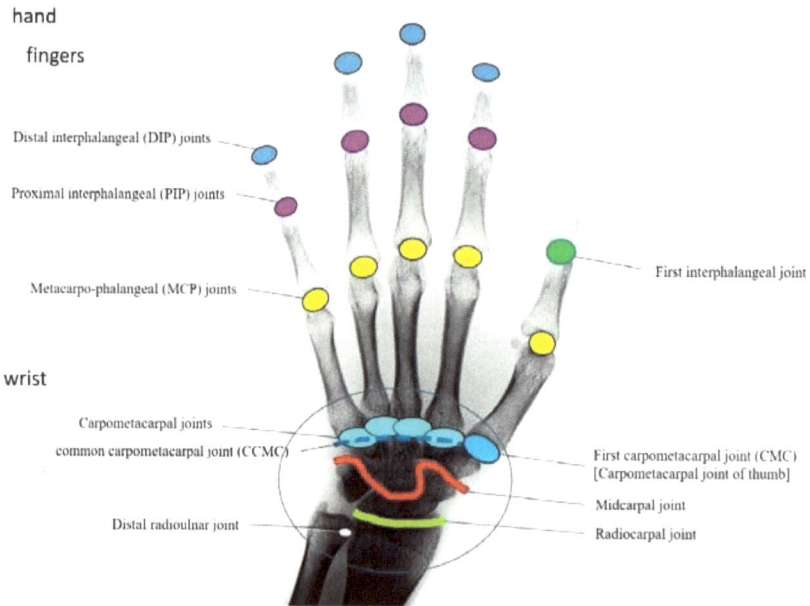

Fig. (16). The joints of the left hand.

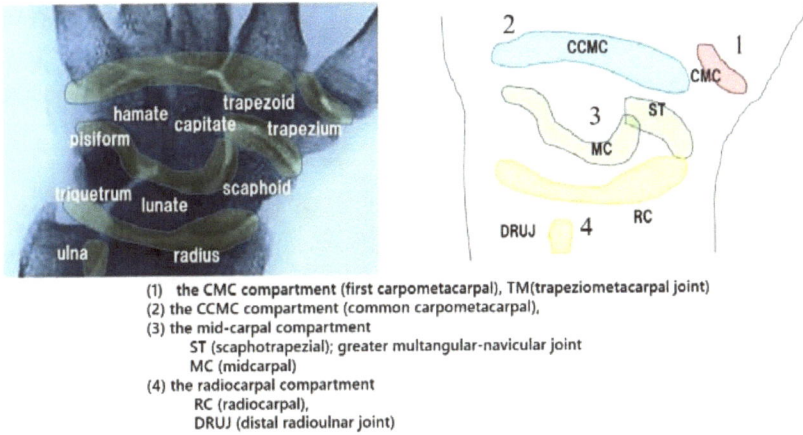

(1) the CMC compartment (first carpometacarpal), TM(trapeziometacarpal joint)
(2) the CCMC compartment (common carpometacarpal),
(3) the mid-carpal compartment
         ST (scaphotrapezial); greater multangular-navicular joint
         MC (midcarpal)
(4) the radiocarpal compartment
         RC (radiocarpal),
         DRUJ (distal radioulnar joint)

Fig. (17). Joint compartments of the wrist.

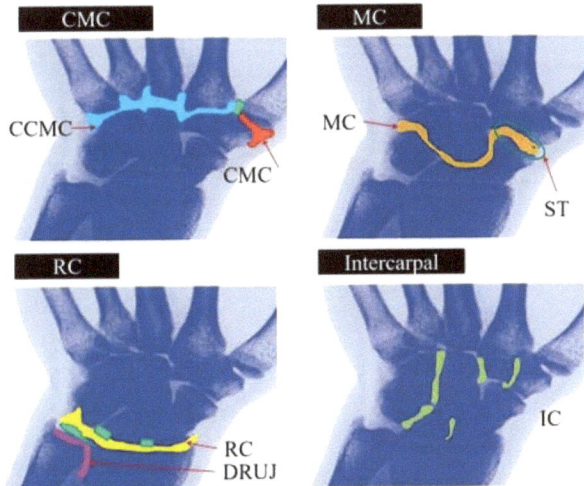

Fig. (18). Joints in the wrist.

Swan-neck Deformities

Swan-neck deformity consists of hyperextension at the PIP joint and flexion at the distal interphalangeal (DIP) joint (Figs. **19 - 22**). The primary cause of the deformity may be the restriction of interphalangeal joint flexion due to tenosynovitis of the flexor tendon.

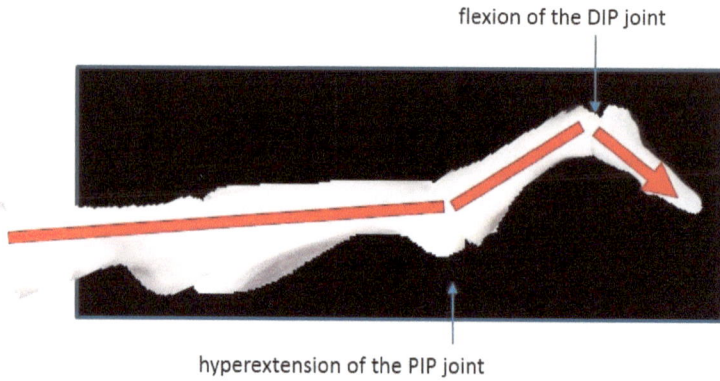

Fig. (19). A simplified schema of swan-neck deformity of the digit. Extension of PIP, flexion of DIP.

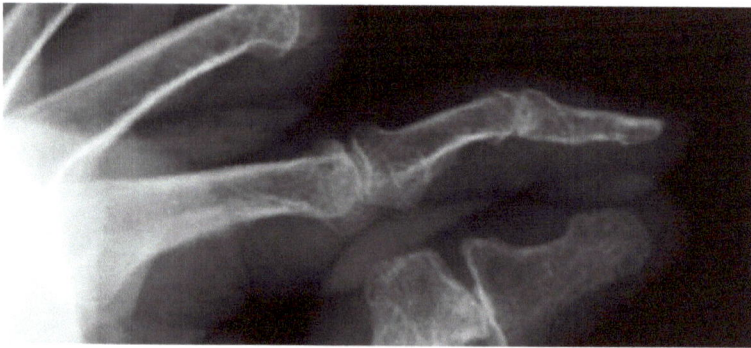

Fig. (20). Mild swan-neck deformity of the digit (the 2nd finger) is observed in a patient with RA.

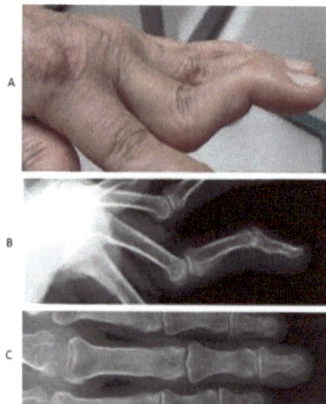

Fig. (21). Severe swan-neck deformities.
A. Severe swan-neck deformities of the third and fourth digits are observed in a patient with RA.
B. Lateral view of the third digit shows severe swan-neck deformity.
C. PA view of the third digit may not illustrate the deformities as the patient is required to press the hands down firmly against the plate.

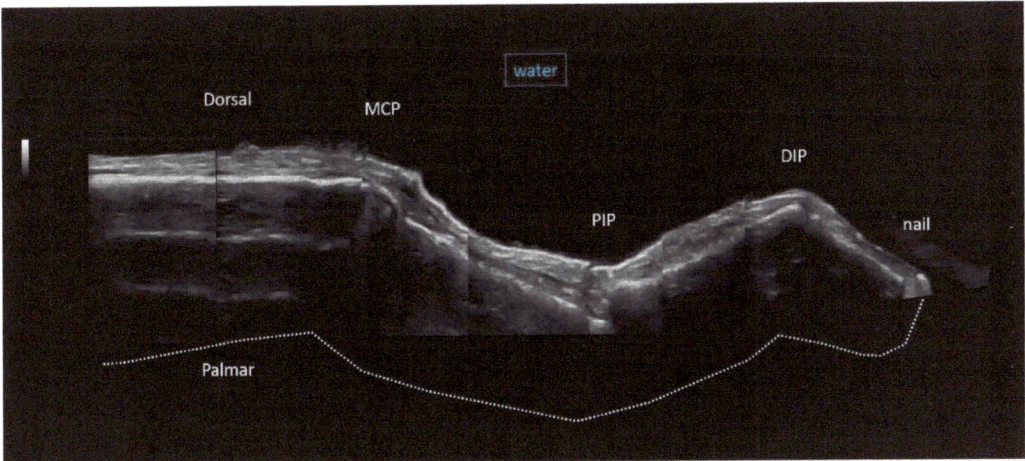

Fig. (22). Longitudinal gray-scale US image over the dorsal aspect of the third digit in water shows the swan-neck deformity.

Button-hole Deformities (boutonnière Deformities)

Button-hole deformity (boutonnière deformity) consists of hyperextension at the DIP joint and flexion at the PIP joint (Figs. **23 - 27**). The dorsal aspect of the PIP joint may have an extensor lag due to the disruption of the central slip. After the central slip disruption, the lateral bands migrate volar side and eventually it may create a pathologic extension of the DIP joint.

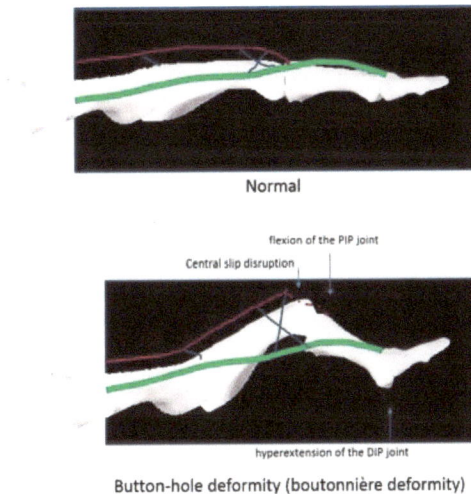

Fig. (23). A simplified schema of button-hole (boutonnière) deformity of the digit. Extension of DIP, flexion of PIP. After central slip (red line) disruption, the lateral bands (green line) migrate volar side.

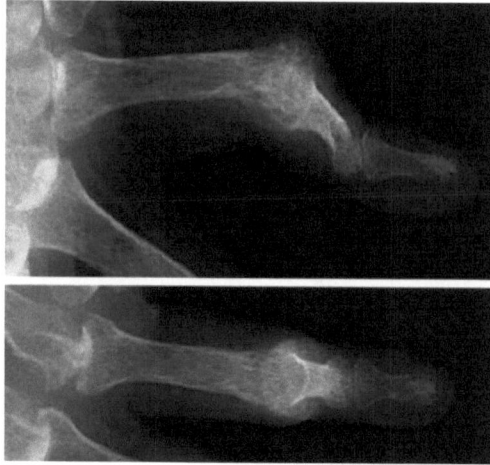

Fig. (24). Typical button-hole (boutonnière) deformity of the digit in a patient with RA.

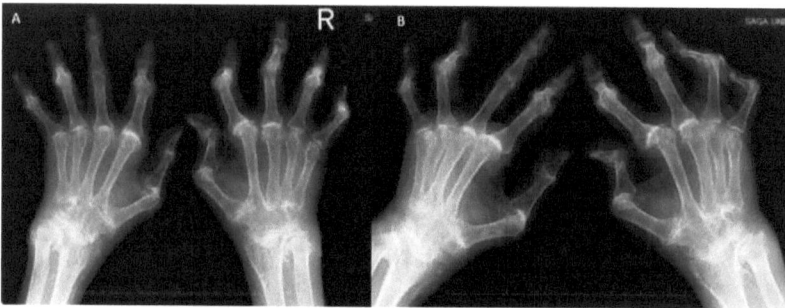

Fig. (25). Moderate button-hole (boutonnière) deformities of the digits. A. PA view of the hands of a patient with RA. Classical button-hole (boutonnière) deformities of the digits are evidently observed. B. Oblique view of the hands of the same patient.

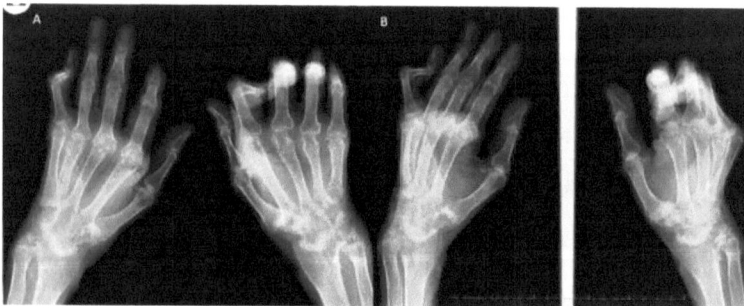

Fig. (26). Severe button-hole (boutonnière) deformities of the digits.
A. PA view of the hands. Button-hole (boutonnière) deformities of the right second and left fifth digits are evident in a patient with RA.
B. Oblique view of the hand of the same patient.

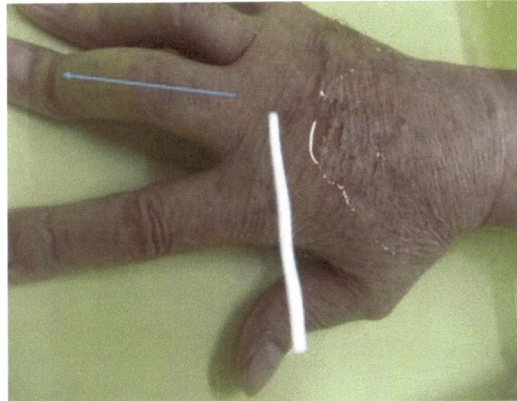

Fig. (27). Button-hole (boutonnière) deformities.

Deformities of the Metacarpophalangeal (MCP) Joints

Ulnar deviations (dislocation, drift), palmar subluxations, and extensor tendon subluxations occur at the MCP joints of the hand in RA. The subluxations at the MCP joints occur in the inflammatory arthritis, especially in RA patients.

Ulnar Deviations of the MCP Joints

Ulnar deviations of the MCP joints are common in 25-65% the hands in patients with RA. The proximal phalanges drift in an ulnar side in relationship to the metacarpal heads due to a possible mechanical compensation for the radial deviation at the wrist (Figs. **28 - 30**).

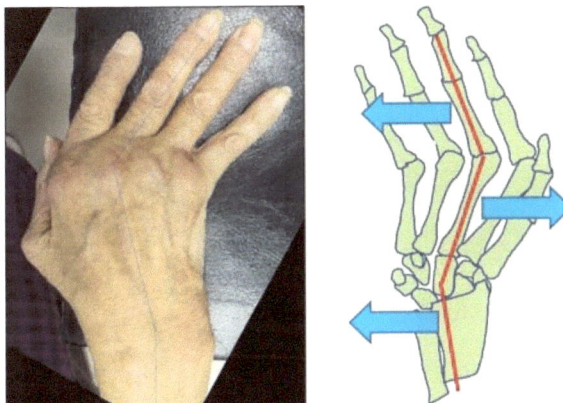

Fig. (28). A simplified schema of ulnar deviations at the MCP joints and the radial deviation at the wrist.

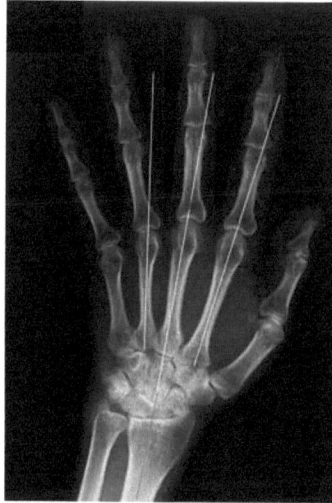

Fig. (29). Mild ulnar deviations at the MCP joints. PA view of the left hand of a patient with RA shows mild ulnar deviations at the MCP joints.

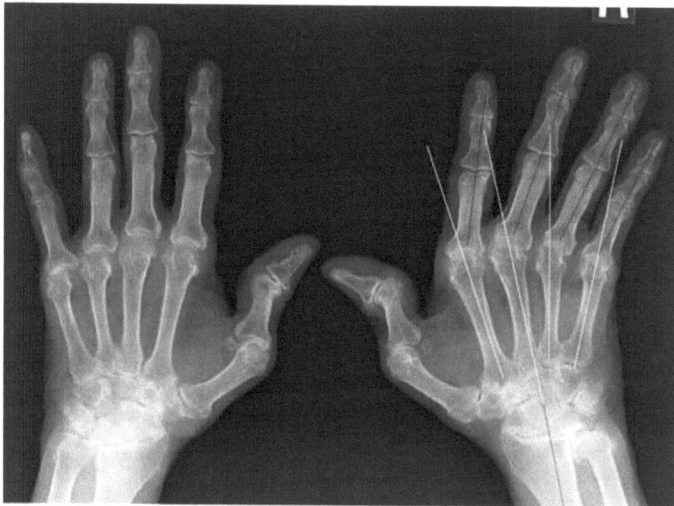

Fig. (30). Severe ulnar deviations of the MCP joints. PA view of the hands of a patient with RA demonstrating severe ulnar deviations at the right MCP joints with erosions.

Palmar Subluxations at the MCP Joints

The palmar subluxations also occur in the hands of patients with RA. The bases of proximal phalanges shift palmar in relationship to the metacarpal heads (Figs. **31 - 33**).

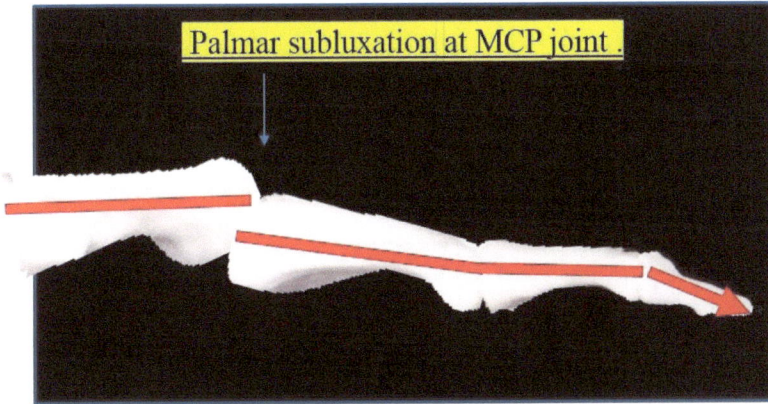

Fig. (31). A simplified schema of the palmar subluxation at the MCP joint.

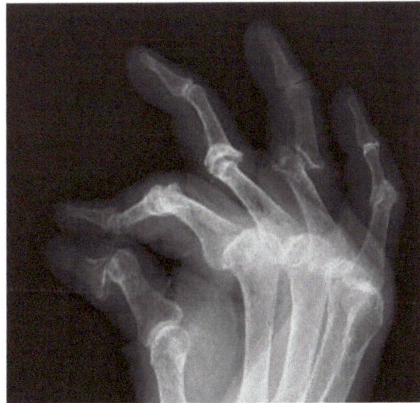

Fig. (32). Oblique view of the right hand of a patient with RA exhibiting the palmar subluxations at the MCP joints. In all fingers, the bases of proximal phalanges move palmar in relationship to the metacarpal heads.

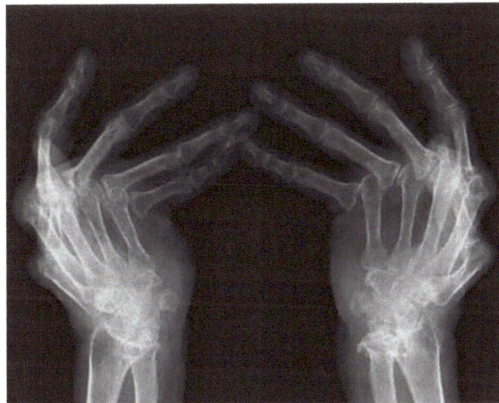

Fig. (33). Nørgaard view of the hands of a patient with RA shows severe subluxations and luxations at the MCP joints.

Zigzag Deformities

The zigzag deformity of the hand and the wrist in RA consists of radial deviation of the wrist and ulnar deviation at the MCP joints due to imbalance of muscles and tendons (Figs. **34 - 37**).

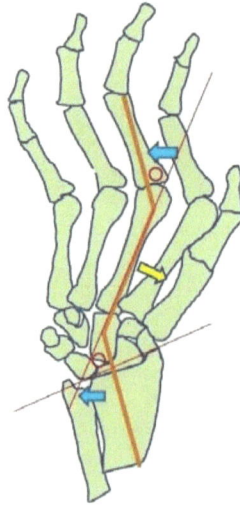

Fig. (34). A simplified schema of zigzag deformity caused by radial deviation at the wrist with ulnar deviation at the MCP joints.

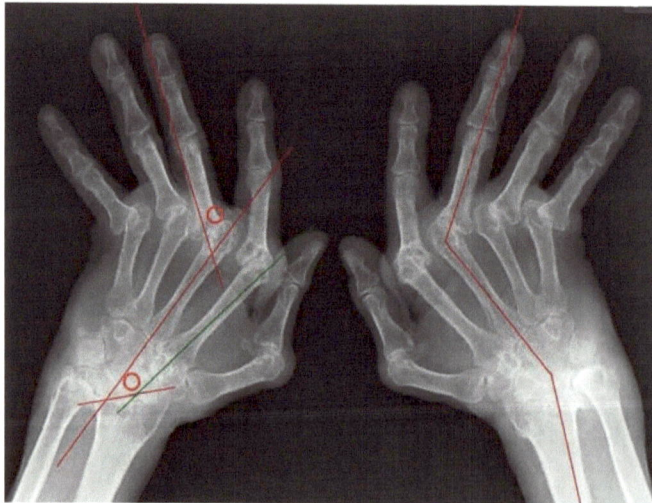

Fig. (35). Severe Zigzag deformities with subluxations. PA view of the hands and wrists shows severe zigzag deformities consisting of the changes of ulnar deviations at the MCP joints and radial deviations at the RC (radiocarpal) joints of the wrists in a patient with RA.

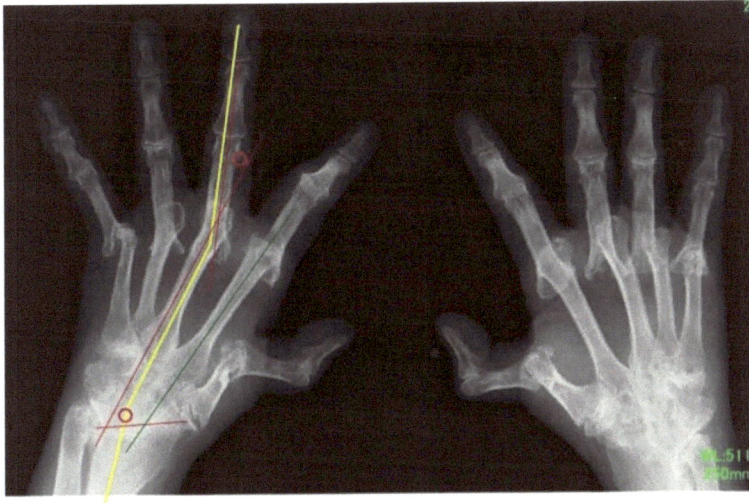

Fig. (36). Moderate zigzag deformities with luxations.PA view of the hands and wrists shows moderate zigzag deformities consisting of the changes of ulnar deviations and luxations at the MCP joints and radial deviations at the RC joints of the wrists in a patient with RA.

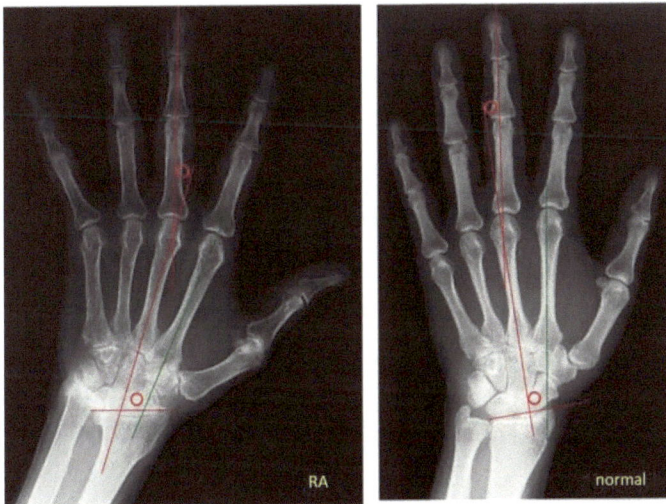

Fig. (37). Mild zigzag deformity without subluxations. PA view of the left hand and wrist shows the mild zigzag deformity in a patient with RA. PA view of a normal person demonstrating normal alignment of the left hand and wrist.

Splaying Laterally of the Digits

The pressure of hypertrophy of synovial membranes and increase fluid accumulation in the MCP joints make metacarpal heads shift laterally and the digits may spread out (Fig. **38**).

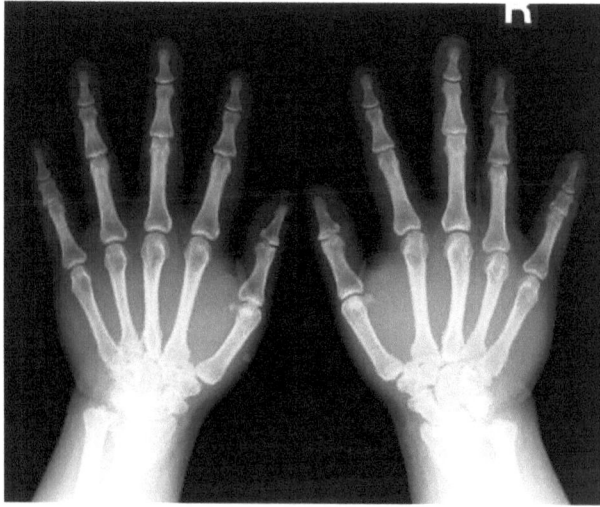

Fig. (38). Splaying laterally of the digits at the MCP joints in a patient with RA.

Cup-and-saucer Deformities

Cup-and-saucer deformity may be found in the late stage of RA. Pointed residual bone of the metacarpal bone (cup) and grooved destruction of the proximal phalanx (saucer) articulate at the MCP joints with each other (Figs. **39** and **40**).

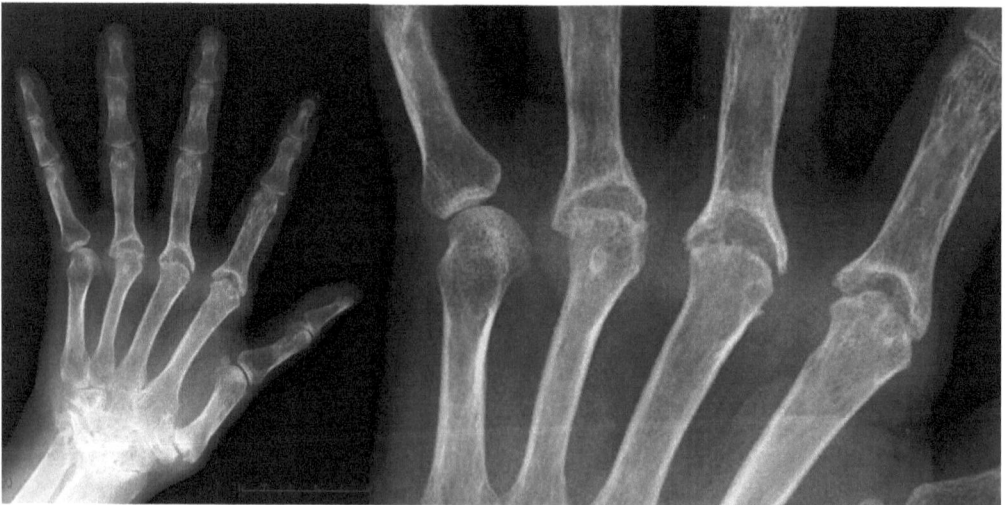

Fig. (39). Cup-and-saucer deformities in a patient with RA.

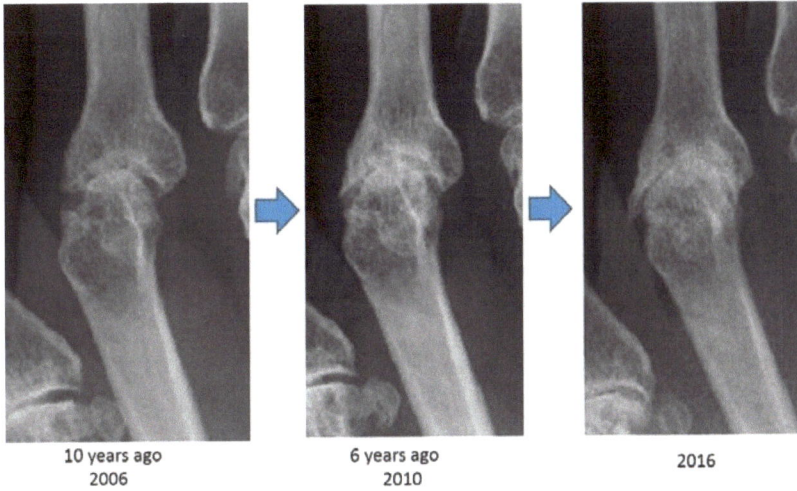

| 10 years ago
2006 | 6 years ago
2010 | 2016 |

Fig. (40). From left to right progressive changes over a 10-year period of cup-and-saucer deformity at the right 2nd MCP joint in a patient with RA.

Deformities of PIP Joints

Lateral Subluxations at the PIP Joints

Sometimes, lateral subluxations may be found in patients with RA (Figs. **41** and **42**).

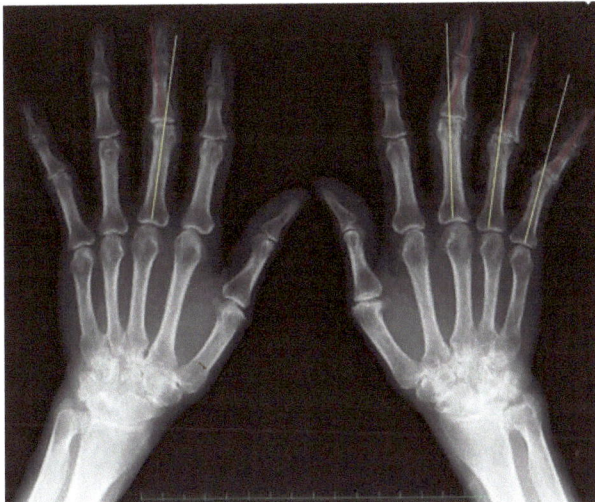

Fig. (41). PA view of the hands shows lateral subluxations of the bases of the middle phalanges in relationship to the proximal phalanges of the digits in a patient with RA.

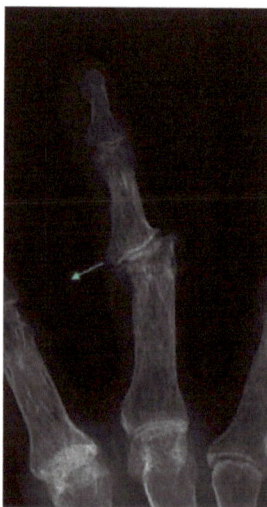

Fig. (42). Subluxation at the third PIP joint of a patient with RA.

Deformities of DIP Joints

Mallet Fingers

Mallet finger is the flexion of the distal phalanx of a finger at the DIP joint due to the disruption or tearing of the extensor tendon (Figs. **43-45**). However, this is not common in patients with RA.

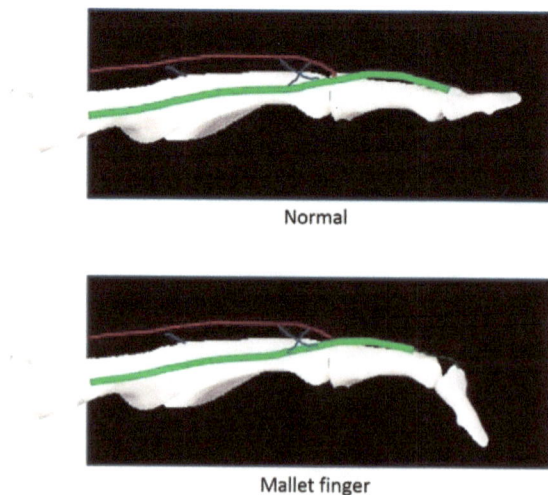

Normal

Mallet finger

Fig. (43). A simplified schema of Mallet finger in RA.

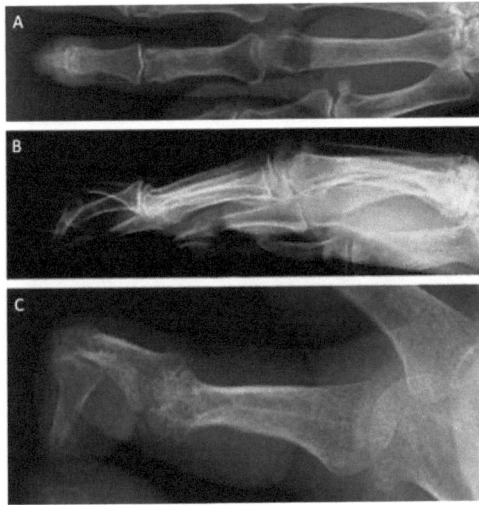

Fig. (44). Severe Mallet finger deformity of the right 2nd digit of a patient with RA. A, PA view; B, lateral view; and C, oblique view of the finger.

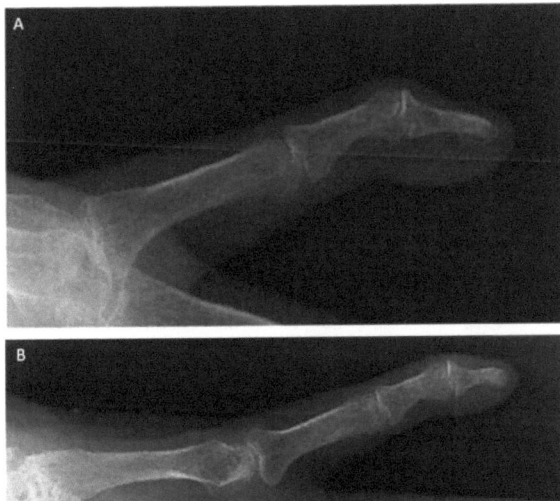

Fig. (45). Mild Mallet finger deformity of the left 5th digit in a patient with RA. A, Lateral view; and B, PA view.

Thumb Deformities

Thumb Deformities are common in patients with RA [1, 2]. Destruction of the joints and stretching of the collateral ligaments and the joint capsules are induced by the synovial hypertrophy at the joints of the thumbs. Then, the joints are unstable and deforming mechanisms of the extensor or flexor tendons act on the joints.

Hitchhiker Thumb Deformities (Boutonnière Deformities, Z-shape Deformities)

Hitchhiker thumb deformity (boutonniere deformity, or Z-shape deformity) is the most common deformity of the thumb in patients with RA. Hitchhiker thumb deformity consists of flexion of the MCP joint and hyperextension of the IP joint (Figs. **46** and **47**).

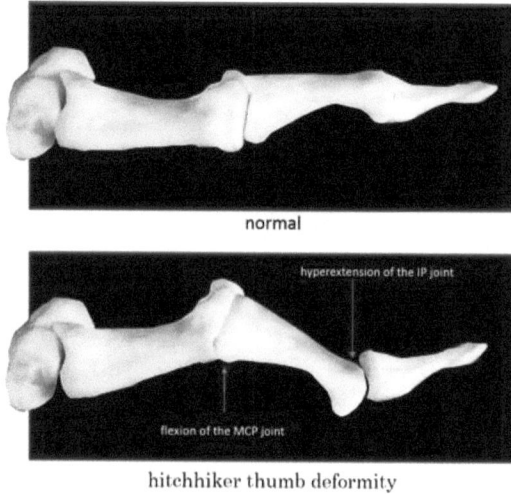

normal

hyperextension of the IP joint

flexion of the MCP joint

hitchhiker thumb deformity

Fig. (46). A simplified schema of hitchhiker thumb deformity in patients with RA.

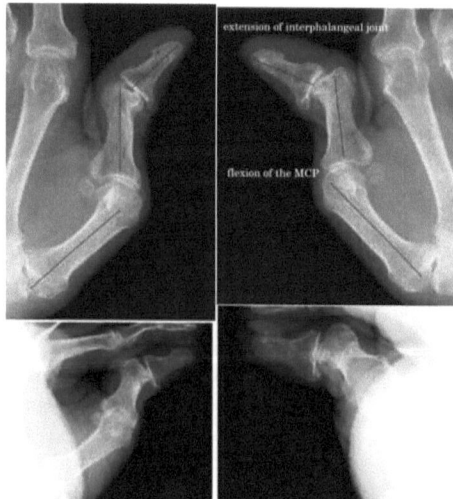

extension of interphalangeal joint

flexion of the MCP

Fig. (47). Radiographs of hitchhiker thumb deformities in a patient with RA.

Swan-neck Deformities of the Thumbs

Swan-neck deformity of the thumb is common. It consists of subluxation at the CMC joint, hyperextension at the MCP joint, and flexion at the IP joint (Figs. **48 - 50**).

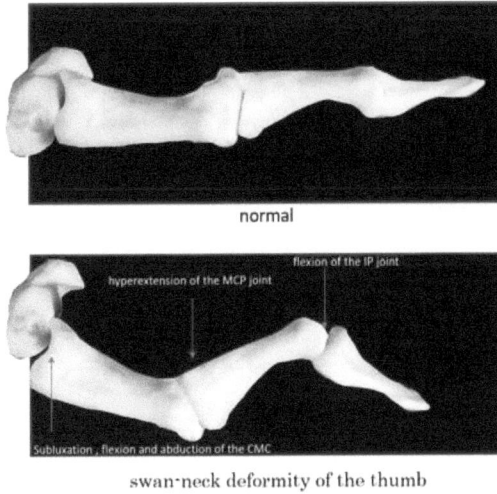

normal

swan-neck deformity of the thumb

Fig. (48). A simplified schema of swan-neck deformity of the thumb in patients with RA.

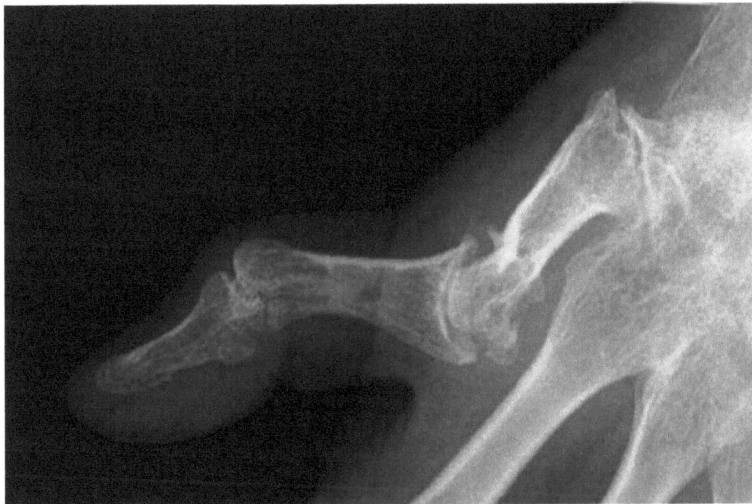

Fig. (49). Swan-neck deformity of the thumb in a patient with RA.

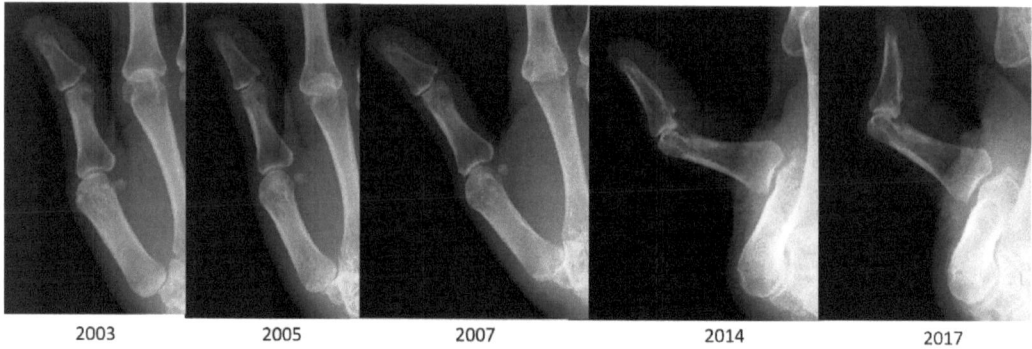

Fig. (50). From left to right the development of over a 14-year period of swan-neck deformity of the right thumb in a patient with RA.

Pencil-in-cup Sign (Pencil-in-cup Appearance)

Bone erosions make the narrowed end of a metacarpal or phalange and the expanded end of the adjacent bone sharing the joint (Fig. **51**). Although the pencil-in-cup sign is typically found in patients with severe psoriasis, it also occurs in RA.

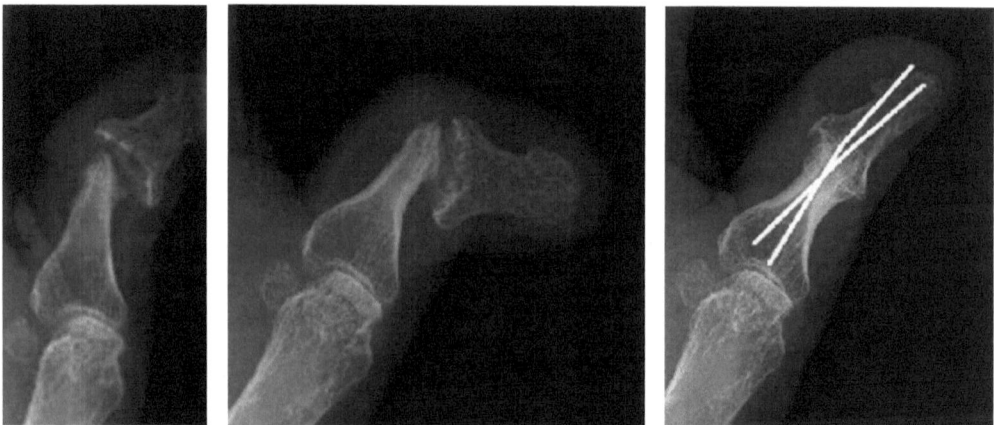

Fig. (51). Plain radiographs of the IP joint show a tapering of the first proximal phalanx and an expansion of the base of the first distal phalanx before and after operation.

Arthritis Mutilans

The deformity may induce structural collapse or loss of bone substance. Then, the affected joints appear to become an arthritis mutilans finally (Figs. **52 - 55**).

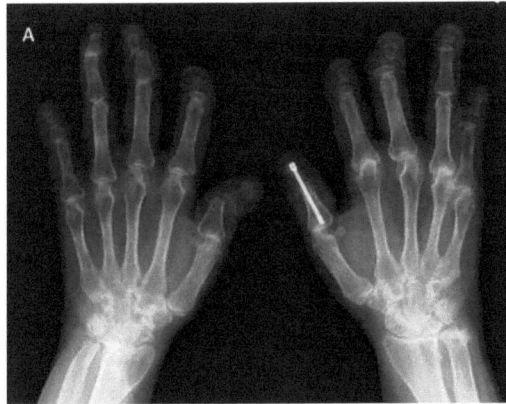

Fig. (52). PA view of the hands of a patient with long-standing RA and psoriatic arthritis show arthritis mutilans.

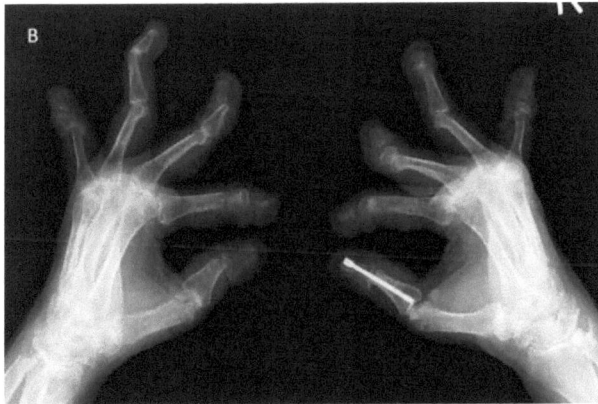

Fig. (53). Oblique view of the hands of a patient with long-standing RA and psoriatic arthritis show arthritis mutilans.

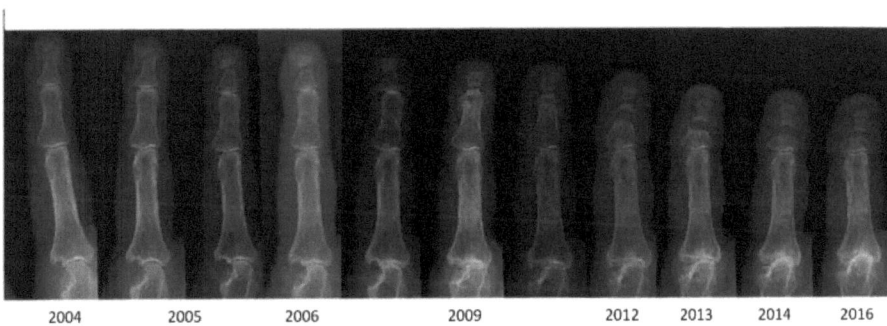

| 2004 | 2005 | 2006 | 2009 | 2012 | 2013 | 2014 | 2016 |

Fig. (54). Radiographs of development of arthritis mutilans in the right second finger of the same patient with RA and PsA (Fig. **53**).

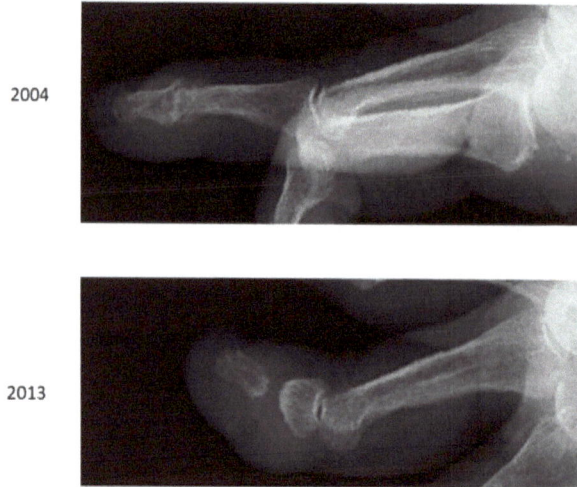

Fig. (55). Oblique radiographs of the third finger of a patient with RA and PsA (arthritis mutilans) obtained 9 years apart.

Wrists

Mal-alignments and deformities of the wrists are various including radial deviation at the radiocarpal compartment, volar translocation of the carpus, and inferior radioulnar and distal ulnar mal-alignment.

Radial Deviation at the Radiocarpal Compartment

The radial deviation at the radiocarpal compartment is common in 70% of patients with RA and may be induced by the medial migration of the scaphoid and lunate bone due to the synovitis and destruction of the ligaments in the wrists (Figs. **56 - 61**). The ulnar side of the wrist becomes a straight line (Fig. **57**).

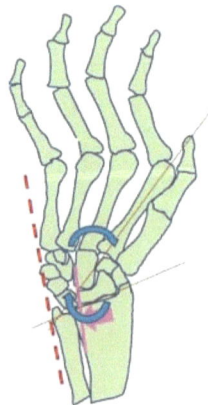

Fig. (56). A simplified schema of the radial deviation at the wrist in RA.

Usually, the line between the scaphoid and the lunate runs at the center of the radius. More than 50% of width of the lunate overlaps the radiocarpal joint. However, in RA, the scaphoid and the lunate migrate in a medial (ulnar) and palmar direction along the inclined articular surface of the distal end of the radius.

The ulnar translocation of the radiocarpal joint produces less than 50% of contact of the lunate with the radius.

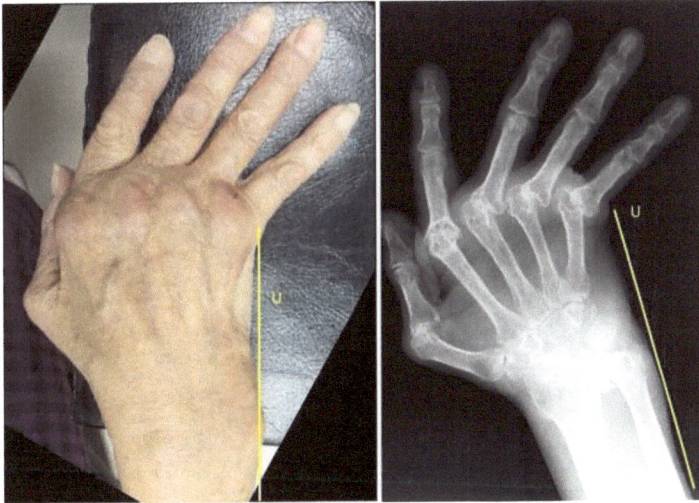

Fig. (57). A straightening of the ulnar border of the wrist [Line U] is observed in a patient with RA. The finding suggests radial deviation at the radiocarpal compartment.

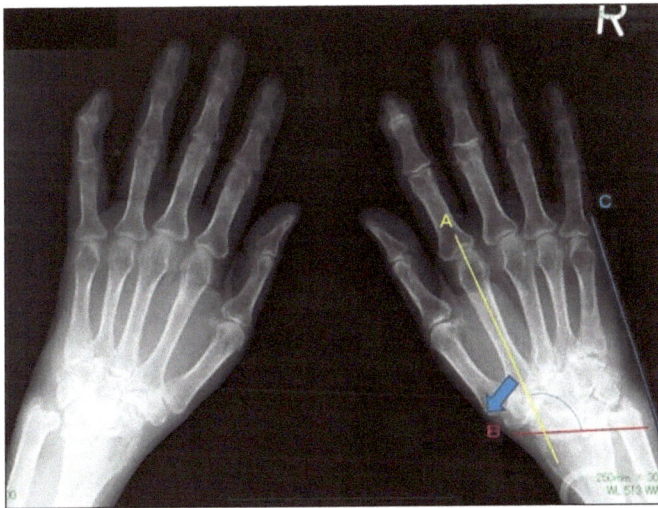

Fig. (58). PA view of the hands shows radial deviation at the right wrist (angle created by the intersection of lines A and B). The radiograph exhibits a straightening of the ulnar side of the wrist (Line C).

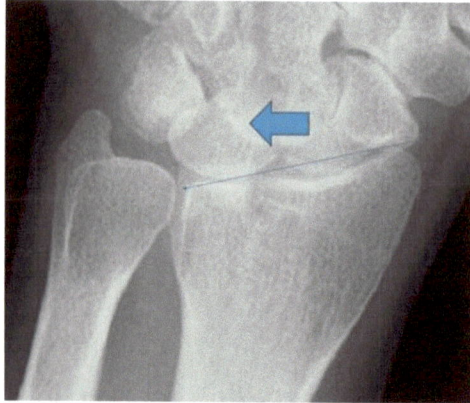

Fig. (59). PA view shows ulnar inclination of the radius. The inclining of the radius towards the ulna may induce the ulnar translocation of the carpal bones.

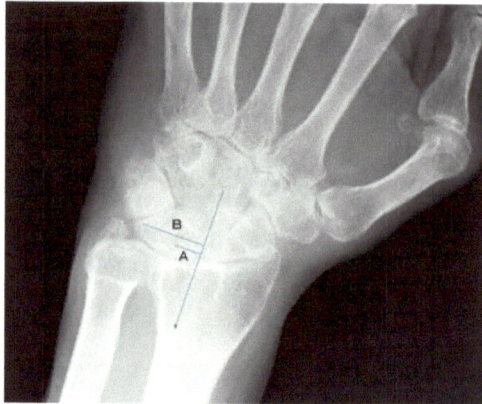

Fig. (60). PA view of the left wrist of a patient with RA shows ulnar translocation of the radiocarpal joint (less than 50% (=A/B) of the lunate contacts with the radius). Also, the line between the scaphoid and the lunate shifts from the center of the radius to ulnar side, and then it induces radial deviation at the RC joint.

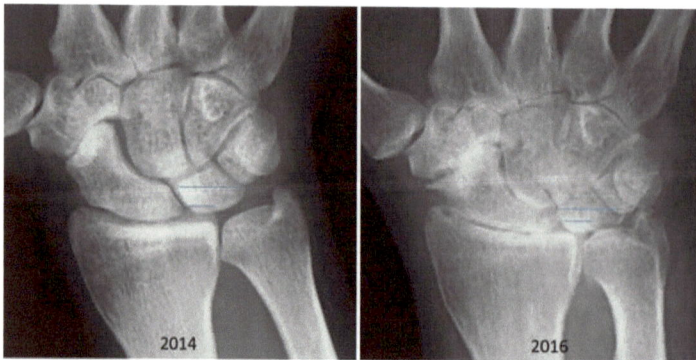

Fig. (61). PA views of the right wrist in a patient with RA obtained 2 years apart show development of ulnar translocation of the RC joint.

Volar Translocation of the Carpus (Palmar (Sub)Luxation in the Radiocarpal Joint)

Volar translocation at the radiocarpal compartment induces palmar subluxations of the lunate and scaphoid bones (Figs. **62 - 64**).

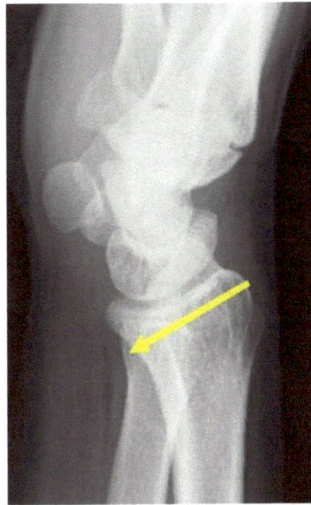

Fig. (62). Lateral view of the wrist shows palmar inclination of the radius. The inclining of the radius towards the palmar induces the palmar subluxation in the radiocarpal joint.

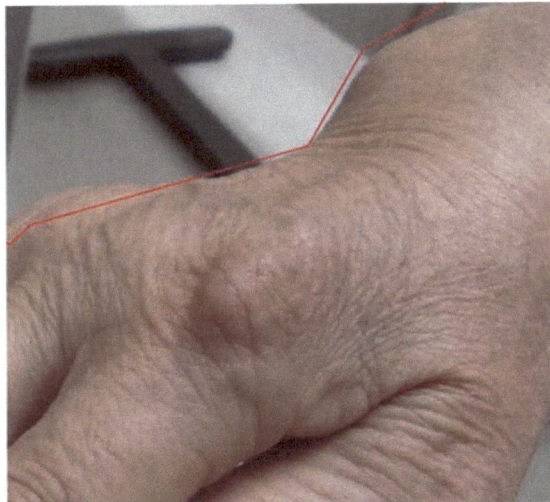

Fig. (63). Photograph of the right wrist shows volar translocation of the carpus (palmar (sub)luxation at the RC joint) (stepped transformation).

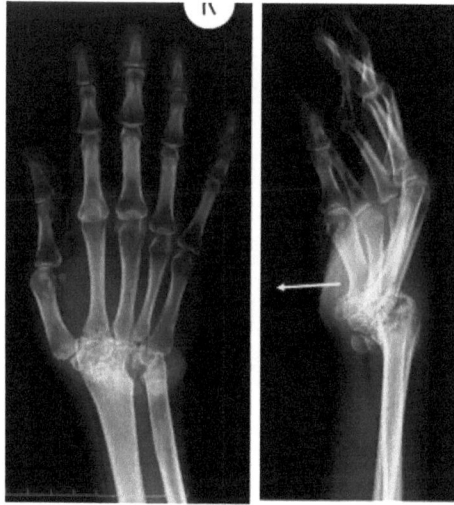

Fig. (64). PA view and lateral view of the right wrist in a patient with advanced RA show destruction of the carpus and volar translocation.

Inferior Radioulnar and Distal Ulnar Malalignment

Dorsal subluxation of the distal portion of the ulna is one of inferior radioulnar and distal ulnar mal-alignments (Figs. **65 - 67**). The eroded head of the ulna projects into the compartments of the extensor tendons at the wrist and produces wear of the tendon surfaces.

The caput-ulnae syndrome has symptoms of pain, limited motion, and dorsal prominence of the distal end of the ulna. Mechanical attrition with tenosynovitis sometimes leads to rupture of the tendons. The extensor tendons on the dorsum of the wrist may rupture and be operated.

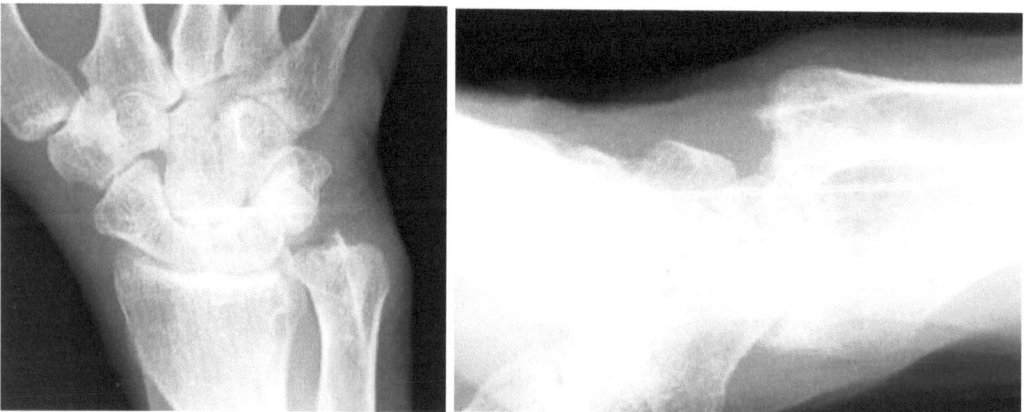

Fig. (65). PA view and lateral view of the right wrist show dorsal prominence of the distal end of the ulna and projection of eroded head of the ulna into the compartments of the extensor tendons at the wrist.

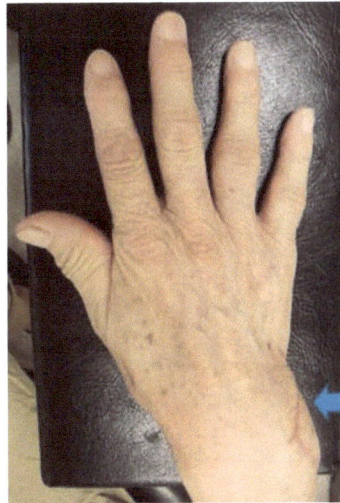

Fig. (66). Photograph of the hand of a patient with RA illustrates dorsal prominence of the distal end of the ulna. The extensor tendons on the dorsum of the wrist ruptured and were operated.

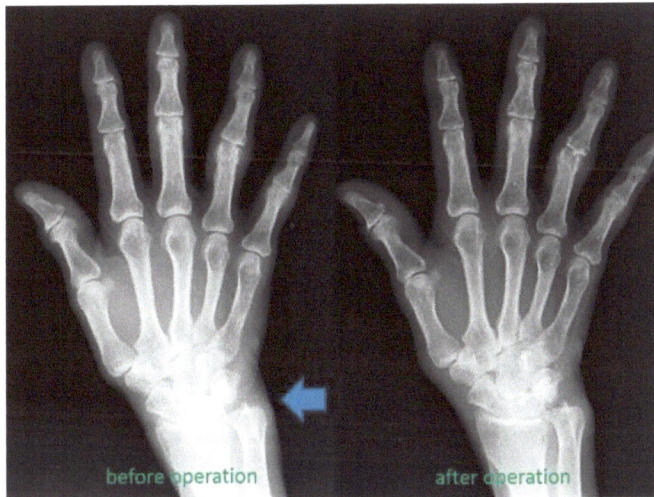

Fig. (67). The radiographs show the rupture of extensor tendon(s) at the distal end of the ulna before and after operation.

Carpal Bones

Measurement of the carpal height is useful to assess the severity of carpal collapse of RA. The carpal height is the distance between the base of third metacarpal and the subchondral cortex of the distal radius. The carpal height ratio is calculated by dividing the carpal height by the length of the third metacarpal [3]. Its normal range is over 0.54 (0.51-0.57) (Fig. **68**). The carpal height ratio decreases in patients with RA (Figs. **69** and **70**).

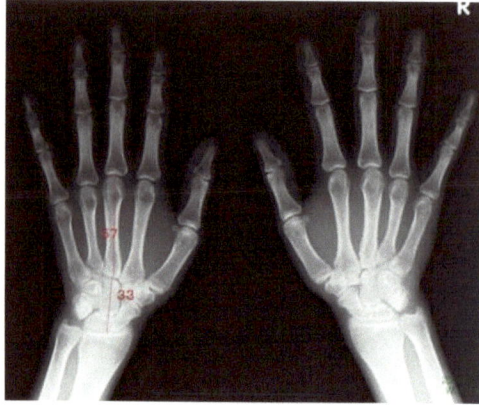

Fig. (68). The carpal height ratio = the carpal height / the length of the third metacarpal = 33 mm/ 57 mm= 0.579 > 0.54; normal.

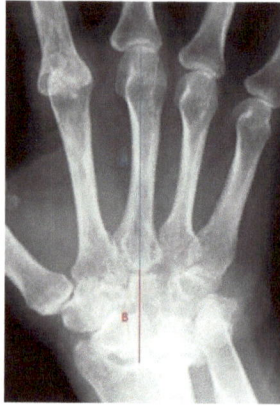

Fig. (69). The carpal height ratio (=0.42) suggests the carpal collapse in a patient with RA.

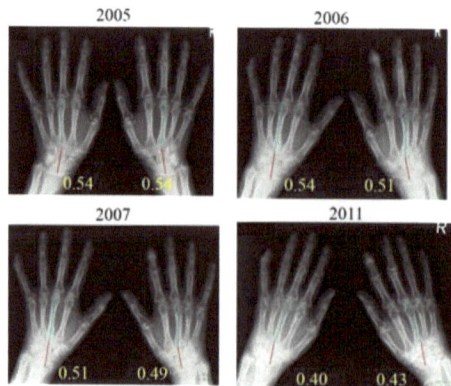

Fig. (70). The carpal height ratio has progressively decreased in a patient with RA.

Elbows

Radiographic anatomy of the skeleton of the elbow in a normal person (Figs. **71** - **74**).

There may be limitation of both flexion and extension of the elbows. In late RA, extensive destruction of the humeroulnar joint may occur due to proximal migration of the trochlear notch of olecranon into deficient trochlea of the humerus. Then, finally, total joint destruction of complete loss of normal articular surface and the luxation of the elbow joint may be observed in patients with RA (Figs. **75** and **76**).

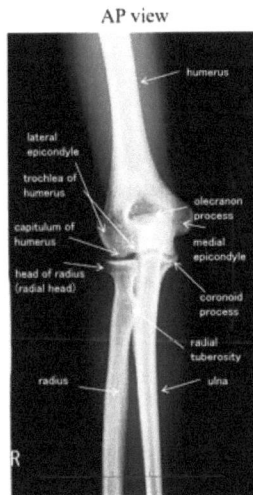

Fig. (71). Radiographic anatomy of the skeleton of the elbow: AP view.

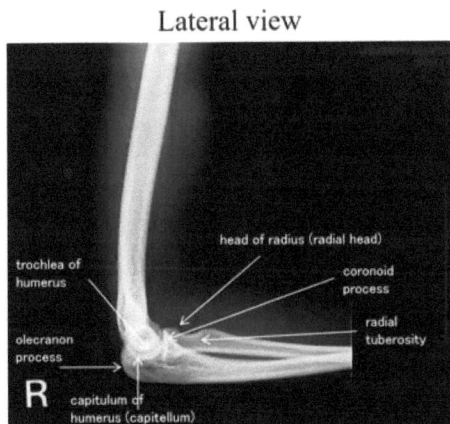

Fig. (72). Radiographic anatomy of the skeleton of the elbow: lateral view.

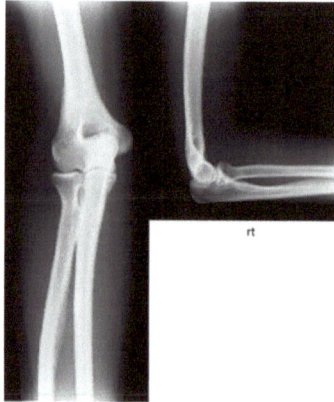

Fig. (73). AP view and lateral view of the elbow of a normal person.

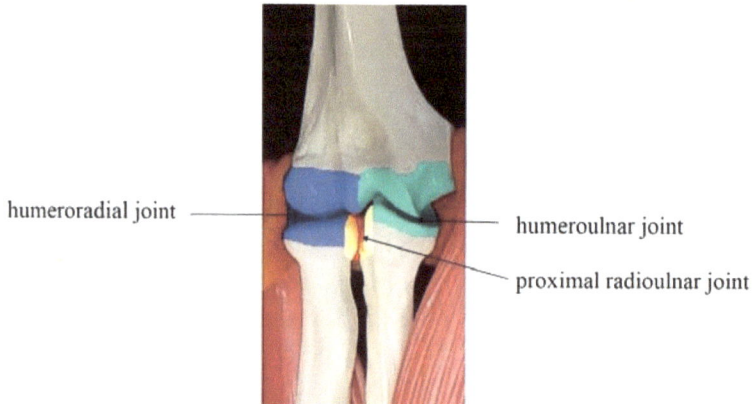

humeroradial joint

humeroulnar joint

proximal radioulnar joint

Fig. (74). Joints of the elbow. There are three joints in the elbow, the humeroradial joint, the humeroulnar joint and the proximal radioulnar joint.

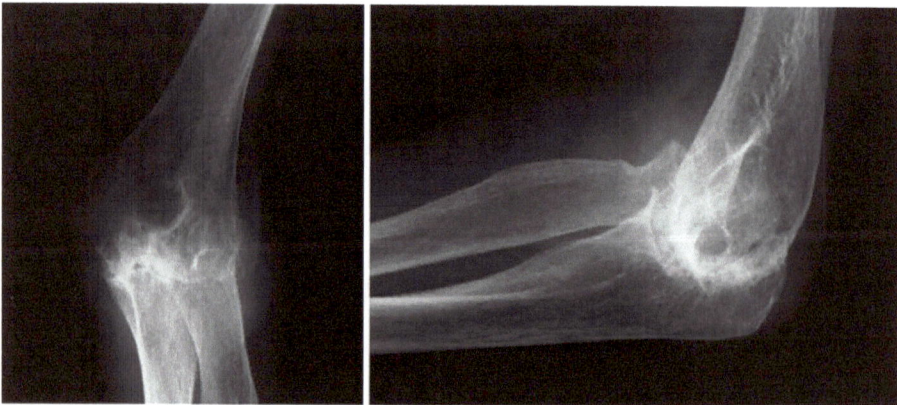

Fig. (75). AP view and lateral view of the elbow of a patient with RA show destruction and complete loss of normal articular surface of the joints.

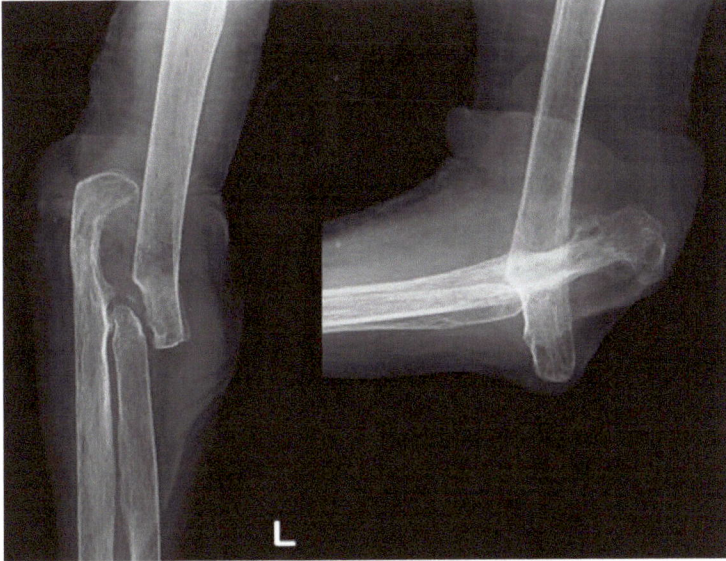

Fig. (76). The luxation of the elbow joint is observed in a patients with RA.

Shoulders

The shoulder joint consists of the glenohumeral, the acromial humeral, and the acromioclavicular (AC) joint (Figs. **77 - 79**). Uniform narrowing may be found in the compartments of the shoulder joint.

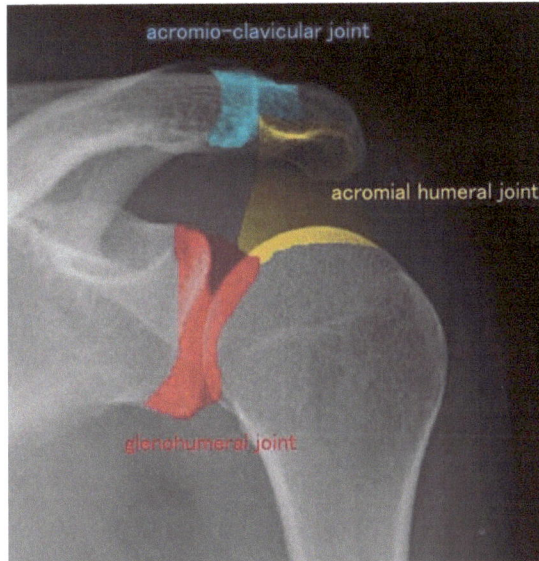

Fig. (77). There are three joints in the shoulder, the glenohumeral, the acromial humeral, and the acromioclavicular (AC) joint.

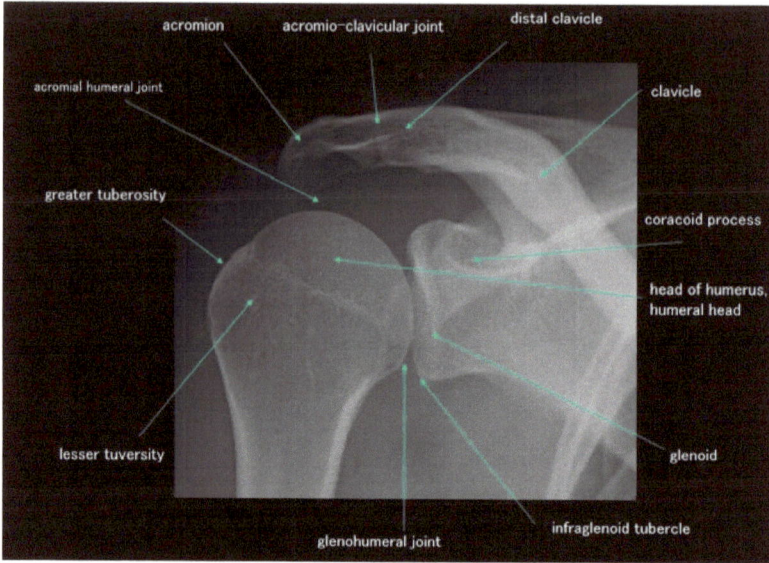

Fig. (78). Radiographic anatomy of the skeleton of the shoulder: AP view.

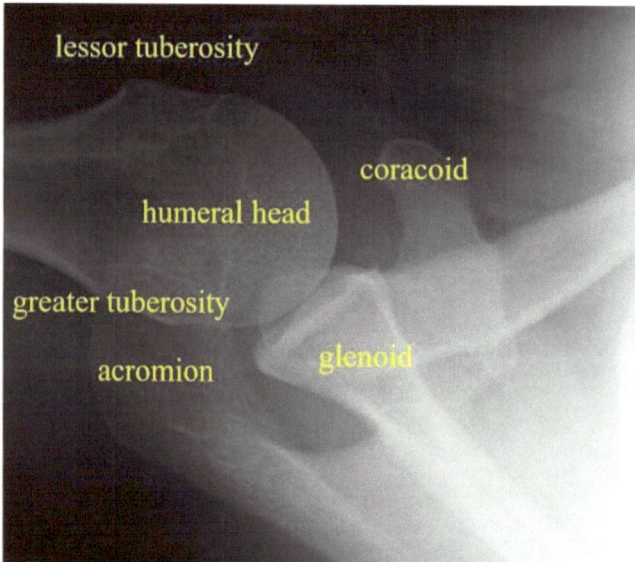

Fig. (79). Radiographic anatomy of the skeleton of the shoulder: axillary view.

Glenohumeral Joints

Proximal Migration of Humeral Head

The humeral head migrates proximally with respect to the glenoid cavity (Figs. **80** and **81**).

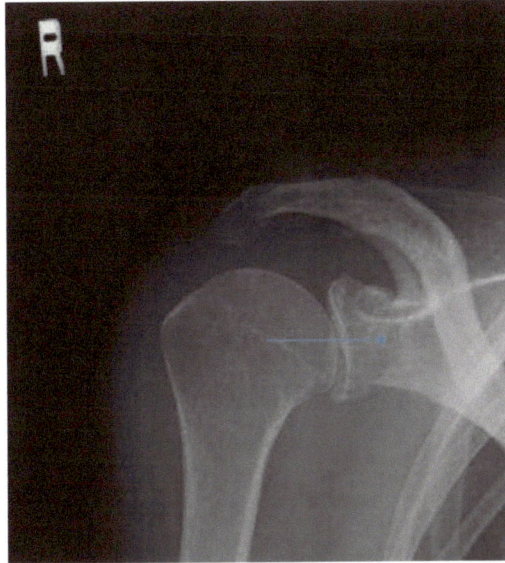

Fig. (80). AP view of the right shoulder of a patient with RA. The humeral head has migrated inward.

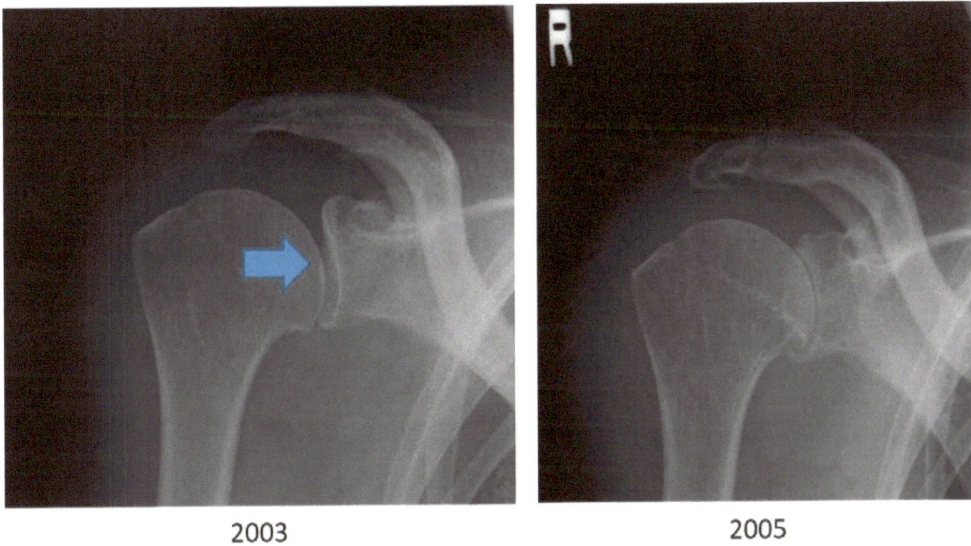

2003   2005

Fig. (81). Newly diagnosed rheumatoid arthritis and its follow-up. AP views of the right shoulder obtained in 2003 and 2005. They show that the humeral head has migrated proximally due to loss of the cartilage in the glenohumeral joint.

Superior Migration of Humeral Head

The humeral head elevates in relationship to the glenoid. Superior migration of the humeral head may occur secondary to rotator cuff atrophy (Figs. **82** and **83**).

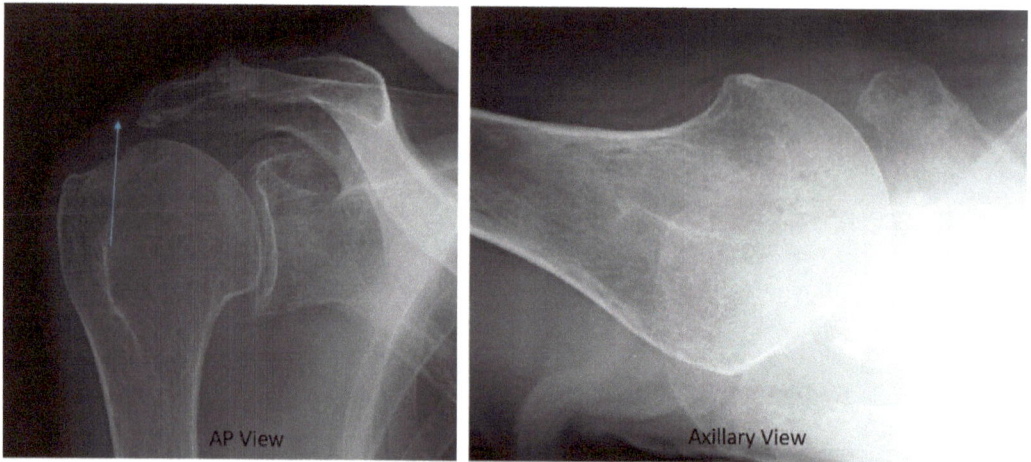

Fig. (82). AP view and axillary view of the right shoulder of a patient with RA show that the right humeral head migrates upward.

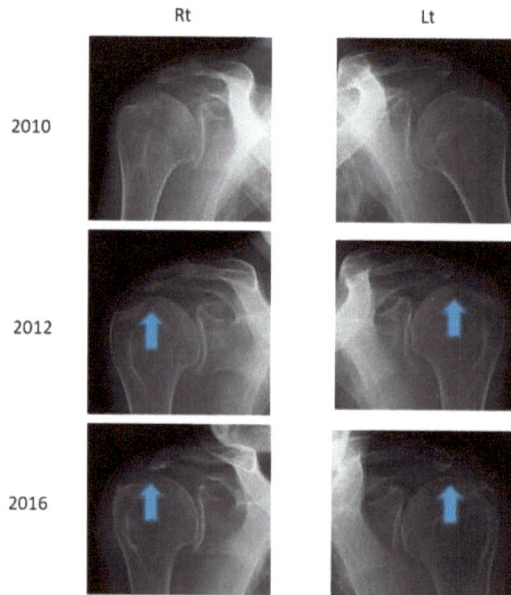

Fig. (83). Radiographs show development of superior migration of the shoulders in a patient with RA.

Proximal and Superior Migration of Humeral Head

The humeral head migrates proximally due to loss of the cartilage in the glenohumeral joint and superiorly in relationship to the glenoid cavity due to a tear of the rotator cuff (Figs. **84 - 86**).

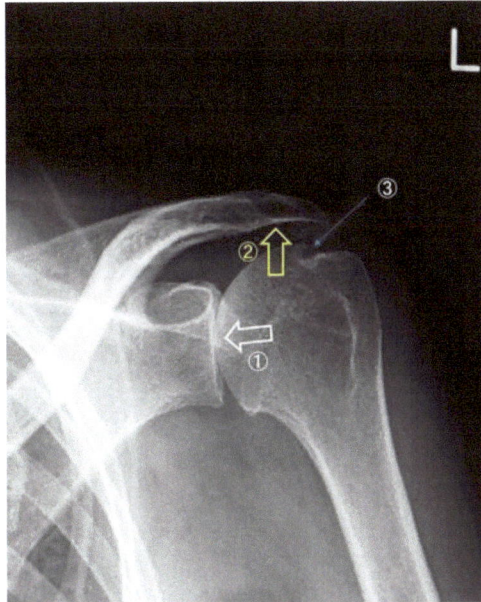

Fig. (84). AP view of the shoulder of a patient with RA shows that the left humeral head migrates inward (1) and upward (2). It also shows an erosion of the proximal humerus with thin sclerotic margination (3).

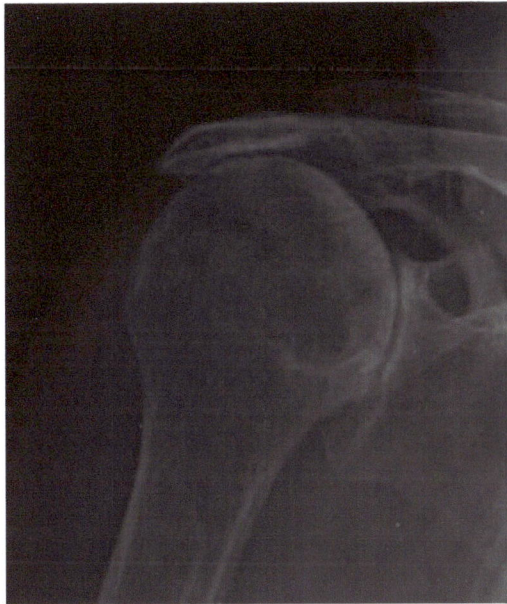

Fig. (85). AP view of the right shoulder of a patient with longstanding RA shows that the humeral head severely migrates inward and upward.

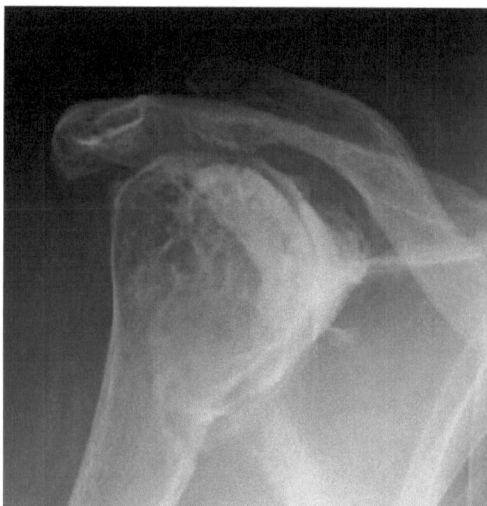

Fig. (86). AP view of the right shoulder of a patient with advanced RA shows destruction of the humeral head and deformity of the shoulder joint. The humeral head migrates inward and upward.

Inferior Migration of Humeral Head

Sometimes, in patients with RA, the humeral head may migrate downward (Fig. 87).

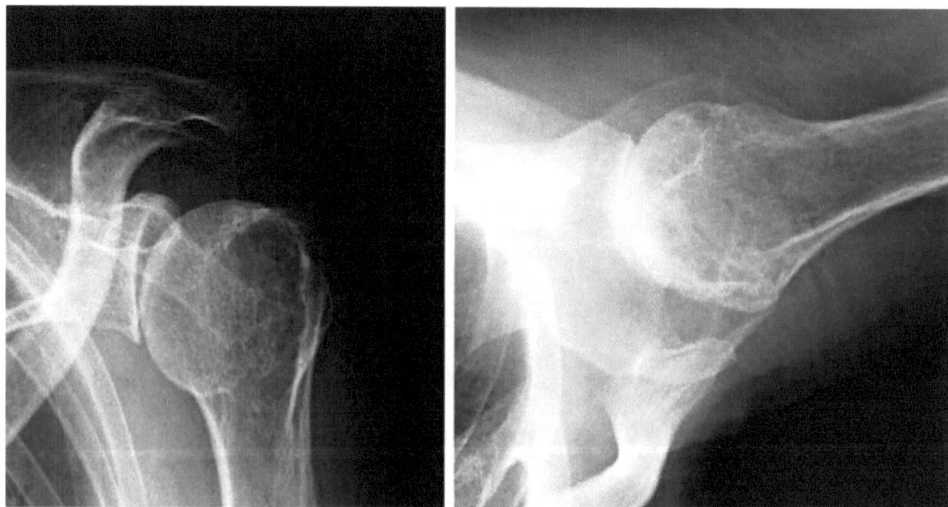

Fig. (87). AP view and axillary view of the right shoulder of a patient with RA show that the humeral head migrates downward.

Acromial Humeral Joints

In the acromial humeral joint, narrowing between the humerus and the acromion is associated with rotator cuff tear (Figs. **88** and **89**).

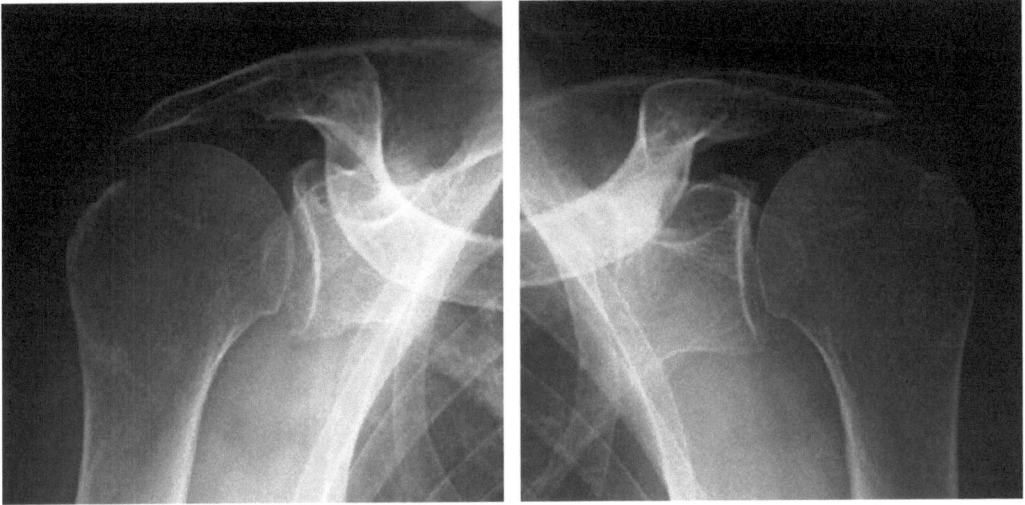

Fig. (88). AP views of the bilateral shoulders show mild superior migration of the humeral heads. The humeral heads slightly elevate and narrowing between the humerus and the acromion occurs due to rotator cuff tears in the acromial humeral joints.

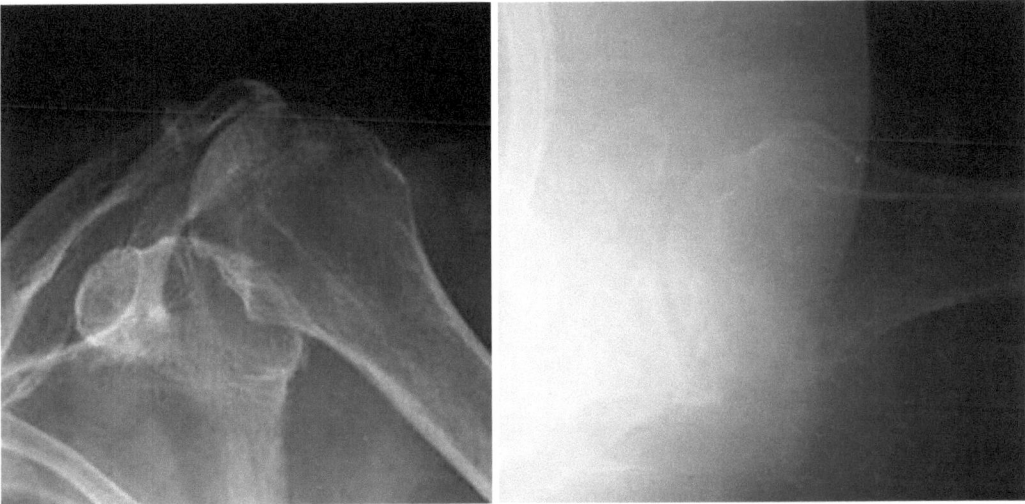

Fig. (89). AP view and axillary view of the left shoulder show severe superior migration of the left humeral head. The humeral head elevates and narrowing between the humerus and the acromion due to a rotator cuff tear is observed at the acromial humeral joint.

Acromioclavicular Joint

In RA, erosions may be found at the acromioclavicular joint and they may progress to osteolysis of the distal clavicle. There is also subluxation due to disruption of the adjacent ligaments and capsule of the joint (Fig. **90**).

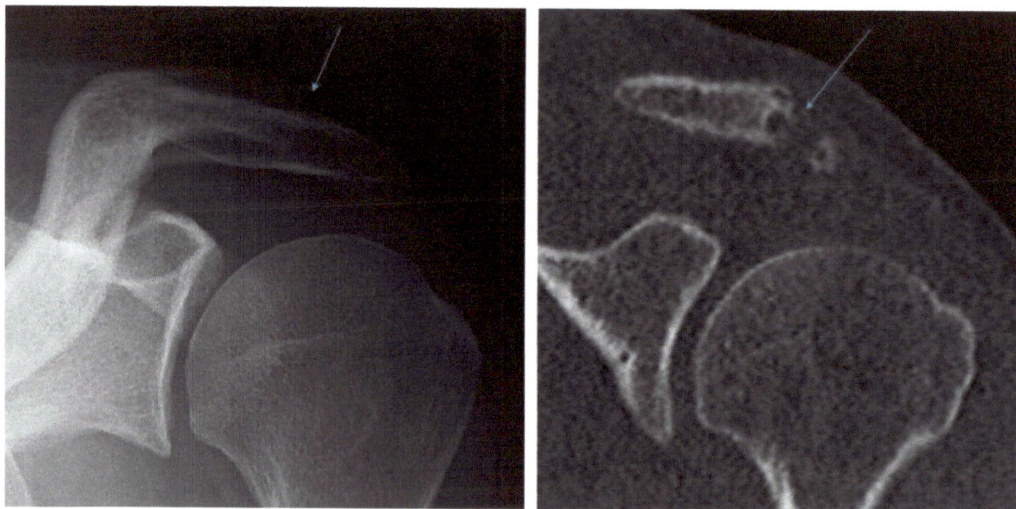

Fig. (90). AP view and CT image of the left shoulder of a patient with RA. Erosions and subluxation are found at the acromioclavicular joint.

Hips

Radiographic anatomy of the skeleton of the hips in a normal person (Figs. **91 - 93**).

In RA, at the hip joint, the cartilage is uniformaly lost and then the femoral head migrates in an axial (superior medial) direction.

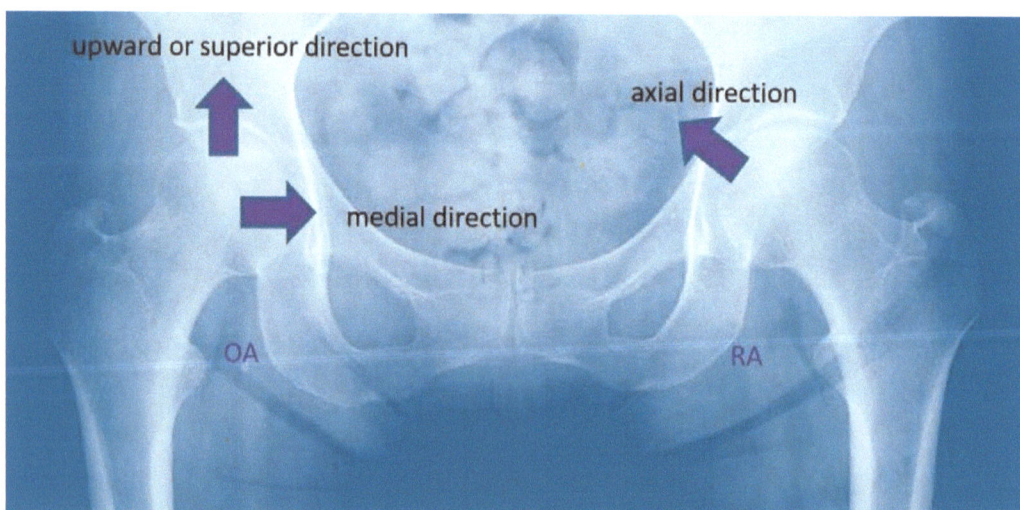

Fig. (91). In OA, the cartilage at the hip joint is not uniformaly lost and the femoral head migrates in an upward or a medial direction. However, in RA, the cartilage is uniformaly lost and then the femoral head migrates in an axial (superior medial) direction.

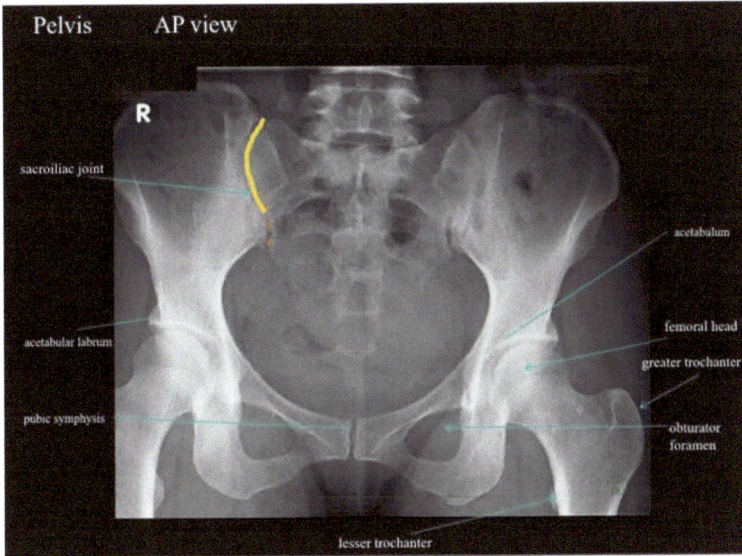

Fig. (92). Radiographic anatomy of the skeleton of the hip: AP view.

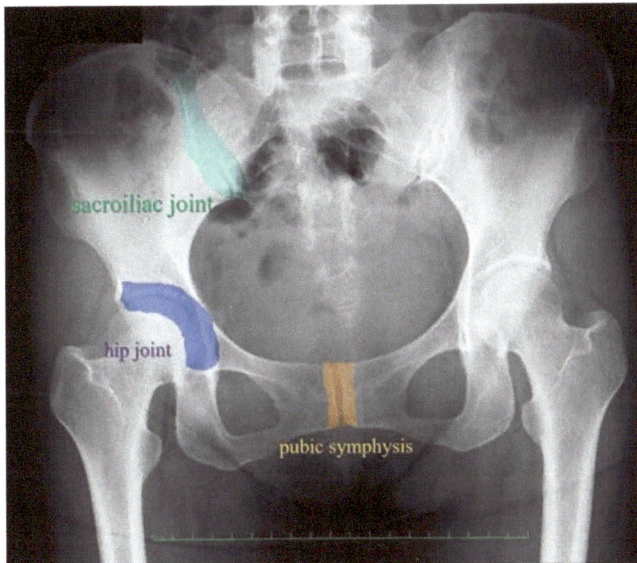

Fig. (93). There are three joints in the pelvis, the hip joint, the pubic symphysis, and the sacroiliac joint.

Axial Migration

In RA, the femoral head migrates centrally with respect to the acetabulum along axis of the femoral neck due to diffuse loss of articular space (Fig. **94**).

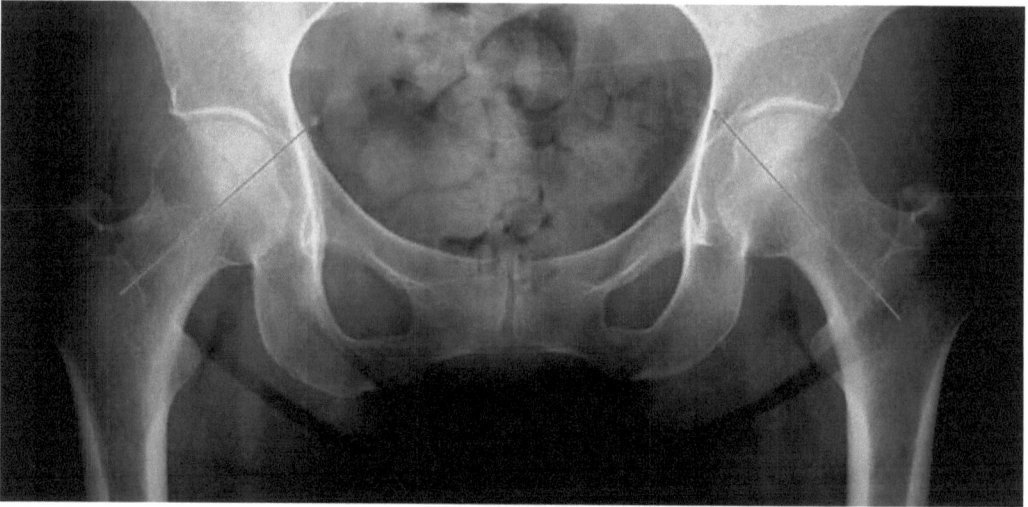

Fig. (94). AP view of the hips of a patient with RA shows bilateral axial migration with mild uniform cartilage loss.

Superior or Medial Migaration of Femoral Head

Rarely, the femoral head may migrate to superior or medial direction with respect to the acetabulum, like osteoarthritis, due to loss of space on superior or medial aspect of the hip joint (Fig. **95**).

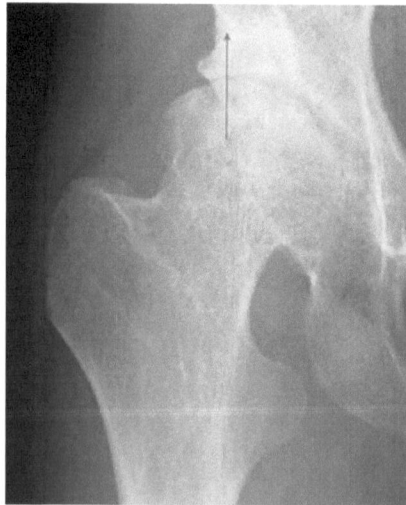

Fig. (95). AP view of the right hip shows superior migration of the femoral head in a patient with RA.

Acetabular Protrusion

Axial migration of the femoral head finally induces to protrude into the pelvis. Acetabular protrusion is a characteristic finding of RA (Figs. **96 - 98**). The hip joint may accompany deformities with bone cysts and collapse of the acetabular roof and the femoral head.

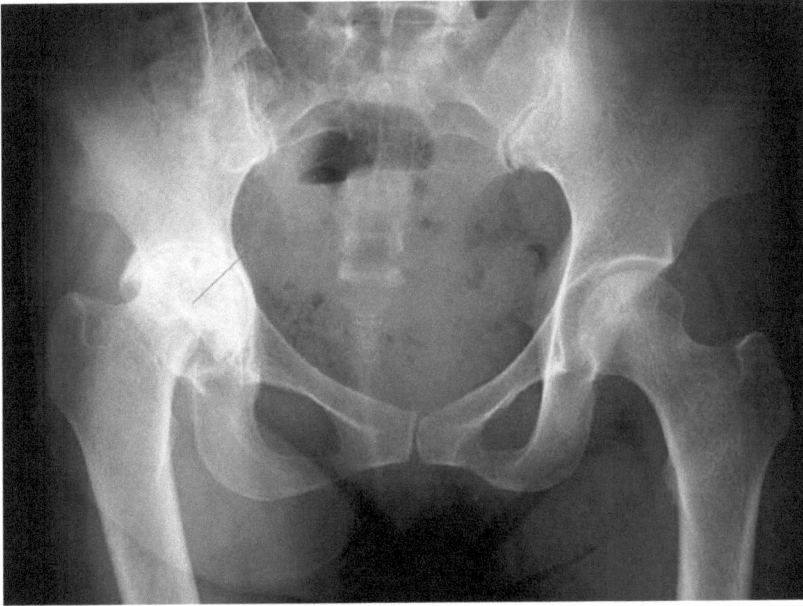

Fig. (96). AP view of the pelvis in a patient with RA shows protrusio acetabuli of the right hip joint.

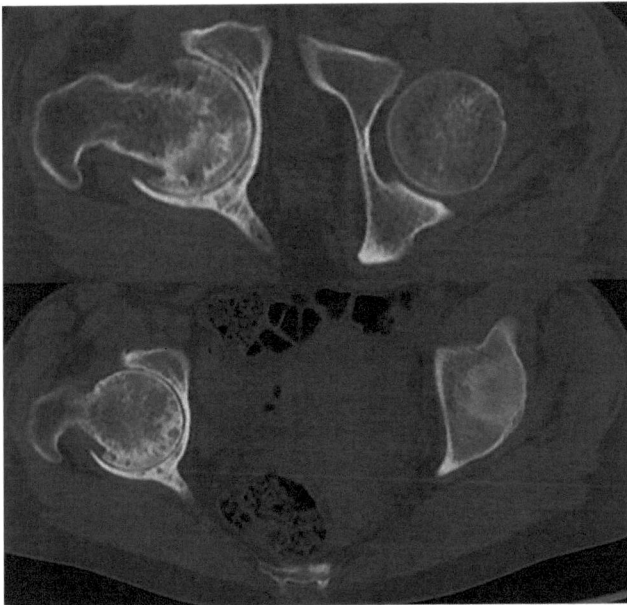

Fig. (97). CT images of the hips in the same patient with RA show protrusio acetabuli of the right hip.

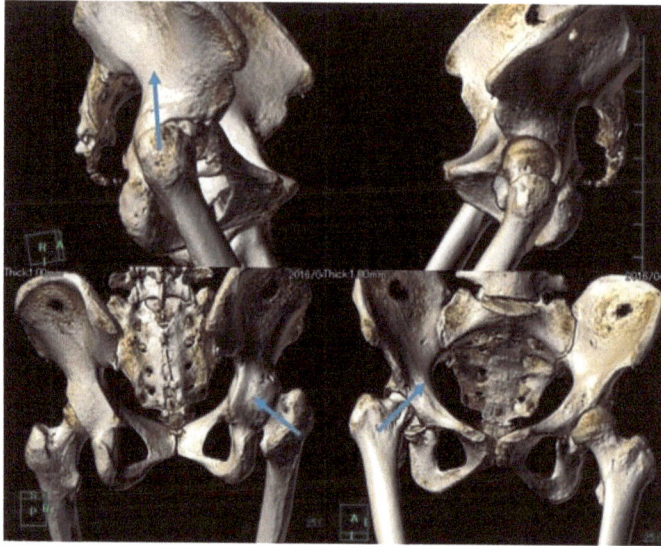

Fig. (98). 3D-CT images of the pelvis in a patient with RA illustrate protrusio acetabuli of the right hip.

Osteonecrosis of Femoral Head

Osteonecrosis of the femoral head occurs generally in patients with RA taking corticosteroids (Figs. **99** and **100**). Although osseous collapse may be found, joint space will be maintained until the end stage.

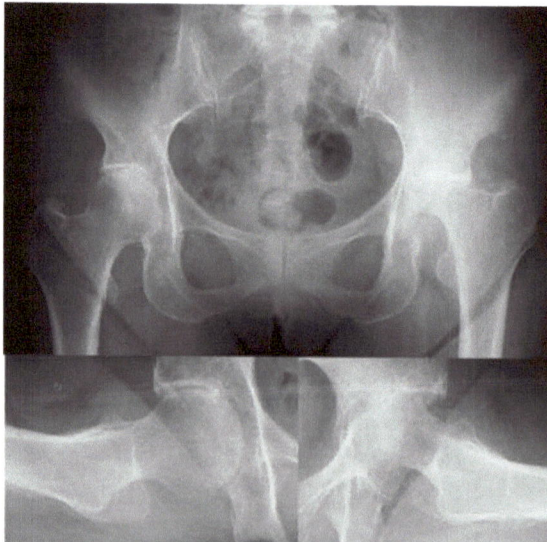

Fig. (99). AP view and frog leg lateral view of the hips in advanced RA. There are bilateral axial migration of the femoral heads and severe destruction of the left hip joint due to osteonecrosis.

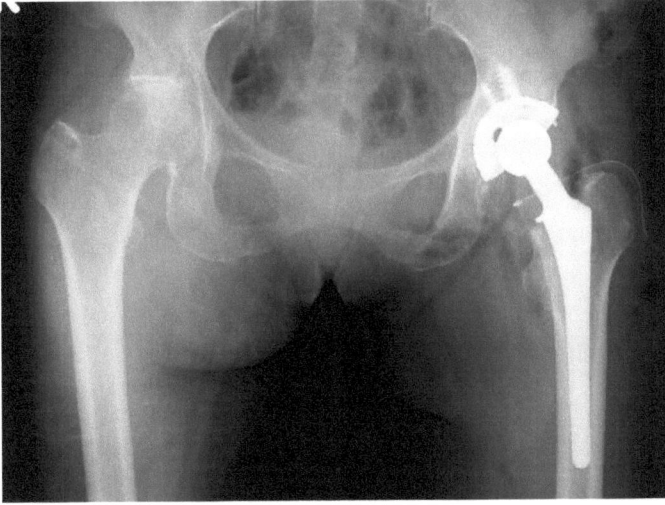

Fig. (100). THA (total hip arthroplasty) was performed in the same patient with RA (Fig. 99).

Pubic Osteolysis

Pubic osteolysis is rare disease (Fig. **101**) and occurs after an insufficiency fracture of the pubic bone [4]. The cases present groin pain and radiographic lesions in the pubic bones. The reported patients are postmenopausal women with a recent history of trauma or increased physical activity. After conservative treatment, it resolves within 6 months [4]. The patients may have had spontaneous groin and gluteal pain for long time. Pubic osteolysis may occur in patients with RA [5].

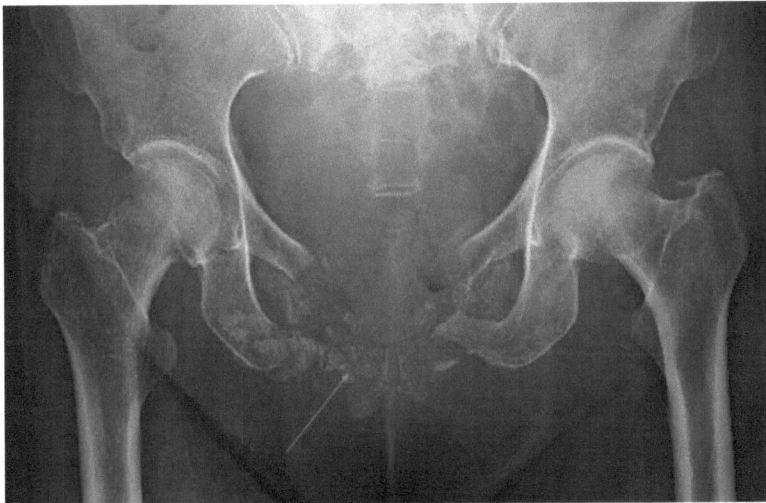

Fig. (101). AP view of the pelvis of a patient with RA shows osteolysis of the pubic bones (pubic osteolysis).

Knees

Radiographic anatomy of the skeleton of the knees in a normal person (Fig. **102**).

Sometimes, the lateral compartment is severely damaged compared to the medial compartment, then a valgus deformity of the knee may occur.

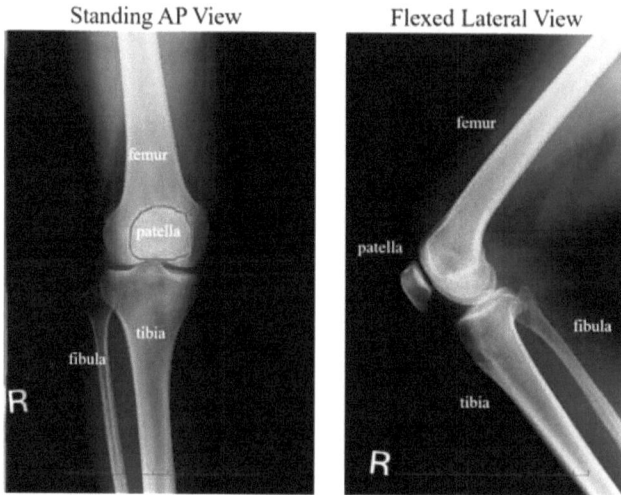

Fig. (102). Radiographic anatomy of the skeleton of the right knee: AP view and lateral view.

Subluxation of Knees

Subluxation of the knees in patients with RA (Fig. **103**).

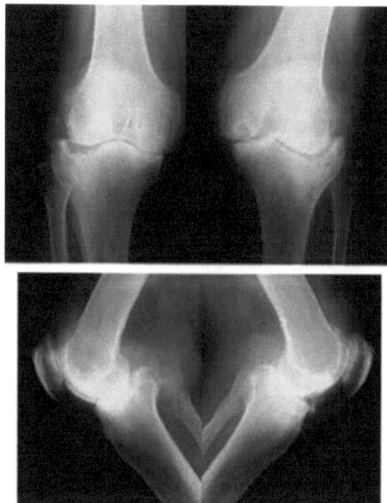

Fig. (103). AP view and lateral view of the knees show subluxation of the knees.

Ankles and Feet

Radiographic anatomy of the skeleton of the ankles and feet in a normal person (Figs. **104 - 107**).

In patients with RA, there are deformities in the foot including pes planovalgus, spreading of the metatarsal bones, hallux valgus, lateral or fibular deviation of the toes (without the fifth digit) at the MTP joints, dorsiflexion and lateral subluxation of the proximal phalanges at the MTP joints, hammer toe, and cock-up toe.

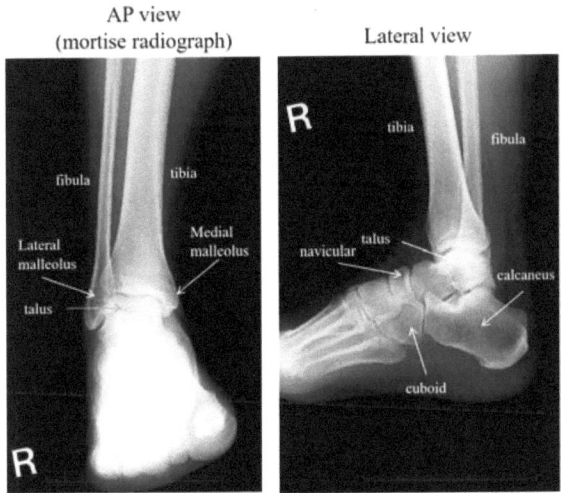

Fig. (104). Radiographic anatomy of the skeleton of the right ankle: AP view and lateral view.

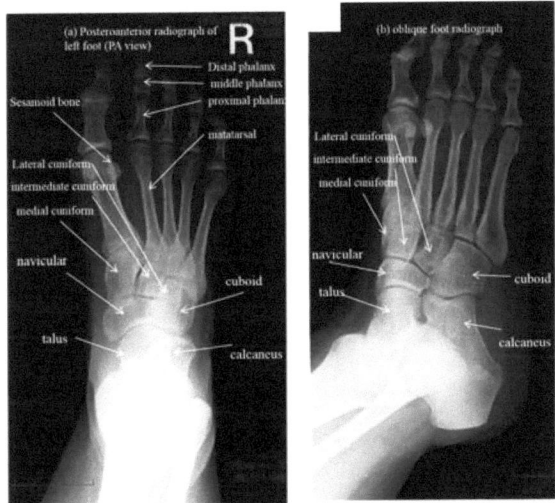

Fig. (105). Radiographic anatomy of the skeleton of the right foot: AP view and oblique view.

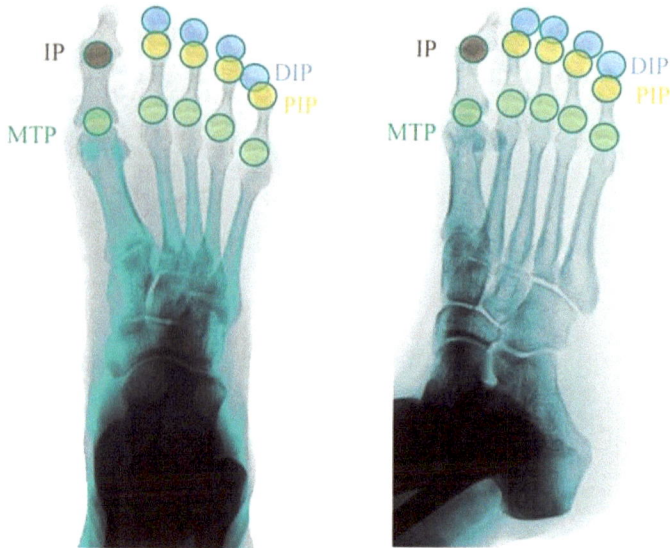

Fig. (106). Joints of the forefoot.

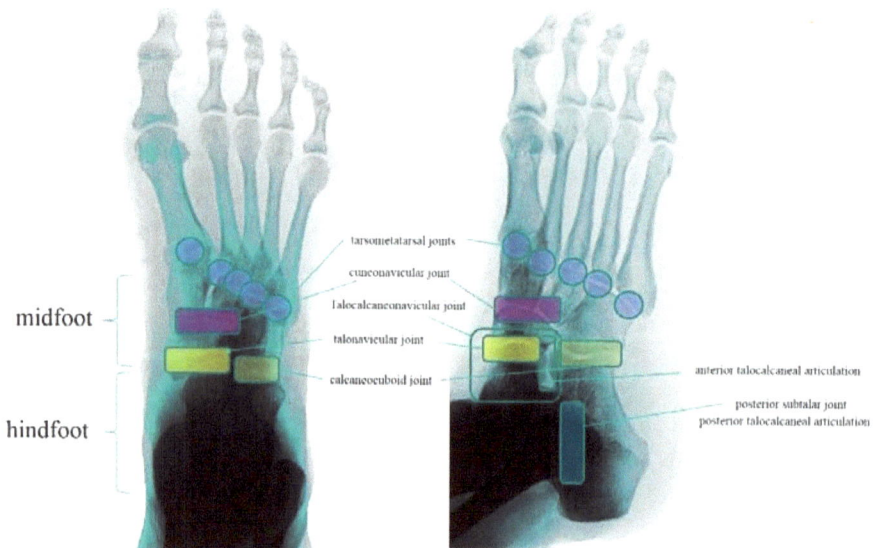

Fig. (107). Joints of the mid- and hindfoot.

Pes Planovalgus

The rupture of a tibialis posterior tendon due to inflammation may induce pes planovalgus in the midfoot (Figs. **108 - 110**).

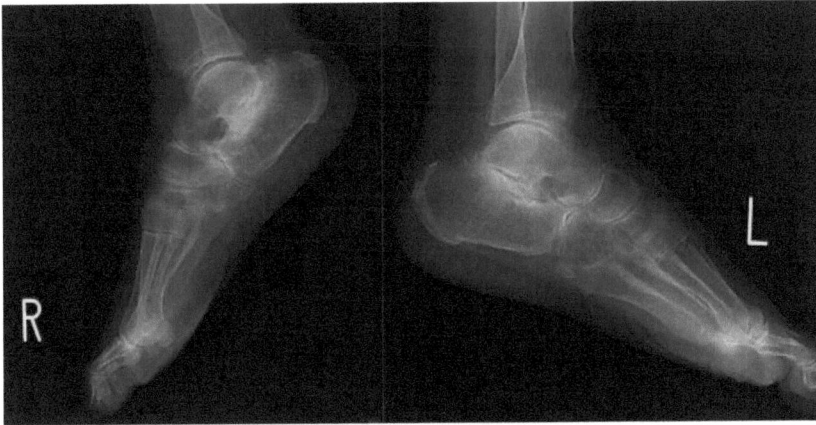

Fig. (108). Lateral views of the feet show mild pes planovalgus in a patient with RA.

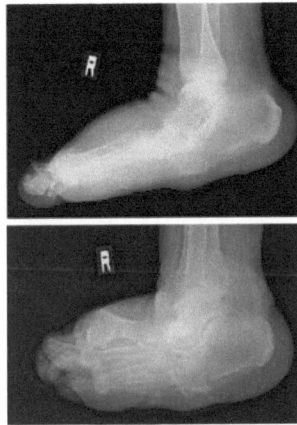

Fig. (109). Pes planovalgus in a patient with arthritis mutilans (RA).

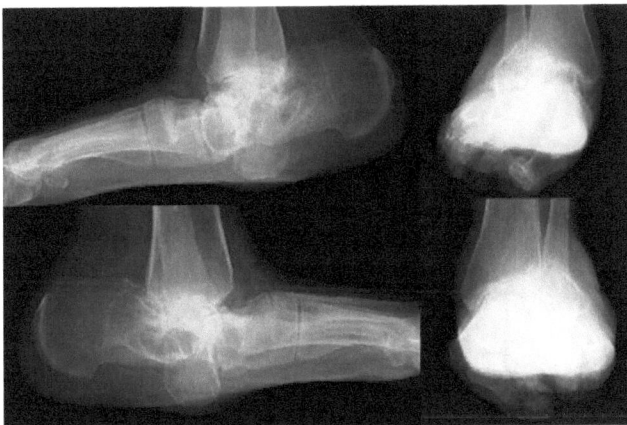

Fig. (110). Severe pes planovalgus in a patient with longstanding RA.

Spreading of Metatarsal Bones (Daylight Sign)

'daylight sign,'

The toes splay laterally and daylight is seen between the toes (daylight sign) (Fig. **111**). Thickened soft tissue and swelling of the joint space due to synovial inflammation cause the heads of metatarsal bones to spread apart.

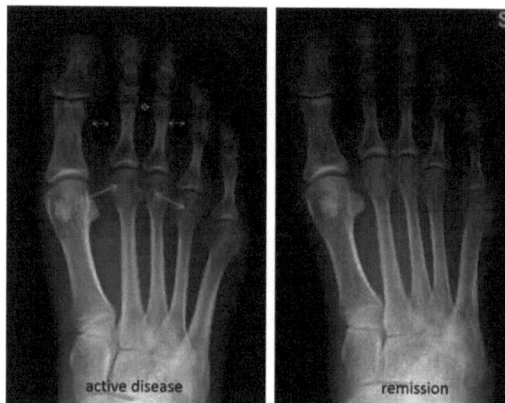

Fig. (111). AP view (left panel) of the right forefoot shows the spreading of the metatarsal bones in active disease of RA compared to those in remission (right panel). There are spaces between the toes (yellow arrow s). Under the condition of remission, the toes of the patient touch each other.

Hallux Valgus

Hallux valgus in RA (Fig. **112**).

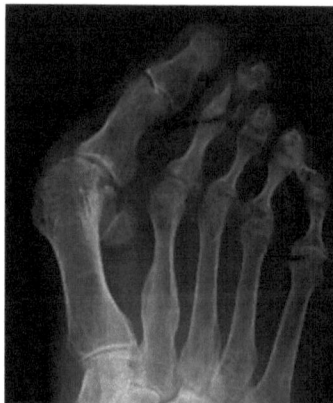

Fig. (112). AP veiw shows hallux valgus in RA. Lateral or fibular deviation of the toes at the first, second, third, and forth MTP joints.

Digitus Minimus Varus

Digitus minimus varus in RA (Figs. **113 - 115**).

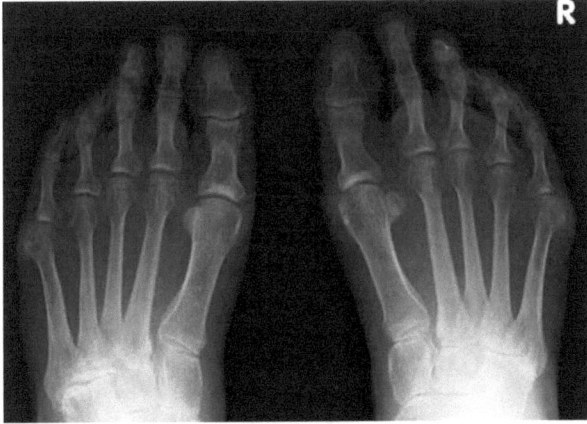

Fig. (113). Digitus minimus varus in a patient with RA.

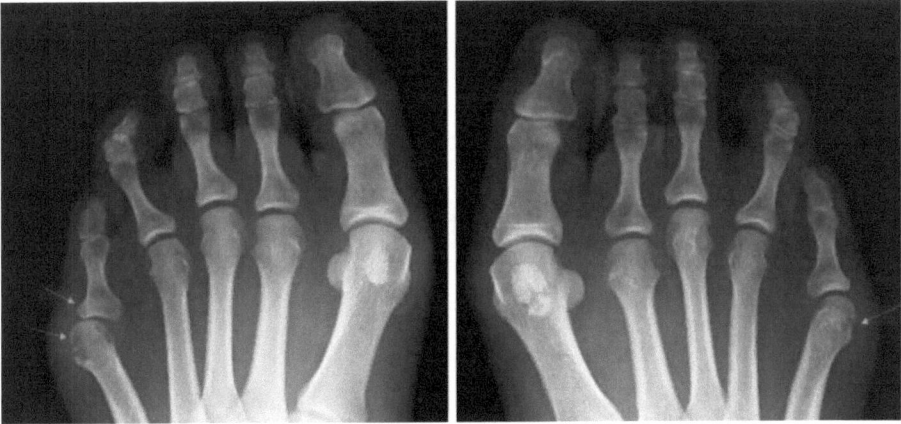

Fig. (114). Digitus minimus varus with subluxation and erosions in a patient with RA.

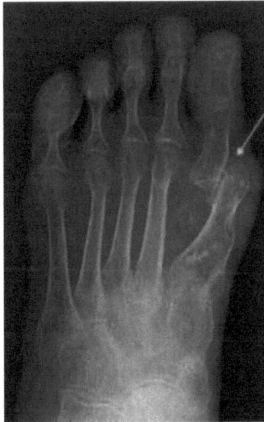

Fig. (115). Luxation at the first MTP joint in a patient with RA.

Dorsiflexion and Lateral Subluxation of Proximal Phalanges at MTP Joints

Dorsiflexion and lateral subluxation of the proximal phalanges at the MTP joints in RA (Fig. **116**).

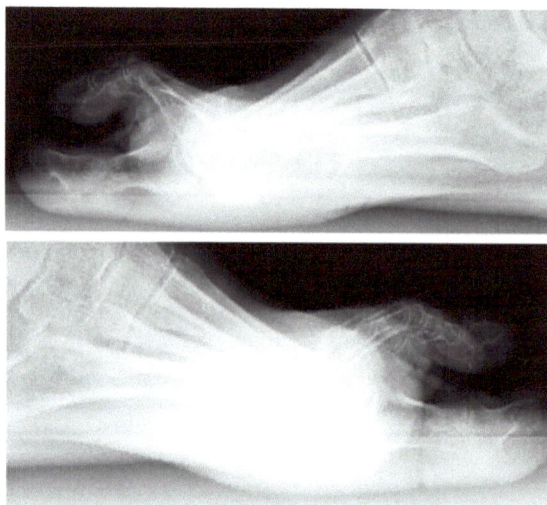

Fig. (116). Lateral views of the foot show dorsiflexion and lateral subluxation of the proximal phalanges at the MTP joints.

Cock-up Toe

Cock-up toe in RA (Fig. **117**).

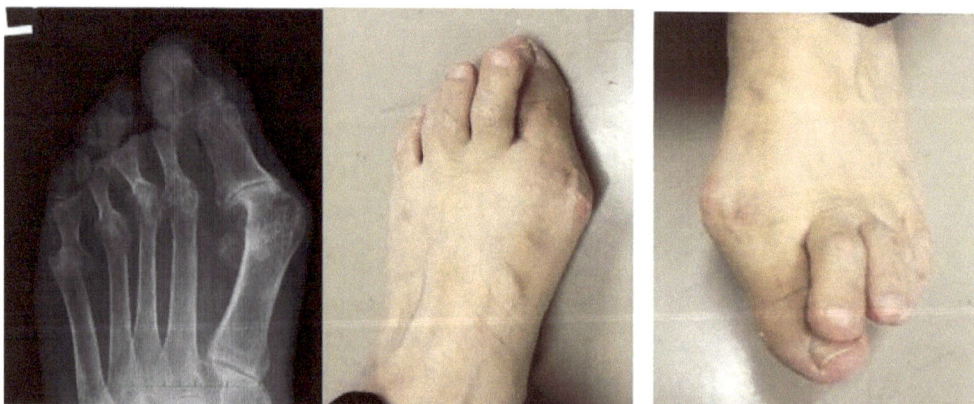

Fig. (117). Cock-up toe in a patient with RA.

Arthritis Mutilans

Destraction of the joints may induce an arthritis mutilans of the foot in RA (Fig. **118**).

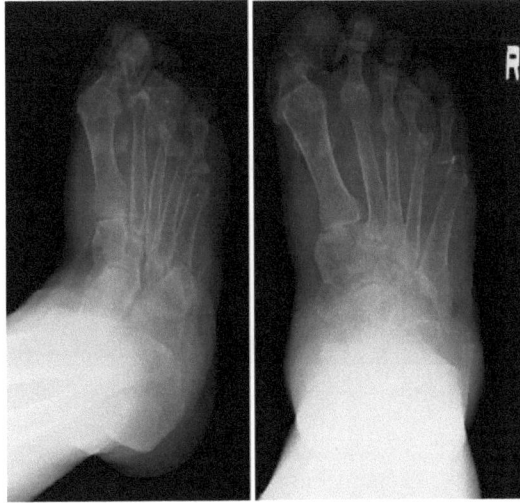

Fig. (118). Arthritis mutilans deformities of the forefoot. Oblique view and AP view of the right foot demonstrate advanced erosive disease of the MTP joints. 'licked candystick' appearance is observed at the distal metatarsals.

Spine

Cervical Spine

Radiographic anatomy of the skeleton of the cervical spine in a normal person (Figs. **119** and **120**).

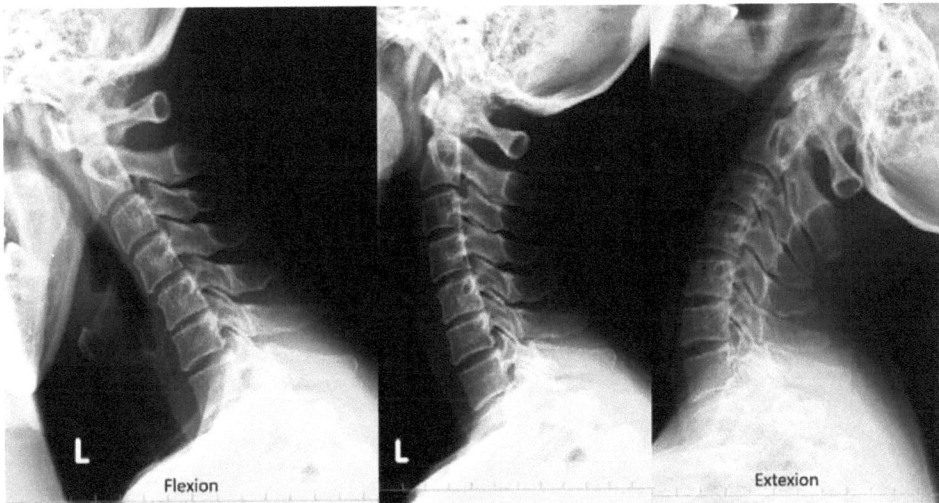

Fig. (119). Radiographic anatomy of the skeleton of the cervical spine: Lateral view.

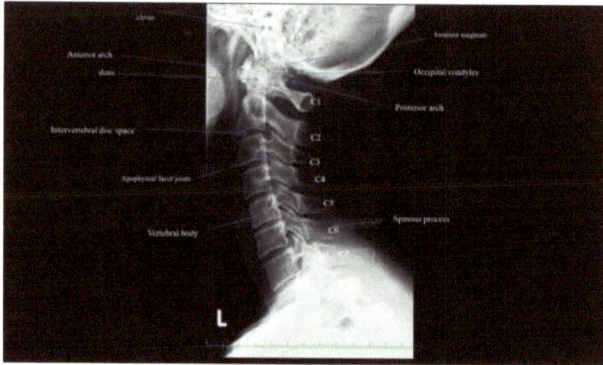

Fig. (120). Flexion and extension lateral radiographs of the cervical spine.

Atlantoaxial Subluxation

The atlantodens interval (ADI) in RA (Figs. **121 - 125**).

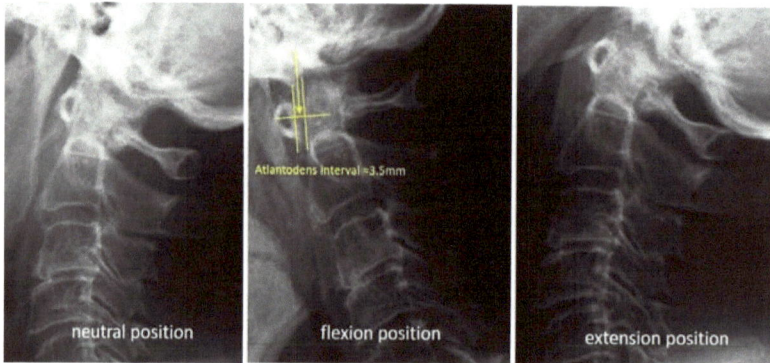

Fig. (121). Radiographs of the cervical spine (neutral position, flexion position, and extension position) show normal atlantodens interval (ADI) in a patient with RA.

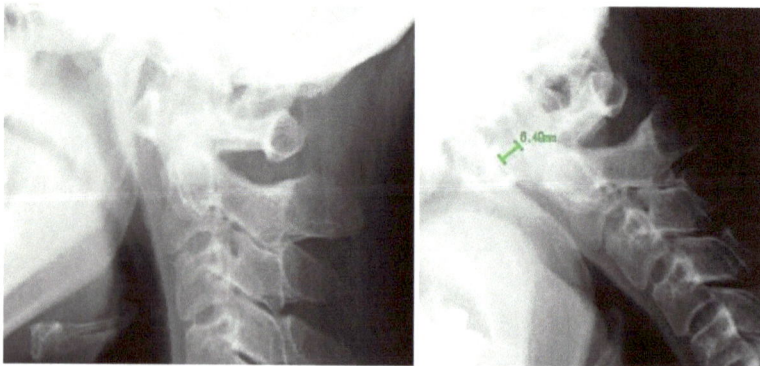

Fig. (122). Radiograph of lateral flexion position of the cervical spine shows mild widening of the atlantodens interval (ADI) in a patient with RA.

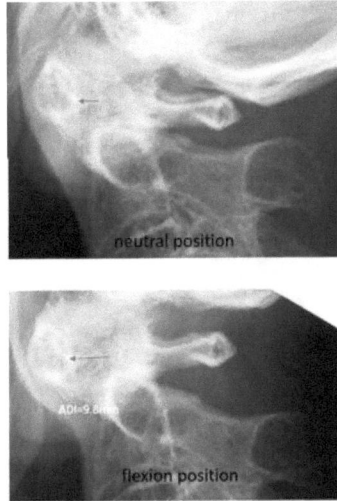

Fig. (123). Severely increased distance between the atlas and the odontoid (arrows). ADI is 9.8mm (>3.5mm). Lateral views of the upper cervical spine show anterior atlantoaxial subluxation in a patient with RA. In a flexed position, increased distance between the atlas and the odontoid (arrows) is evident. This finding suggests the laxity of the transverse ligament.

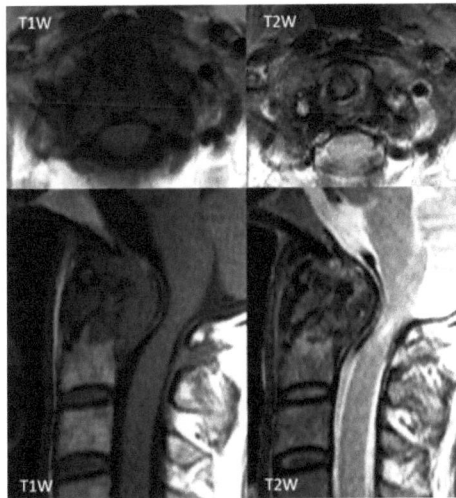

Fig. (124). Sagittal and transverse T1- and T2-weighted MR images show a large-sized nodule at C1/C2 and the compression of the spinal cord between the dens and the posterior arch of C1 (arrows).

Subaxial Articulations

Anterior subluxations at subaxial levels

In RA, subluxation and dislocation can occur at the subaxial levels, especially at the levels of C3-C4 and C4-C5 with erosive changes in the facet joints (Figs. **126** and **127**). Progressive changes at the apophyseal joints may induce osteoporosis, disk space narrowing, and subluxations at multiple levels. Lateral view of the neck shows subluxations at the multiple levels, doorstep or stepladder appearance.

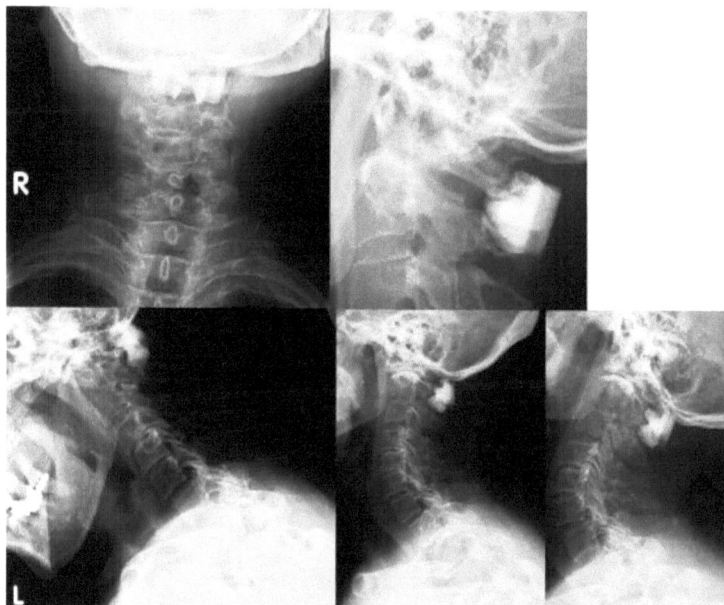

Fig. (125). The same patient with RA (Fig. **124**) required posterior fusion.

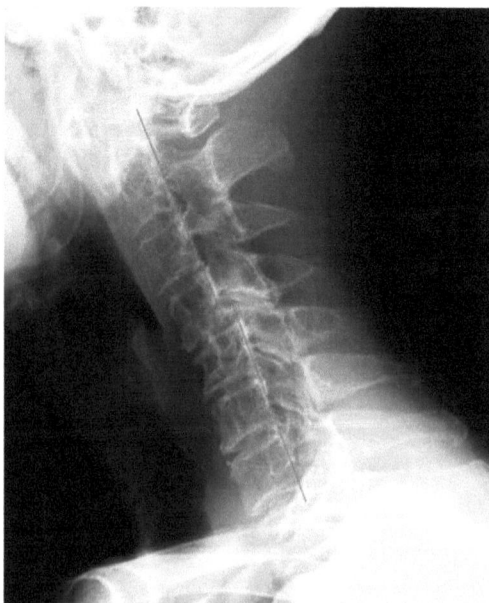

Fig. (126). Lateral view of the cervical spine of a patient with RA shows anterior subluxation and severe erosions of facets at C4-C5 level.

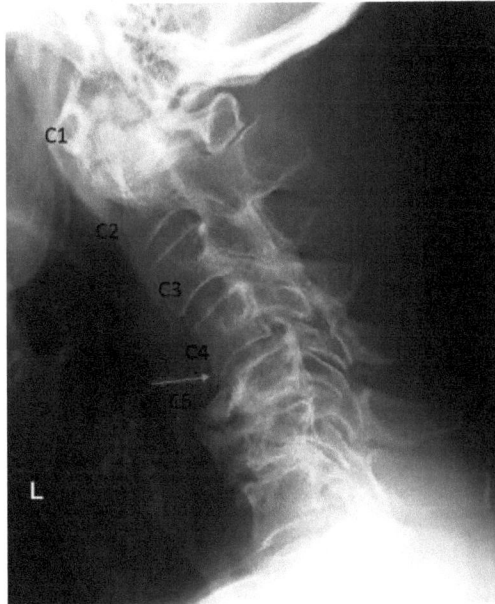

Fig. (127). Lateral view of the cervical spine of a patient with RA shows severe anterior subluxation at C4-C5 level.

Thoracic Spine

Radiography of the skeleton of the cervical spine in a normal person (Fig. **128**).

The thoracic spine is generally not involved in RA. However, spinal compression fracture of the thoracic spine may be seen in patients with RA (Fig. **129**).

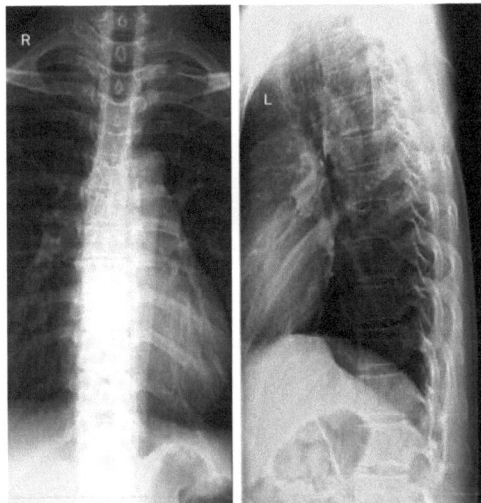

Fig. (128). Thoracic spine in a normal person.

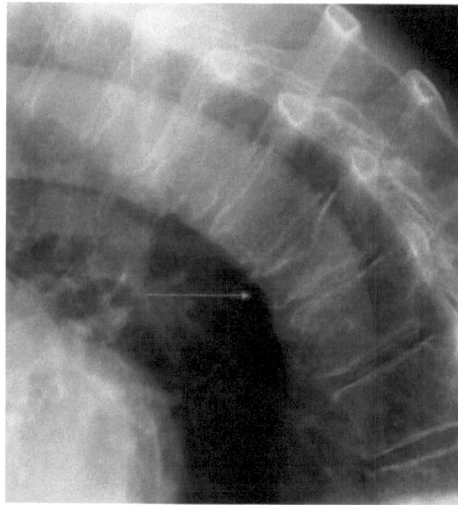

Fig. (129). Lateral radiograph of the thoracic spine demonstrates spinal compression fracture of Th7 in a patient with RA.

Lumbar Spine

Radiographic anatomy of the skeleton of the lumbar spine in a normal person (Figs. **130 - 132**). The lumbar spine is usually not involved in RA. Spinal compression fracture of the lumbar spine is seen in patients with RA (Fig. **133**).

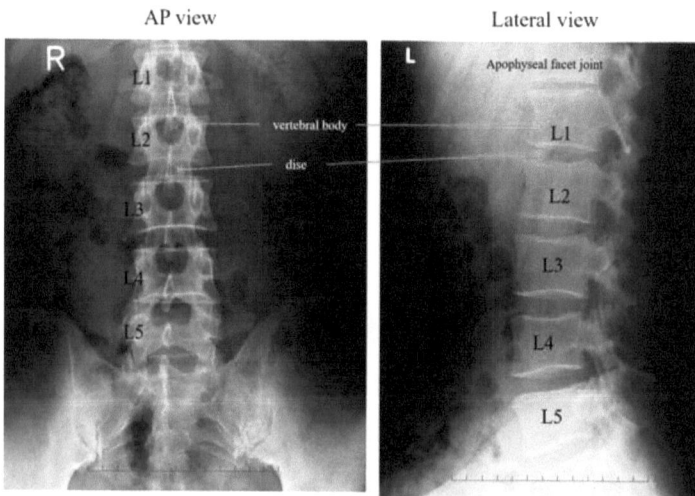

Fig. (130). Lumbar spine 2 views ; AP view and lateral view.

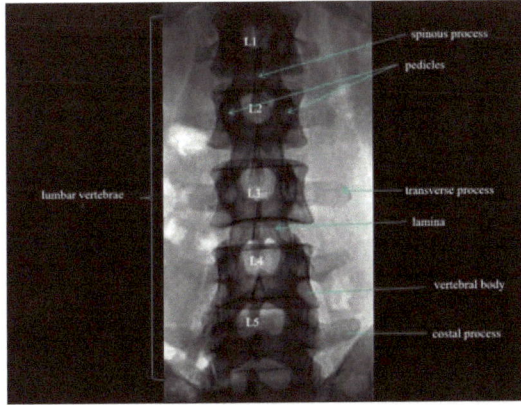

Fig. (131). Radiographic anatomy of the skeleton of the lumbar spine: AP view.

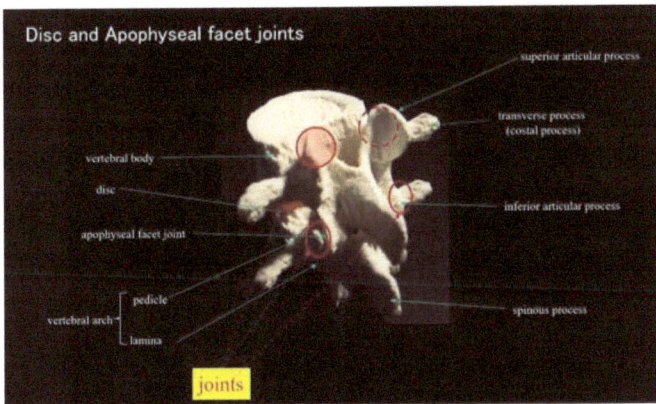

Fig. (132). Disc and apophyseal facet joints.

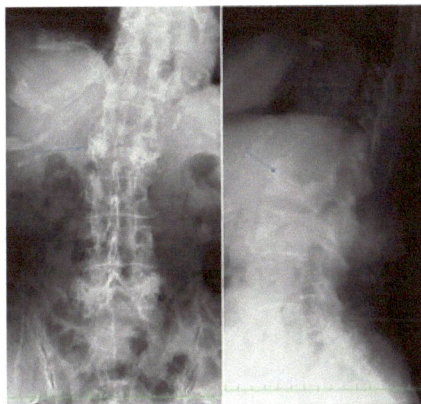

Fig. (133). AP view and lateral view of the lumbar spine of a patient with RA show L2 osteoporotic compression fracture.

BONE FRACTURES

Insufficiency Fractures

Insufficiency fracture is one of the important complications of RA. Insufficiency fracture occurs in a fragile bone because of a minor trauma. It may occur in the sacrum, the femoral neck, the parasymphyseal bone, tubular bones of the lower extremity including the tibia or the fibula, and so on. However, initial plain radiographs may show no definite fracture line of the bone (Figs. **134 - 136**). Therefore, it is difficult to make diagnoses of insufficiency fractures based on the initial plain radiographs. MRI and US are useful for the early diagnosis.

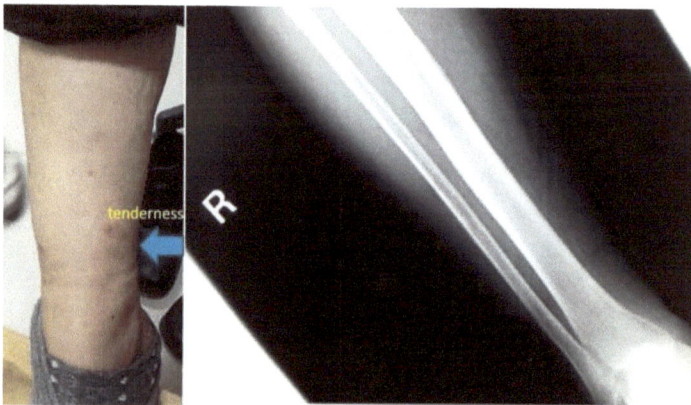

Fig. (134). A 62-year-old woman has history of RA for long years after the diagnosis. She also had pain and tenderness at a few centimeters up the right ankle towards the right knee after her walking. However, a plain radiograph of the right lower leg shows no abnormality in the bone of the tibia. Note the smooth cortical surface of the tibia.

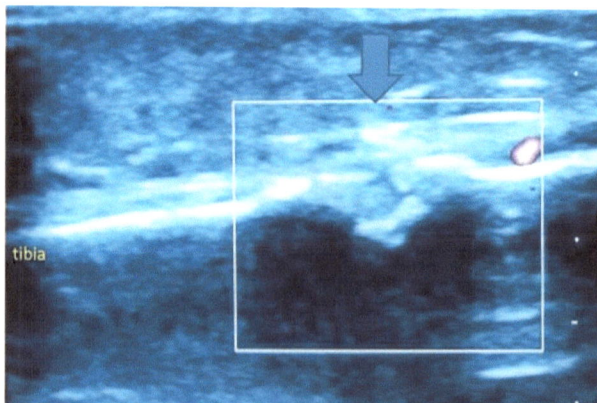

Fig. (135). US imaging shows a fracture of the tibia. The smooth cortical surface of the tibia is Interrupted by the fracture.

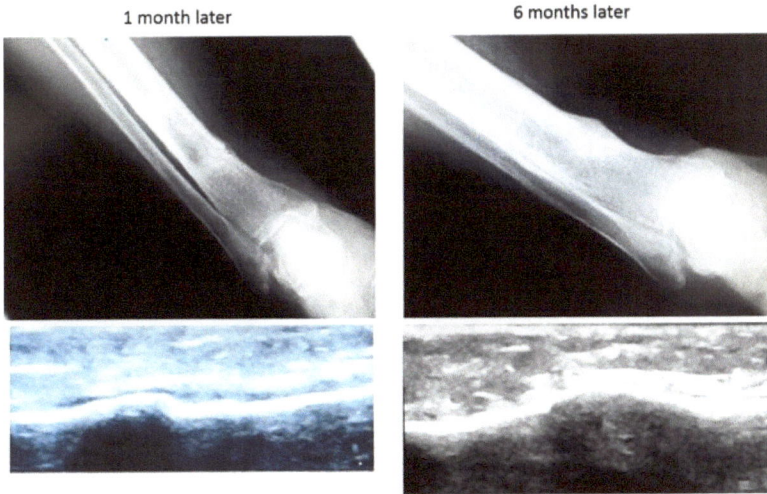

Fig. (136). Plain radiographs and US imaging after 1 and 6 months from the onset show the fracture of the tibia in the same patient (Fig. **135**).

Parasymphyseal Insufficiency Fractures

Parasymphyseal insufficiency fractures of the pubis may occur in patients with RA (Figs. **137** and **138**).

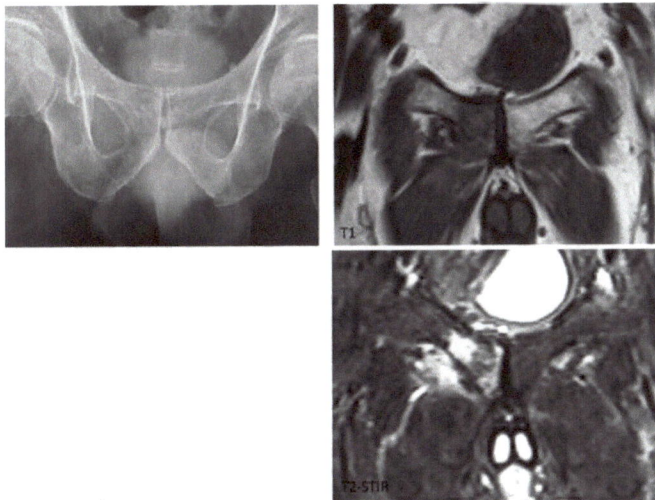

Fig. (137). Although AP view of the pelvis shows no fracture, an insufficiency fracture of the pubis can be detected by MR imaging in a patient with RA.

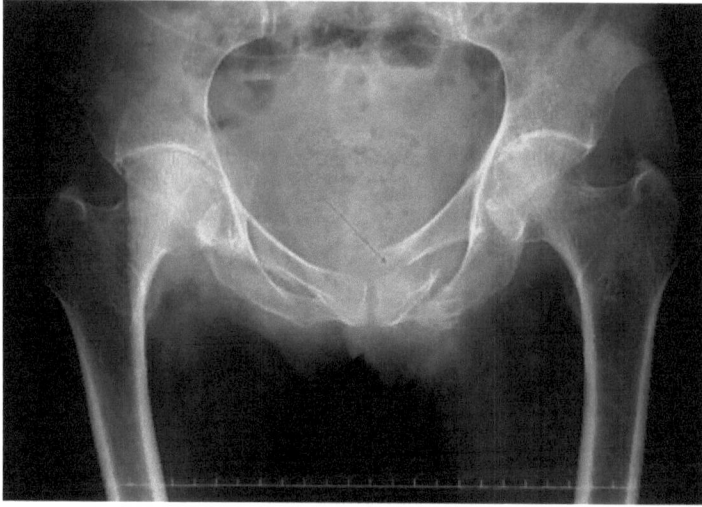

Fig. (138). AP view of the pelvis shows insufficiency fractures of the pubis in a patient with RA.

Compression Fractures of Thoracic and Lumbar Spine

Osteoporotic compression fracture of the lumbar spine in RA (Fig. **139**).

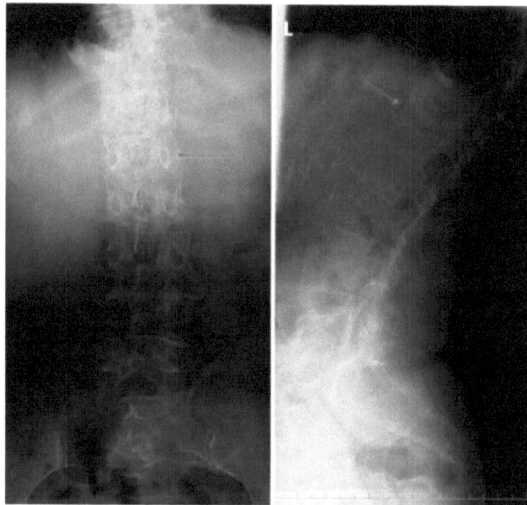

Fig. (139). AP view and lateral view of the lumbar spine of a patient with RA show an osteoporotic compression fracture of L1.

Traumatic Bone Fractures

Traumatic fracture can be seen in patients with RA (Figs. **140 - 143**).

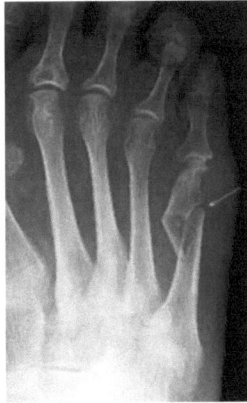

Fig. (140). A fracture of the fifth metatarsal bone in a patient with RA. The patient consulted a doctor as having swelling and pain of the fifth MTP joint due to RA. In actual, the pain was caused by the fracture (not RA).

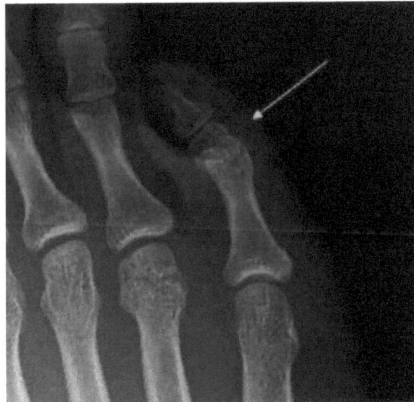

Fig. (141). A fracture of the head of the fifth proximal phalanx in a patient with RA.

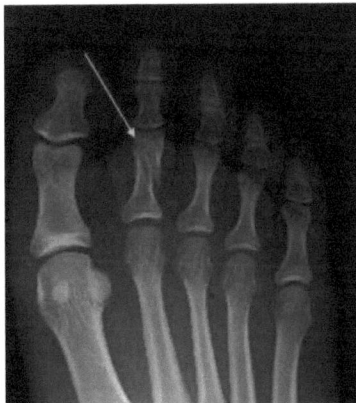

Fig. (142). Bone fracture of the shaft of the second proximal phalanx in a patient with RA.

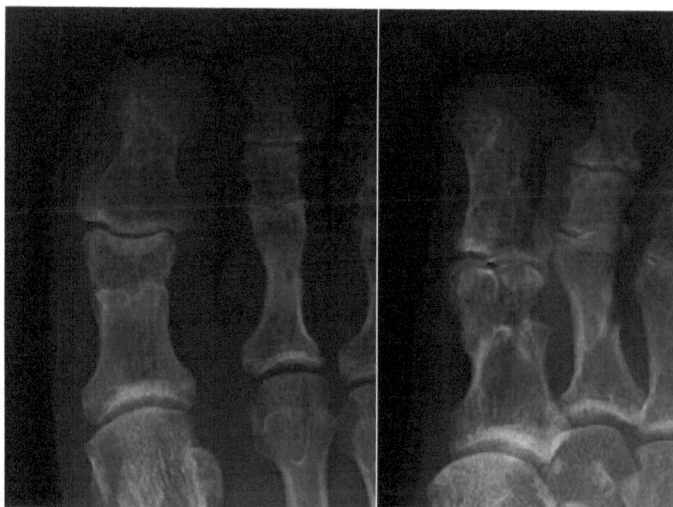

Fig. (143). AP view of the great toe of a patient with RA shows a fracture.

DESTRUCTION OF THE JOINTS

Septic Arthritis

Destructive septic arthritis in a patient with RA (Figs. **144 - 146**).

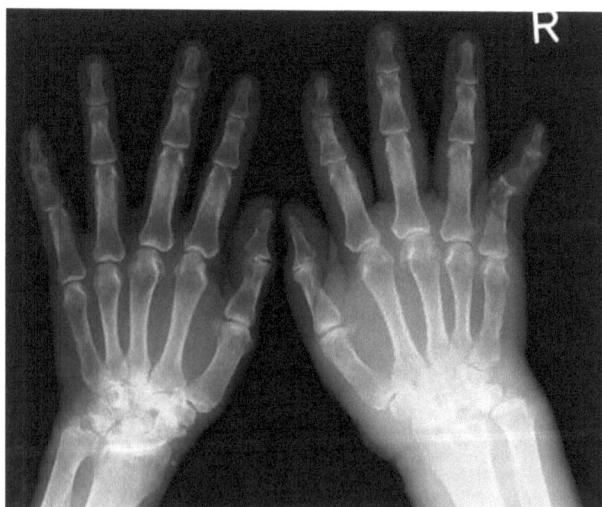

Fig. (144). Septic arthritis in a patient with RA. The right wrist is swelling and bones of the wrist are destroyed.

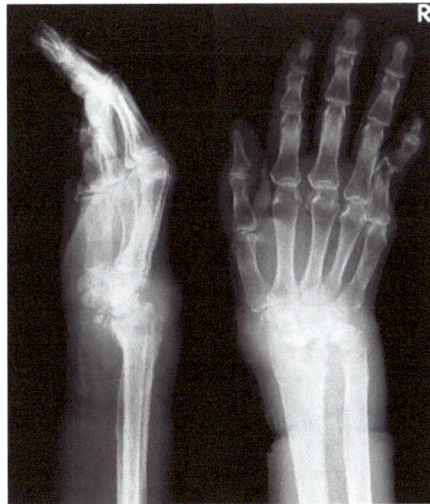

Fig. (145). The progressive destruction of the wrist joint in the same patient with RA and septic arthritis (Fig. 144).

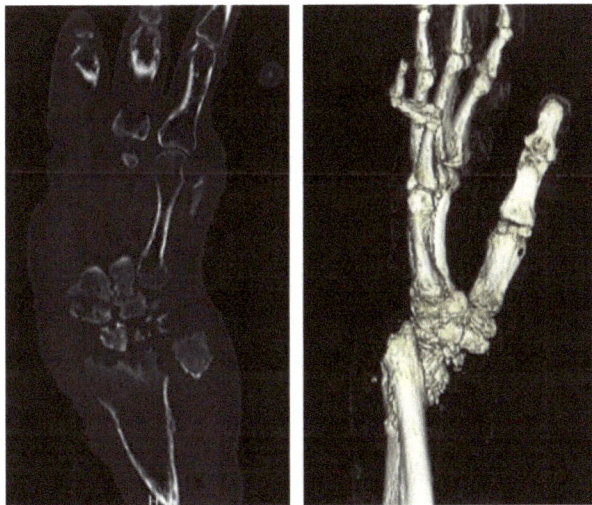

Fig. (146). CT and 3D-CT illustrate the destructed bones of the wrist joint.

CONSENT FOR PUBLICATION

Not applicable.

CONFLICT OF INTEREST

The author (editor) declares no conflict of interest, financial or otherwise.

ACKNOWLEDGEMENTS

The authors thank Ms. K. Eguchi and A. Ibe for secretarial assistance.

REFERENCES

[1]   Brumfield RH, Conaty JP. Reconstructive surgery of the thumb in rheumatoid arthritis. Orthopedics 1980; 3(6): 529-33.
[PMID: 24822776]

[2]   Tubiana R, Toth B. Rheumatoid arthritis: clinical types of deformities and management. Clin Rheum Dis 1984; 10(3): 521-48.
[PMID: 6532642]

[3]   Youm Y, McMurthy RY, Flatt AE, Gillespie TE. Kinematics of the wrist. I. An experimental study of radial-ulnar deviation and flexion-extension. J Bone Joint Surg Am 1978; 60(4): 423-31.
[http://dx.doi.org/10.2106/00004623-197860040-00001] [PMID: 670263]

[4]   Goergen TG, Resnick D, Riley RR. Post-traumatic abnormalities of the pubic bone simulating malignancy. Radiology 1978; 126(1): 85-7.
[http://dx.doi.org/10.1148/126.1.85] [PMID: 619439]

[5]   Tsuzuki K. Insufficiency fracture and post-traumatic osteolysis of the pubic bone. Jap J Rheum Joint Surg 1998; pp. 273-8.

CHAPTER 3

B: Bone Mineralization and Shape

Syuichi Koarada[*] and **Yuri Sadanaga**

Division of Rheumatology, Faculty of Medicine, Saga University, Saga, Japan

Abstract: Category B is the mineralization and shape of the bones. This category includes bone mineralization, erosions, bone cysts, and osteophyte formation. In rheumatoid arthritis (RA), marginal erosion is a hallmark of the disease and occurs in the bare areas of the bone. Especially, juxta-articular osteoporosis is the earliest change in plain radiograph of patients with RA.

Keywords: Bone mineralization, Cone cysts, Erosions, Juxta-articular osteoporosis, Osteopytes, Rheumatoid arthritis.

BONE DENSITY

Normal Mineralization

Bone density is evaluated at the metacarpal shaft of the 2nd or the 3rd digit in PA view of the hand. The sum of the lateral side of cortices of the shaft is more than 50% of width of the bone (Fig. **1**).

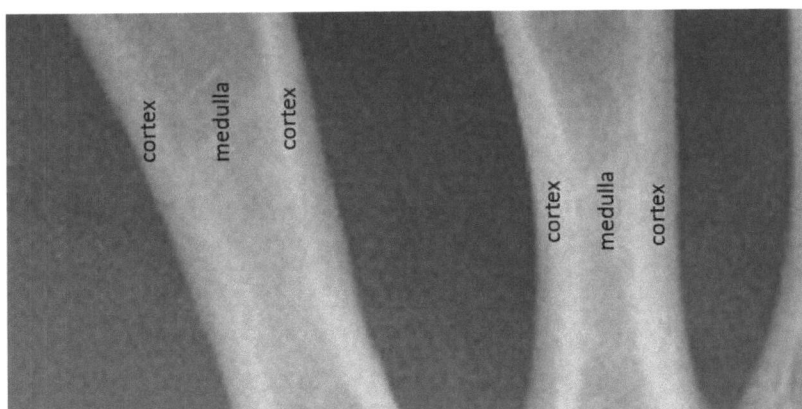

Fig. (1). The cortices (white) of the shaft is clearly more than 50% of width of the bone in a normal person.

[*] **Corresponding author Syuichi Koarada:** Division of Rheumatology, Faculty of Medicine, Saga University, Saga, Japan; Tel: 81-952-31-6511; E-mail: koarada@cc.saga-u.ac.jp

Decreased Mineralization

Diffuse Osteoporosis (Systemic Osteoporosis)

Diffuse osteoporosis (systemic osteoporosis) is shown in Figs. (**2** and **3**).

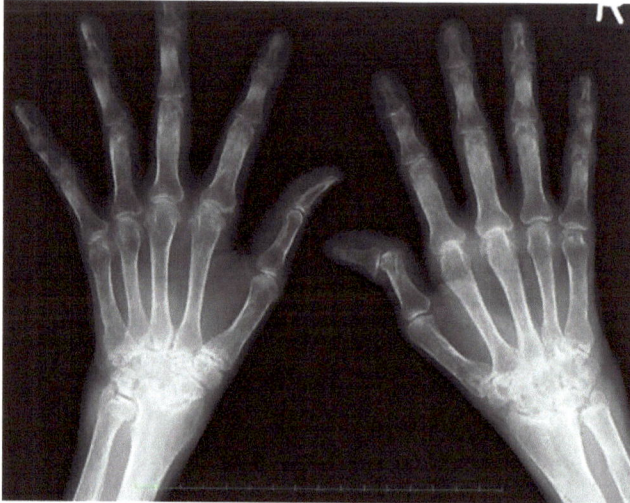

Fig. (2). Radiograph of the hands of a patient with RA shows that white cortices may be less than 50% of width of the shaft in the 2nd metacarpal bone.

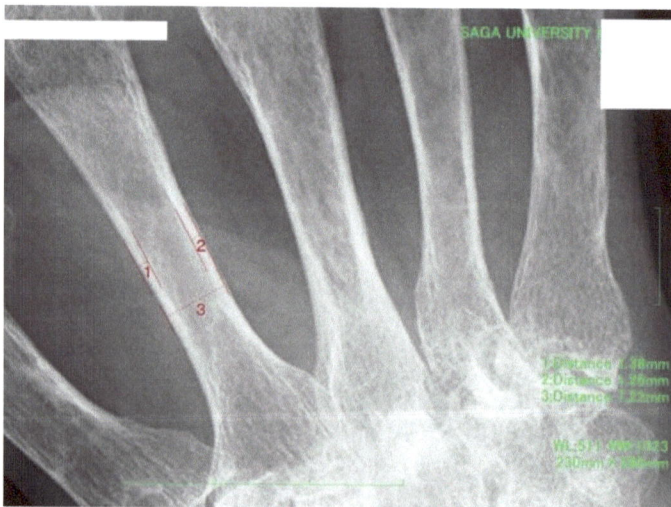

Fig. (3). Cortices/ width of the 2nd shaft=(1.38+1.26)/7.22=□36.5% < 50%.

Osteoporosis of Lumbar Spine

When the diffuse osteoporosis exists in a patient, the evaluation of bone density should be performed (Fig. **4**).

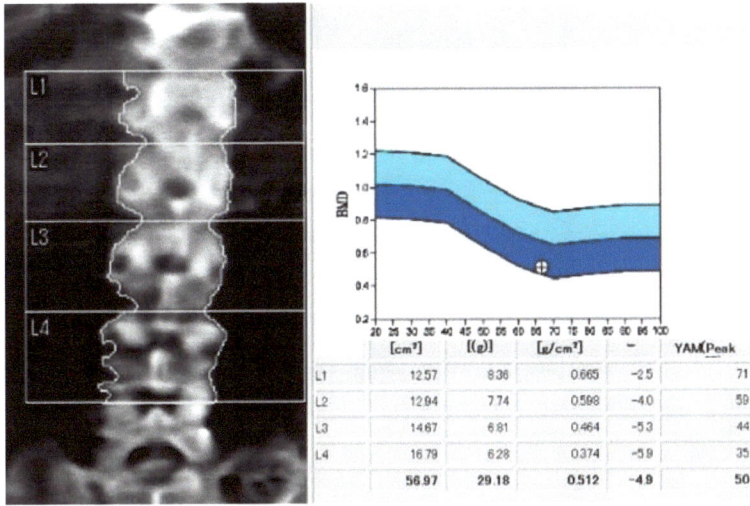

	[cm²]	[(g)]	[g/cm²]	–	YAM(Peak
L1	12.57	8.36	0.665	-2.5	71
L2	12.94	7.74	0.598	-4.0	59
L3	14.67	6.81	0.464	-5.3	44
L4	16.79	6.28	0.374	-5.9	35
	56.97	29.18	0.512	-4.9	50

Fig. (4). Bone densitometry (DEXA; dual energy x-ray absorptiometric scan) shows systemic osteoporosis showing low BMD (bone mineral density) in a 66-year-old female with RA. Bone fractures should be evaluated.

Juxta-articular Osteoporosis, Periarticular Osteoporosis

In normal condition, the metaphyseal-epiphyseal part of the digits is darker than the diaphysis because of the thinner cortical bone in the metaphysis and epiphysis (Fig. **5**). The blacked bones and their dramatic differences may be found in inflammatory joints in patients with RA (Figs. **6 - 9**) [1].

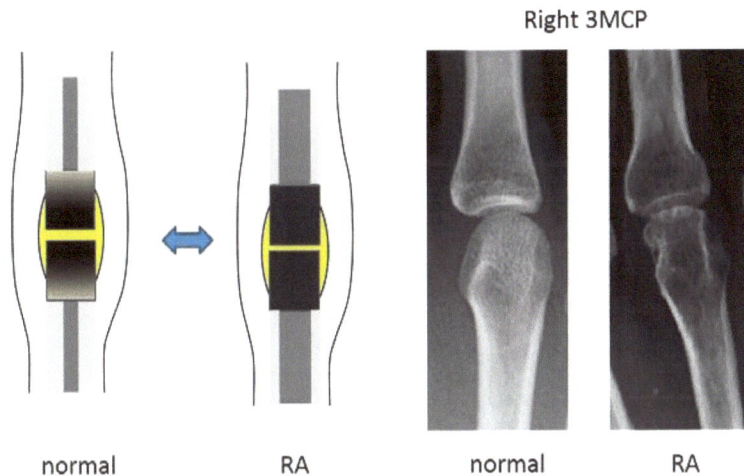

Fig. (5). Juxta-articular osteoporosis is the earliest change in plain radiograph of patients with RA. It suggests an inflammation of the joint, but it is nonspecific.

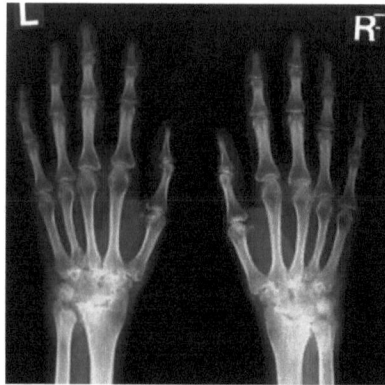

Fig. (6). PA view of the hands in a 25-year-old woman with RA shows juxta-articular osteoporosis of the MCP, PIP, and IP joints of the all digits. The left carpal bones and the distal radius are also osteoporotic. However, there is no systemic osteoporosis.

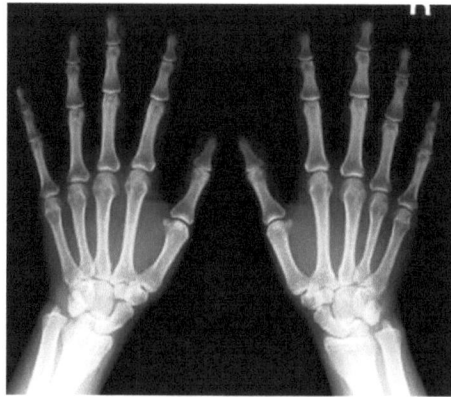

Fig. (7). PA view of the hands in a patient with RA shows juxta-articular osteoporosis at the MCP and PIP joints of the all digits, but not at the wrist.

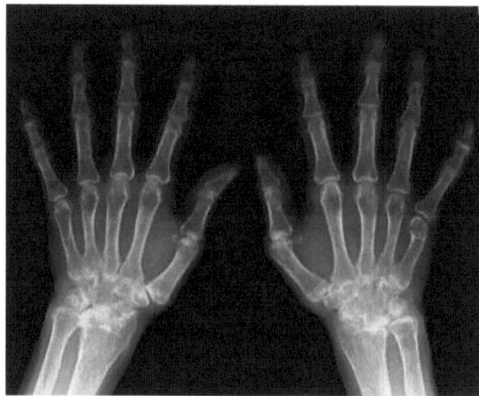

Fig. (8). PA view of the hands in a patient with advanced RA shows juxta-articular osteoporosis at the joints of all the digits and both the wrists with systemic osteoporosis.

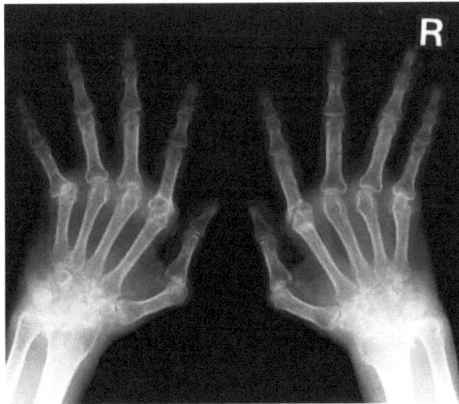

Fig. (9). PA view of the hands in a patient with late RA shows osteoporosis with osteosclerosis.

Fingers and Thumbs

IPs

Juxta-articular osteoporosis of the 1st IP joints (Figs. **10** and **11**).

Juxta-articular Osteoporosis of the right 1ˢᵗ IP

normal   RA

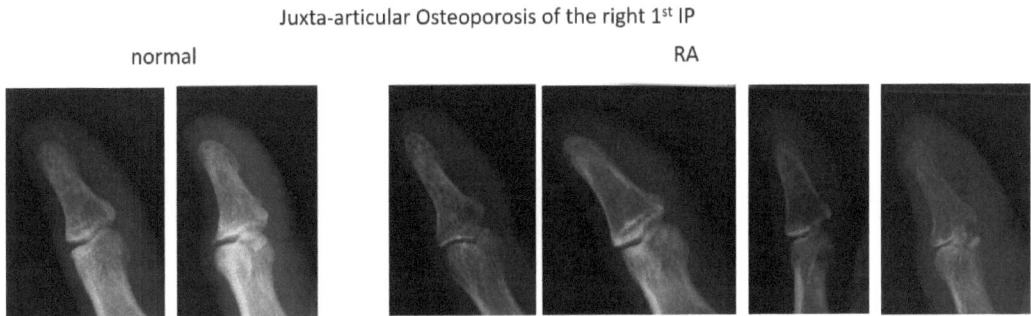

Fig. (10). Juxta-articular osteoporosis of the right 1st IP joints.

Juxta-articular Osteoporosis of the left 1ˢᵗ IP

normal   RA

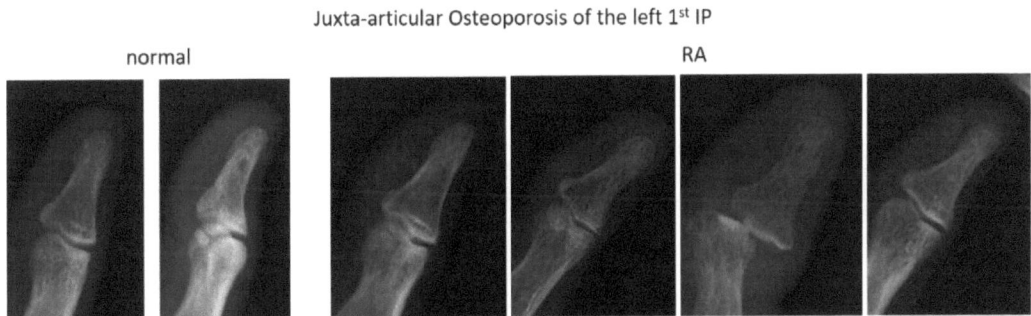

Fig. (11). Juxta-articular osteoporosis of the left 1st IP joints.

PIPs

Juxta-articular osteoporosis of the PIP joints (Figs. **12 - 19**).

Juxta-articular Osteoporosis of the right 2nd PIP

normal   RA

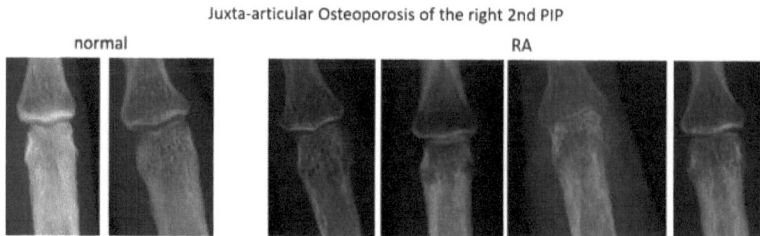

Fig. (12). Juxta-articular osteoporosis of the right 2nd PIP joints.

Juxta-articular Osteoporosis of the left 2nd PIP

normal   RA

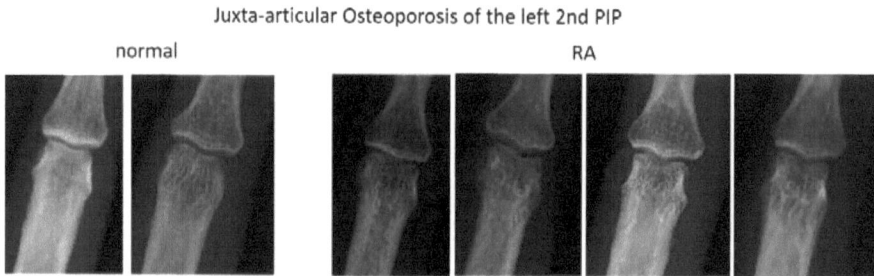

Fig. (13). Juxta-articular osteoporosis of the left 2nd PIP joints.

Juxta-articular Osteoporosis of the right 3rd PIP

normal   RA

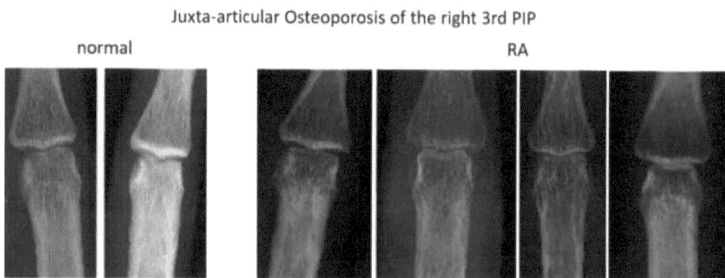

Fig. (14). Juxta-articular osteoporosis of the right 3rd PIP joints.

Juxta-articular Osteoporosis of the left 3rd PIP

normal   RA

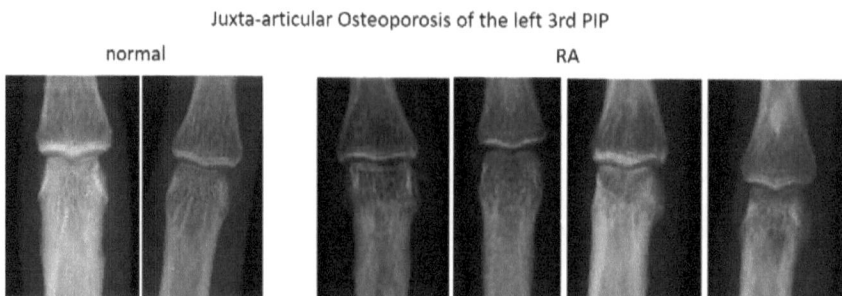

Fig. (15). Juxta-articular osteoporosis of the left 3rd PIP joints.

Juxta-articular Osteoporosis of the right 4th PIP

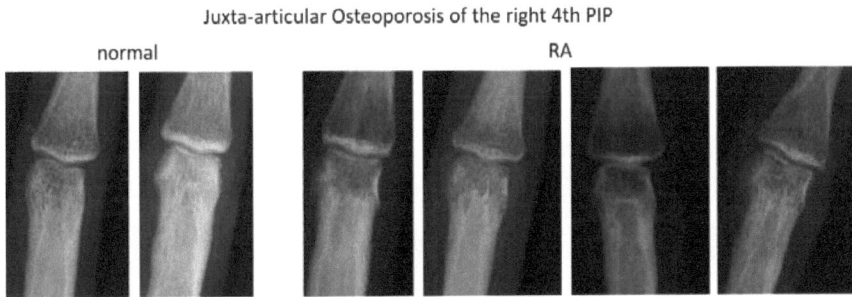

Fig. (16). Juxta-articular osteoporosis of the right 4th PIP joints.

Juxta-articular Osteoporosis of the left 4th PIP

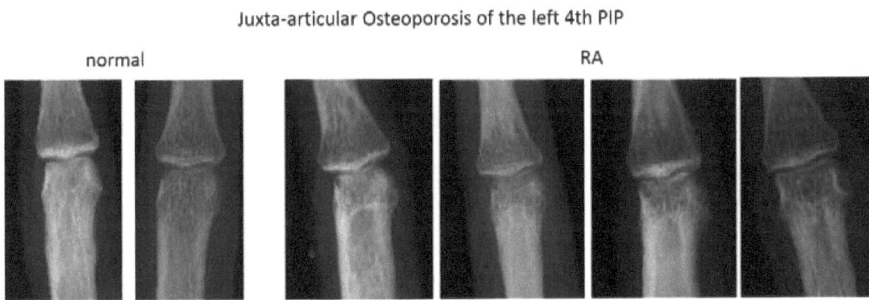

Fig. (17). Juxta-articular osteoporosis of the left 4th PIP joints.

Juxta-articular Osteoporosis of the right 5th PIP

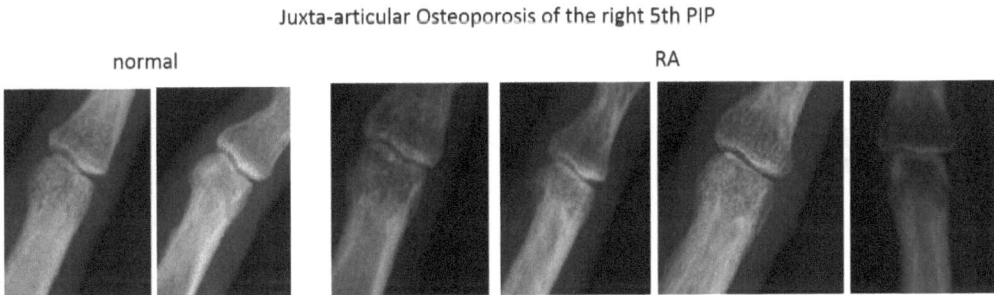

Fig. (18). Juxta-articular osteoporosis of the right 5th PIP joints.

Juxta-articular Osteoporosis of the left 5th PIP

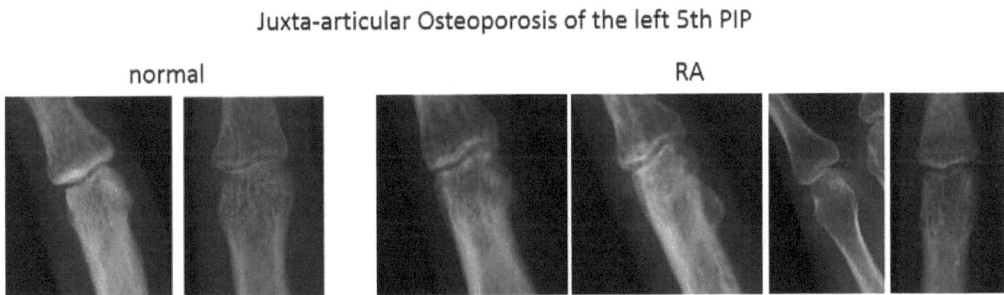

Fig. (19). Juxta-articular osteoporosis of the left 5th PIP joints.

MCPs

Juxta-articular osteoporosis of the MCP joints (Figs. **20 - 29**).

Juxta-articular Osteoporosis of the right 1st MCP

normal   RA

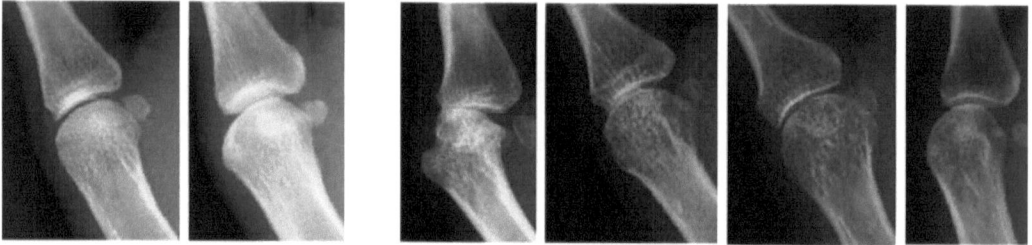

Fig. (20). Juxta-articular osteoporosis of the right 1st MCP joints.

Juxta-articular Osteoporosis of the left 1st MCP

normal   RA

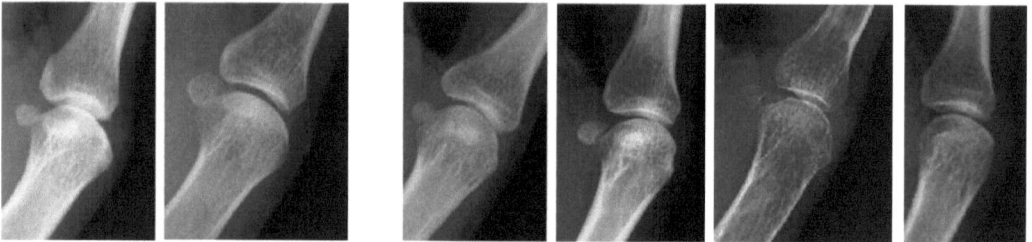

Fig. (21). Juxta-articular osteoporosis of the left 1st MCP joints.

Juxta-articular Osteoporosis of the right 2nd MCP

normal   RA

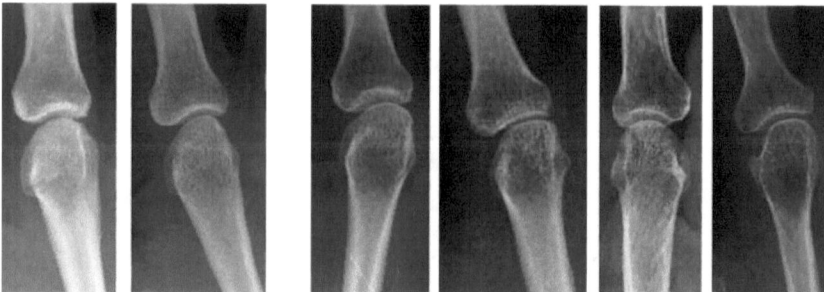

Fig. (22). Juxta-articular osteoporosis of the right 2nd MCP joints.

Juxta-articular Osteoporosis of the left 2nd MCP

normal   RA

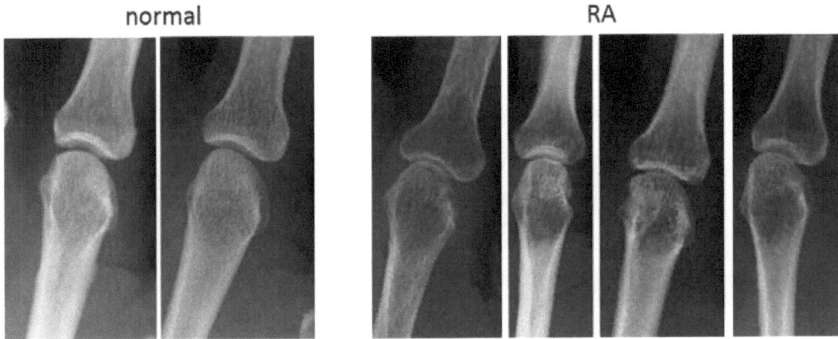

Fig. (23). Juxta-articular osteoporosis of the left 2nd MCP joints.

Juxta-articular Osteoporosis of the right 3rd MCP

normal   RA

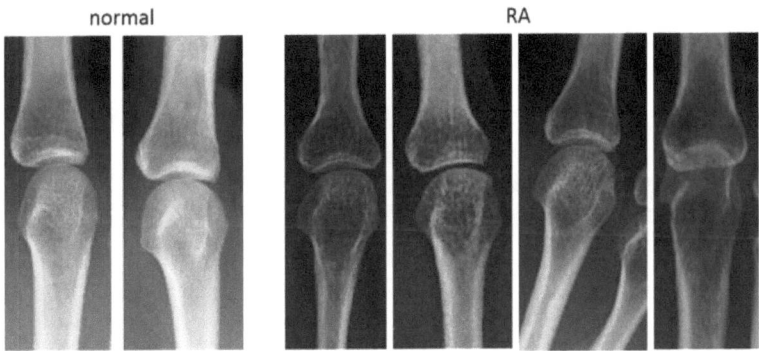

Fig. (24). Juxta-articular osteoporosis of the right 3rd MCP joints.

Juxta-articular Osteoporosis of the left 3rd MCP

normal   RA

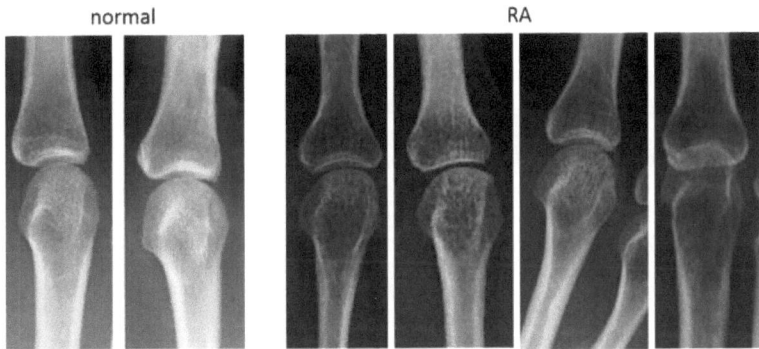

Fig. (25). Juxta-articular osteoporosis of the left 3rd MCP joints.

Juxta-articular Osteoporosis of the right 4th MCP

normal   RA

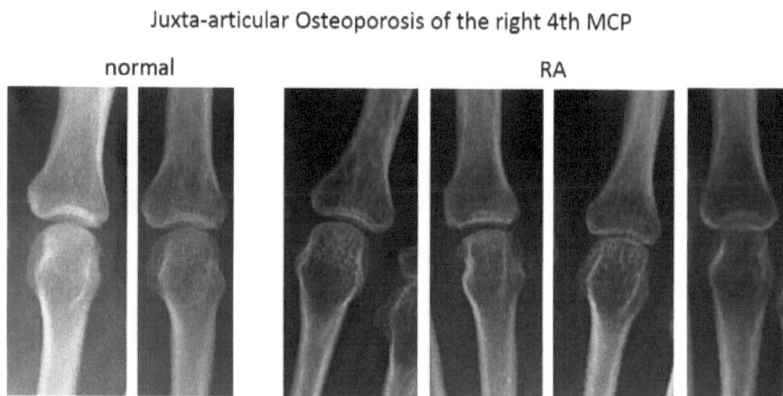

Fig. (26). Juxta-articular osteoporosis of the right 4th MCP joints.

Juxta-articular Osteoporosis of the right 4th MCP

normal   RA

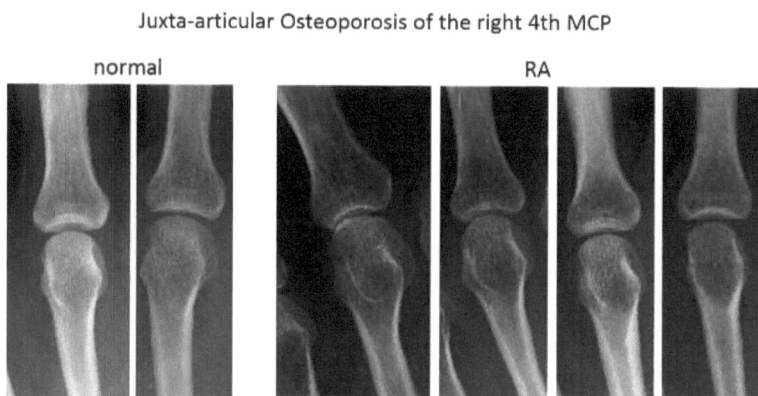

Fig. (27). Juxta-articular osteoporosis of the left 4th MCP joints.

Juxta-articular Osteoporosis of the right 5th MCP

normal   RA

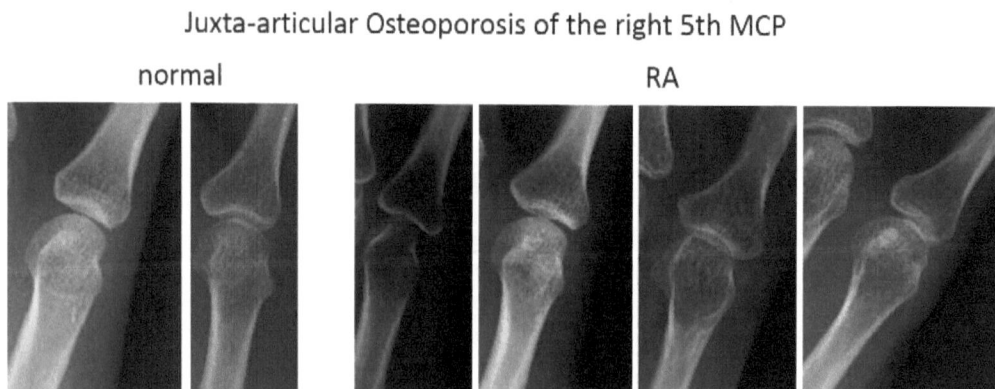

Fig. (28). Juxta-articular osteoporosis of the right 5th MCP joints.

Juxta-articular Osteoporosis of the left 5th MCP

normal   RA

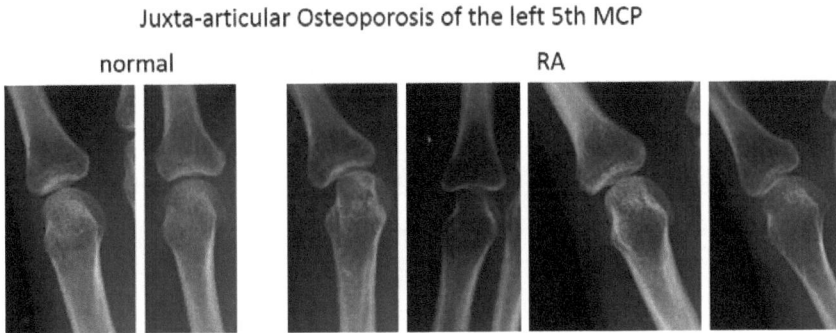

Fig. (29). Juxta-articular osteoporosis of the left 5th MCP joints.

CMCs

Juxta-articular osteoporosis of the CMC joints (Figs. **30 - 34**).

Juxta-articular Osteoporosis of the 1st CMC

normal   RA

Rt

Lt

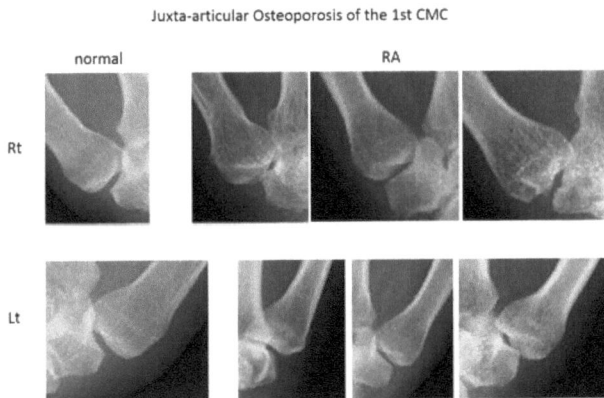

Fig. (30). Juxta-articular osteoporosis of the 1st CMC joints.

Juxta-articular Osteoporosis of the 2nd CMC

normal   RA

Rt

Lt

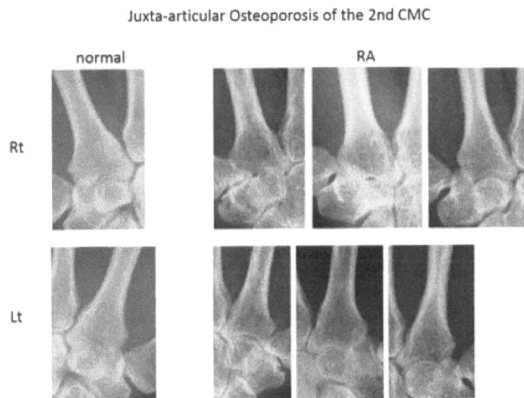

Fig. (31). Juxta-articular osteoporosis of the 2nd CMC joints.

Juxta-articular Osteoporosis of the 3rd CMC

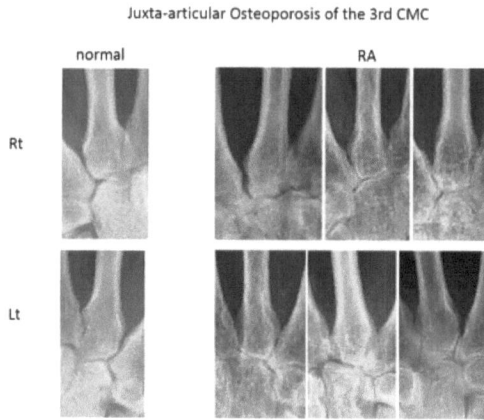

Fig. (32). Juxta-articular osteoporosis of the 3rd CMC joints.

Juxta-articular Osteoporosis of the 4th CMC

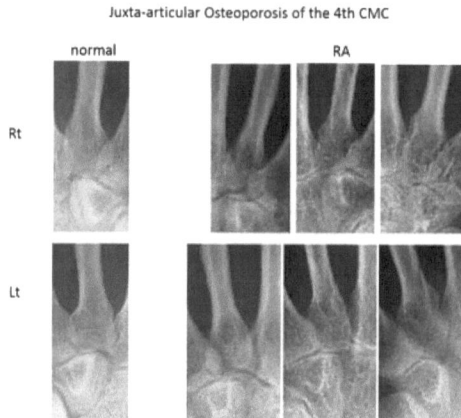

Fig. (33). Juxta-articular osteoporosis of the 4th CMC joints.

Juxta-articular Osteoporosis of the 5th CMC

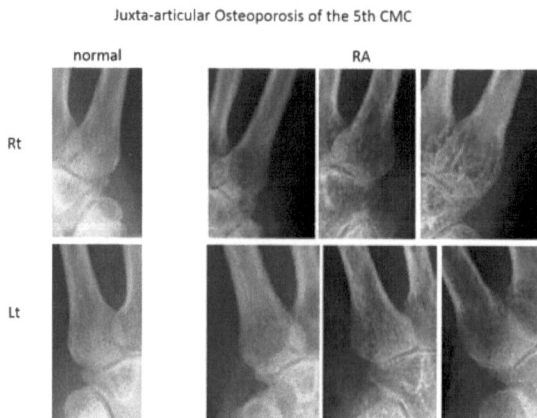

Fig. (34). Juxta-articular osteoporosis of the 5th CMC joints.

Wrists

Juxta-articular osteoporosis of the wrists (Figs. **35** and **36**).

Juxta-articular Osteoporosis of RC joints

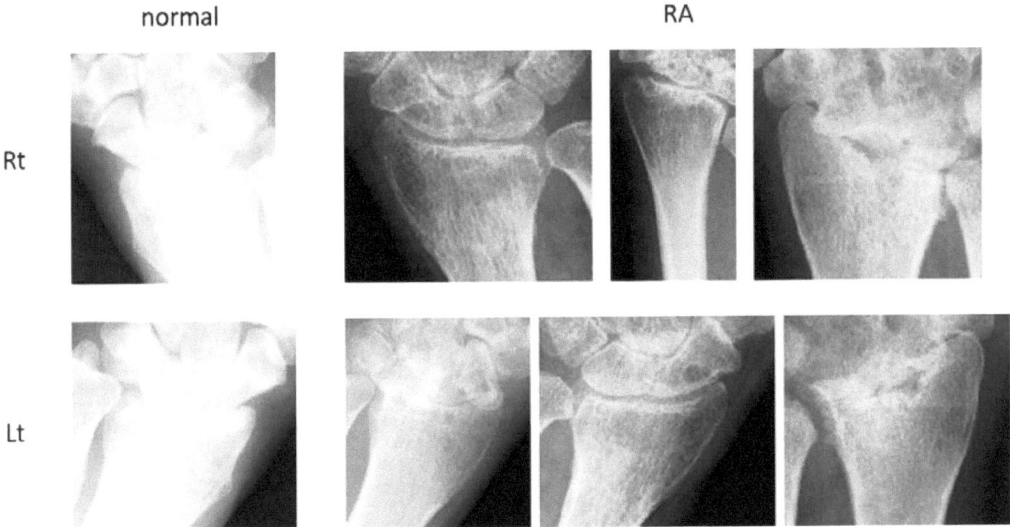

Fig. (35). Juxta-articular osteoporosis of the RC joints.

Juxta-articular Osteoporosis of the Ulna

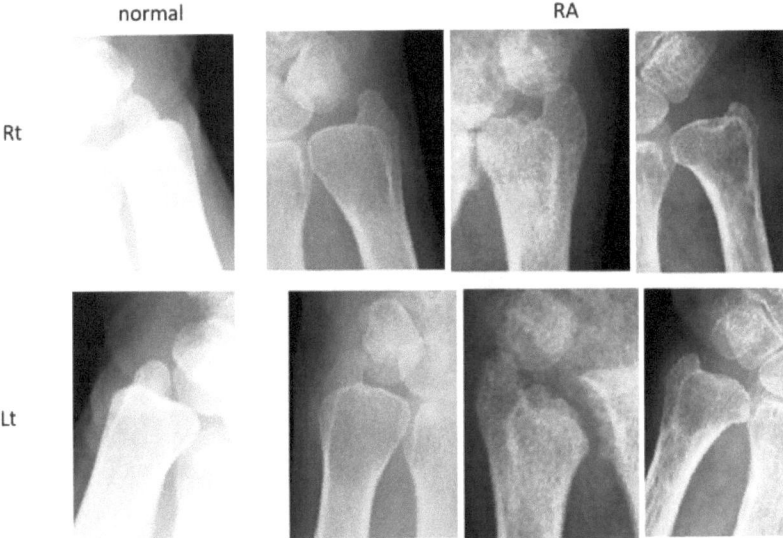

Fig. (36). Juxta-articular osteoporosis of the ulnae.

Elbows

Juxta-articular osteoporosis of the elbows (Figs. **37** and **38**).

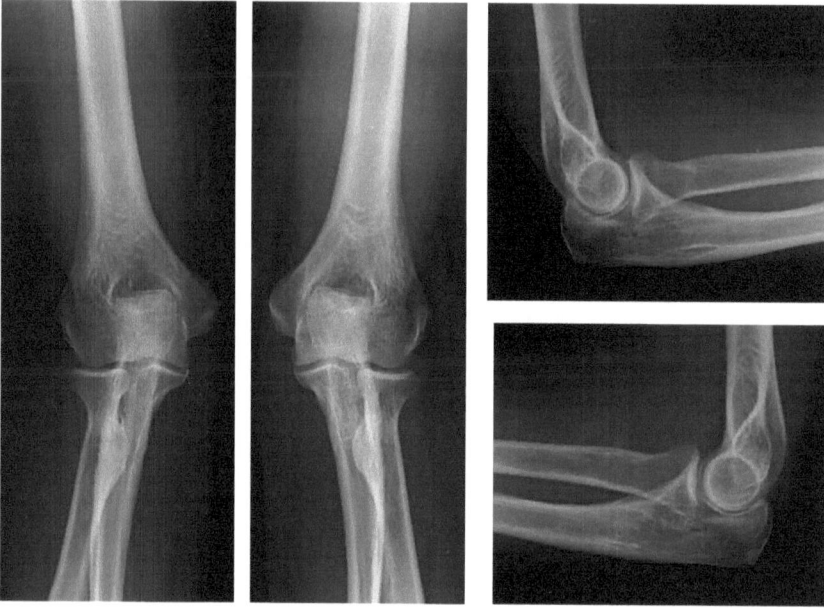

Fig. (37). Juxta-articular osteoporosis of the elbows.

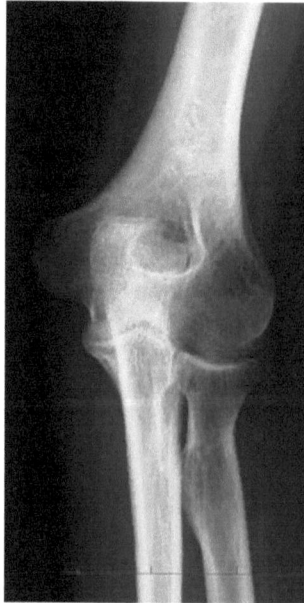

Fig. (38). AP view of the elbow shows juxta-articular osteoporosis of the humeroradial joint in the elbow.

Knees

Juxta-articular osteoporosis of the knees (Fig. **39**).

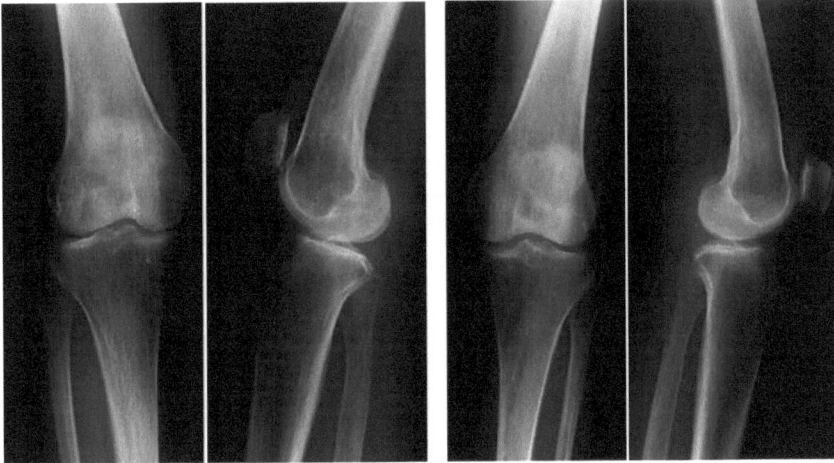

Fig. (39). Juxta-articular osteoporosis of the knees.

Increased Mineralization

Osteosclerosis

A simplified schema of osteosclerosis shows that the subchondral bone has proliferative change that is white (Fig. **40**). Secondary osteosclerosis of the joints may be seen in patients with RA (Figs. **41** and **42**).

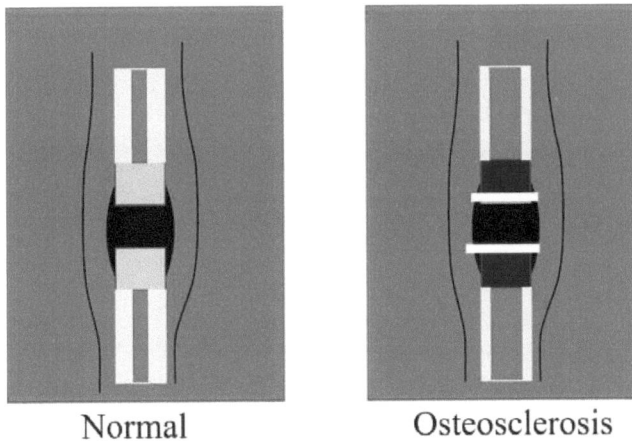

Normal   Osteosclerosis

Fig. (40). A simplified schema of osteosclerosis. The subchondral bone has proliferative change that is white.

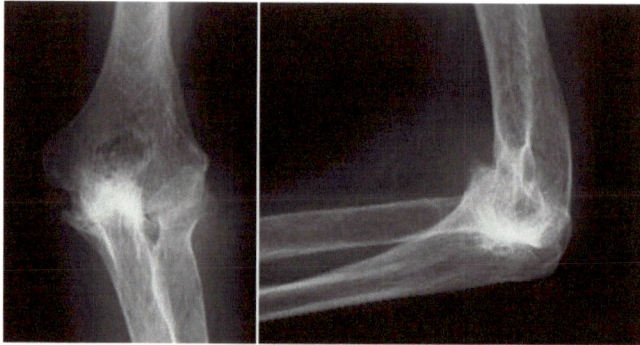

Fig. (41). AP view and lateral view of the right elbow show osteosclerosis of the humeroradial joint.

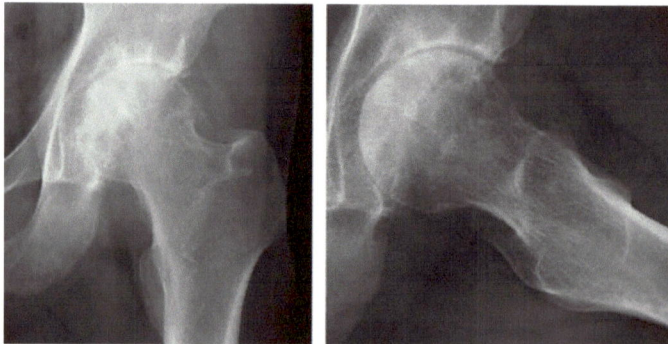

Fig. (42). AP view and frog leg view of the left hip show osteosclerosis of the femoral head and the acetabulum.

EROSIONS

In RA, marginal erosions occur in the bare areas of the bone (Fig. **43**). An early change of the erosion is the loss of the continuity of the white cortical line (Figs. **44** and **45**). It causes marginal erosion in the bare area (Fig. **46**).

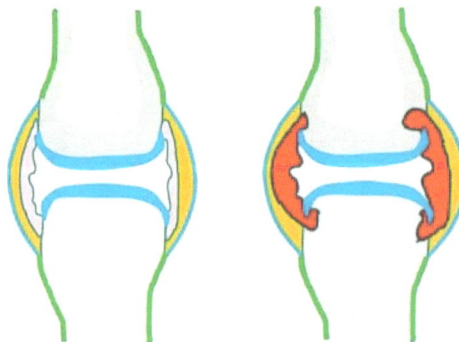

Fig. (43). In RA, marginal erosions occur in the bare areas of the bone. In the bare areas, the cartilage does not cover the bone, then proliferated synovium directly touches the bones.

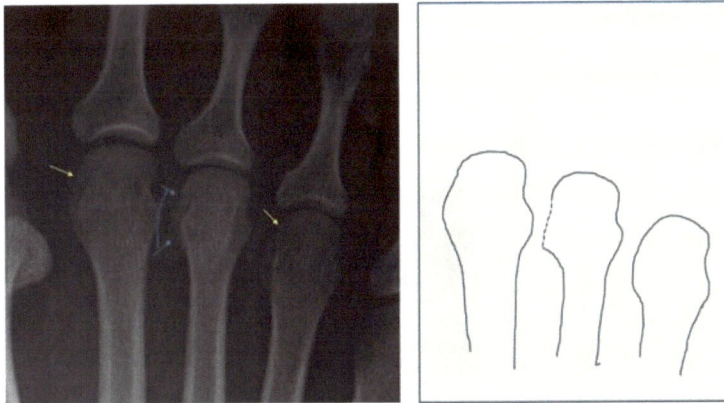

Fig. (44). An early change of the erosion is observed at the head of the third metacarpal bone of the right foot in a patient with RA. Loss of the continuity of the white cortical line is found (blue arrows) at the third metacarpal bone. However, there is no discontinuation at the second and the fourth metacarpal bones.

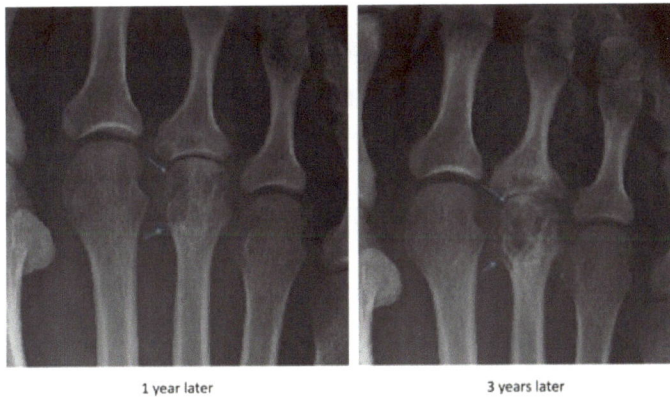

1 year later   3 years later

Fig. (45). The plain radiographs of 1 year and 3 years later show the development of the erosions in the same patient with RA.

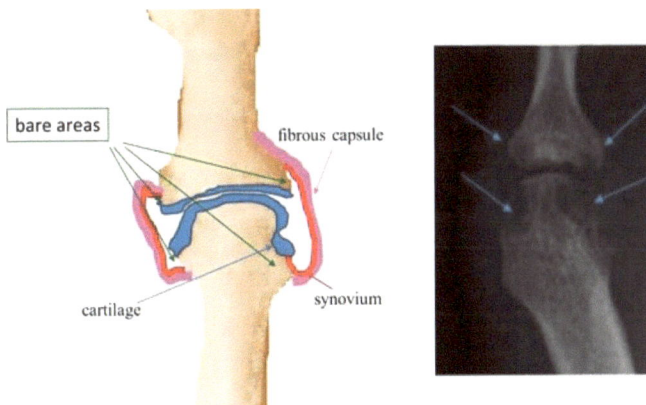

Fig. (46). Marginal erosions at the bare areas are characteristic for RA.

Fingers and Thumbs

IPs

Erosions of the first IP joint in RA (Fig. **47**).

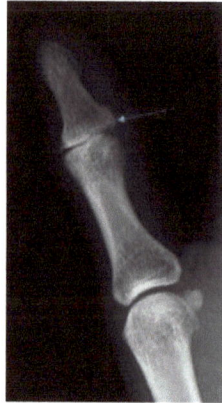

Fig. (47). An erosion at the right first IP joint in a patient with RA.

PIPs

Erosions occur at the bare areas on the head of the proximal phalanx and the base of the middle phalanx (Fig. **48**). In many cases, the erosions are larger on the head of the proximal phalanx than on the base of the middle phalanx.

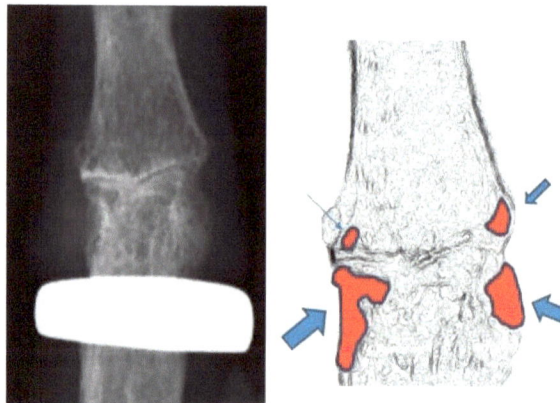

Fig. (48). Erosions on the head of the proximal phalanx are larger than those on the base of middle phalanx in a patient with RA.

Second PIPs

Erosions of the second PIP joints (Figs. **49** and **50**).

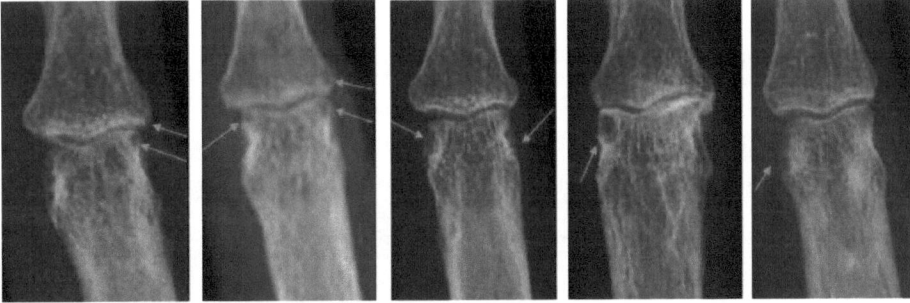

Fig. (49). Erosions of the right 2nd PIP joints.

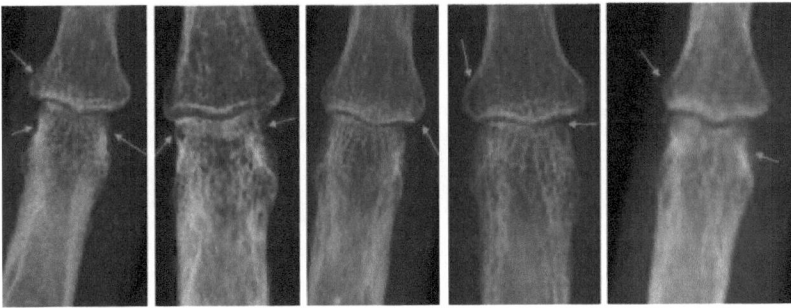

Fig. (50). Erosions of the left 2nd PIP joints.

Third PIPs

Erosions of the third PIP joints (Figs. **51** and **52**).

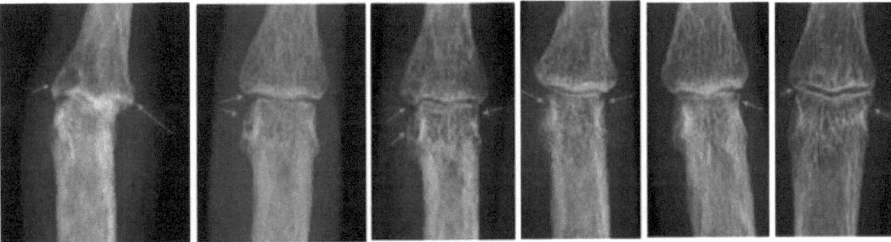

Fig. (51). Erosions of the right 3rd PIP joints.

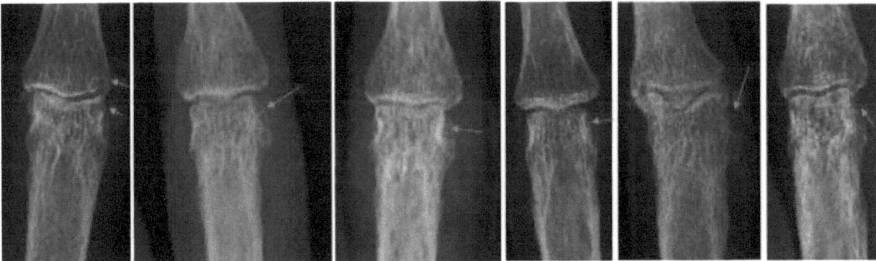

Fig. (52). Erosions of the left 3rd PIP joints.

Fourth PIPs

Erosions of the fourth PIP joints (Figs. **53** and **54**).

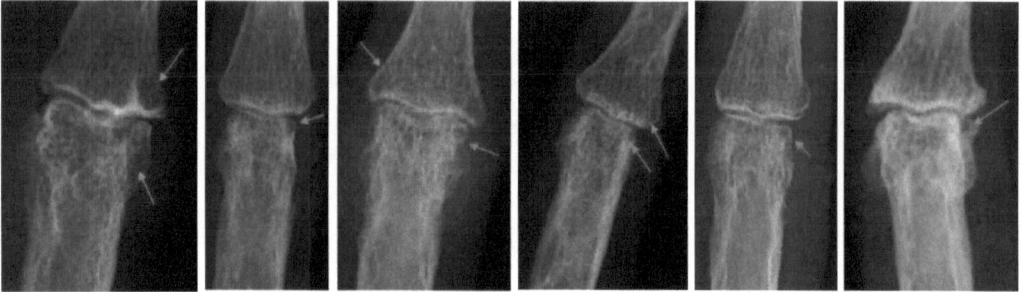

Fig. (53). Erosions of the right 4th PIP joints.

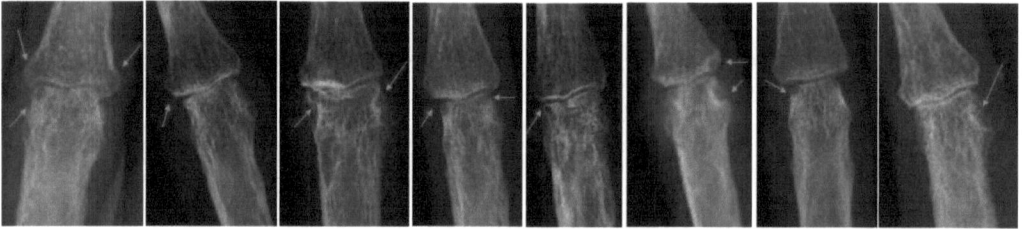

Fig. (54). Erosions of the left 4th PIP joints.

Fifth PIPs

Erosions of the fifth PIP joints (Fig. **55**).

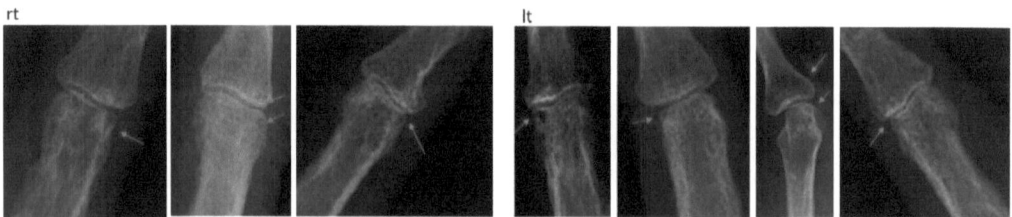

Fig. (55). Erosions of the 5th PIP joints.

MCPs

First MCPs

Erosions of the first MCP joints (Figs. **56 - 60**).

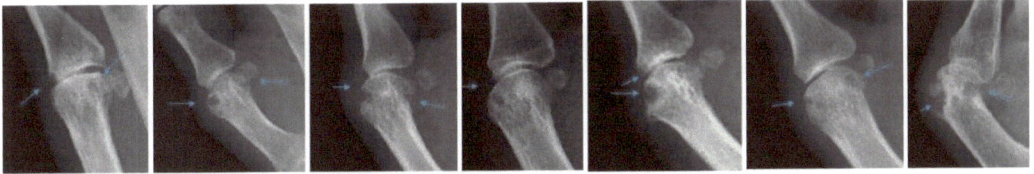

Fig. (56). Erosions of the right 1st MCP joints.

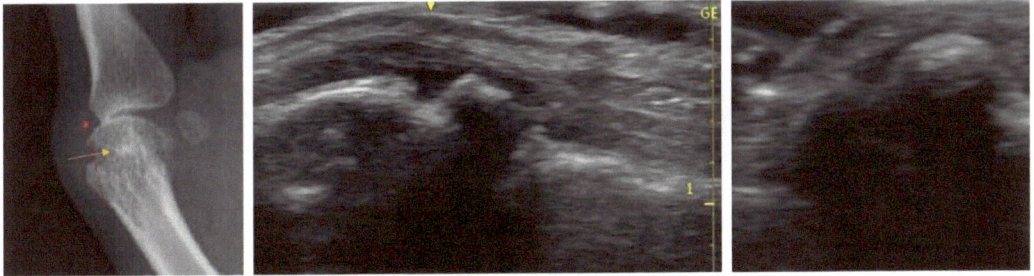

Fig. (57). Longitudinal and transverse gray-scale US images of the right first MCP joint show an erosion in a patient with RA. Also, plain radiograph shows the same erosion.

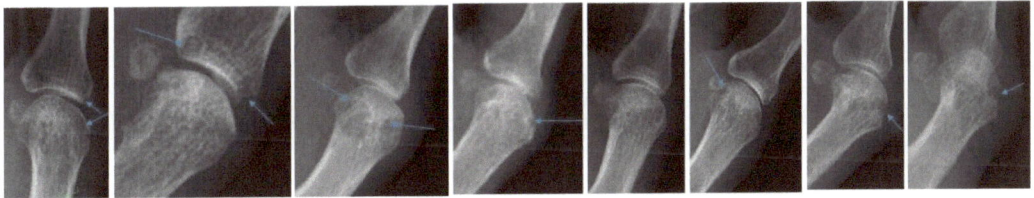

Fig. (58). Erosions of the left 1st MCP joints.

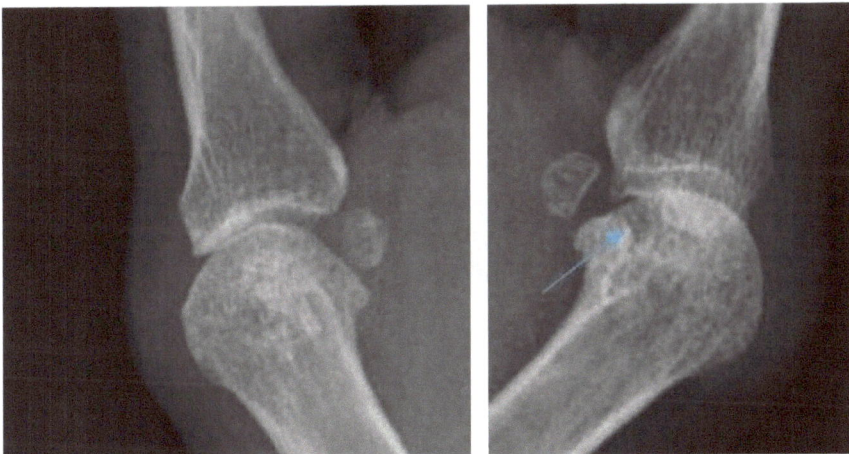

Fig. (59). PA view (left panel) of the first MCP joint does not show an erosion, but ball-catch view illustrates the erosion.

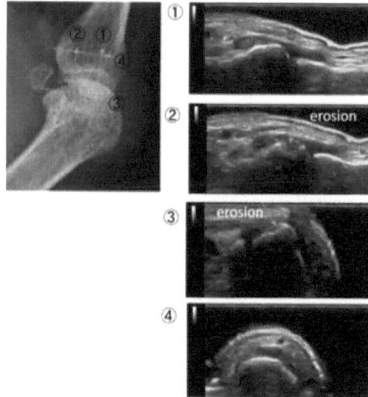

Fig. (60). US images show the erosion of the head of the metacarpal at the first MCP joint in the same patient with RA.

Second MCPs

Erosions of the second MCP joints (Figs. **61 - 63**).

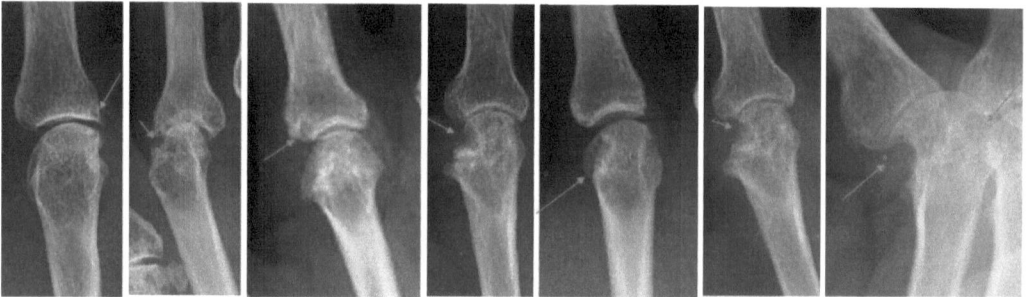

Fig. (61). Erosions of the right 2nd MCP joints.

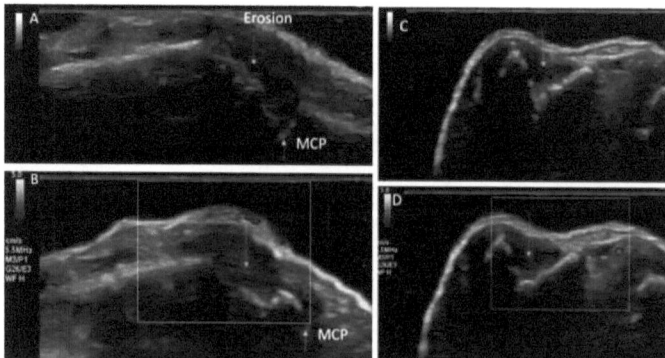

Fig. (62). A, B: Longitudinal gray-scale and power Doppler hydro-US images show a large erosion of the second metacarpal head at the second MCP joint in a patient with RA. There is no PD signal. C, D: Transverse gray-scale and power Doppler hydro-US images show the erosion.

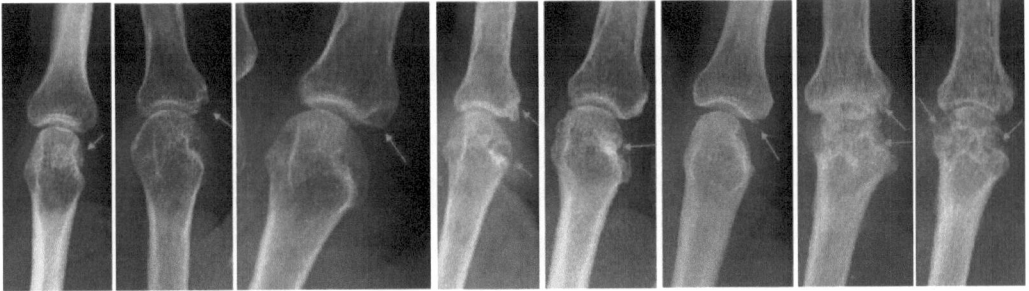

Fig. (63). Erosions of the left 2nd MCP joints.

Third MCPs

Erosions of the third MCP joints (Figs. **64 - 68**).

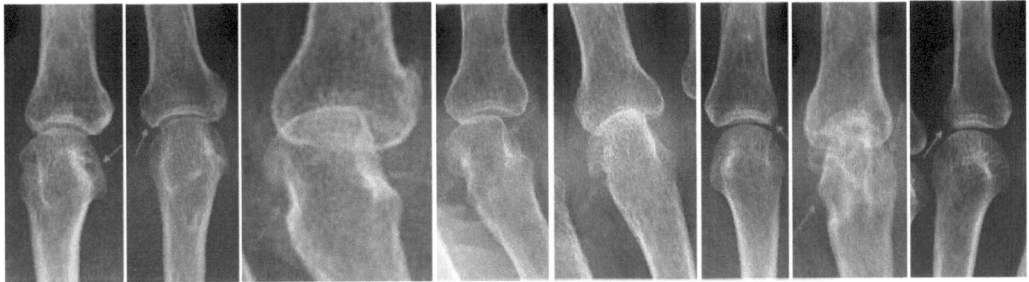

Fig. (64). Erosions of the 3rd MCP joints.

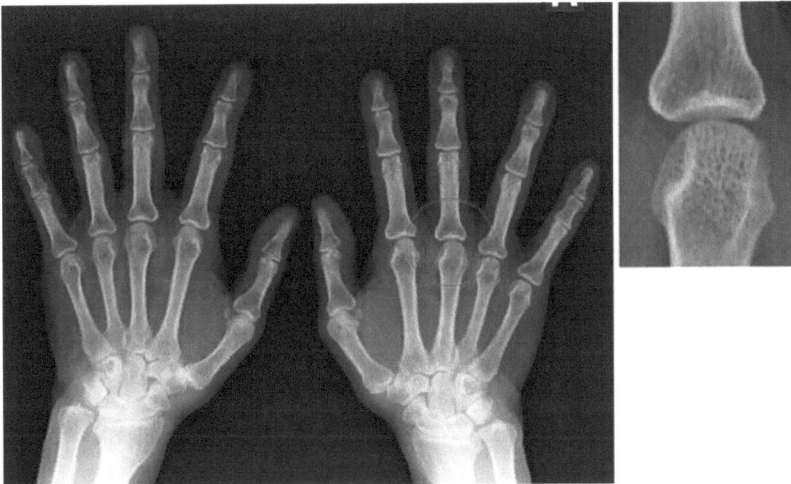

Fig. (65). PA view of the hands cannot clearly illustrate an erosion of the base of the proximal phalanx at the third MCP joint in a patient with RA.

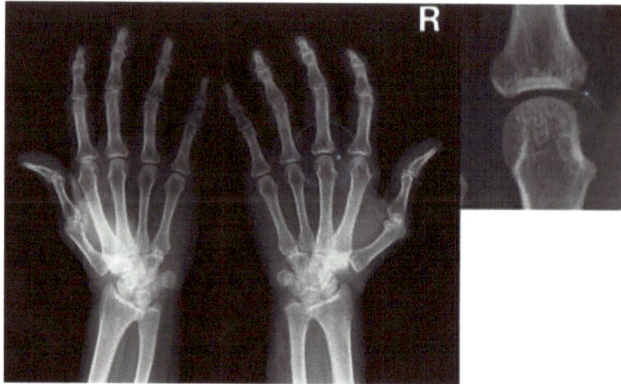

Fig. (66). Nørgaard view (ball-catch view) shows the erosion of the base of the proximal phalanx in the same patient with RA.

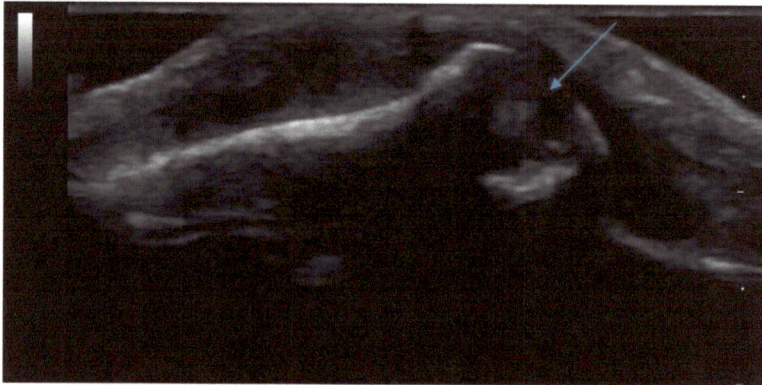

Fig. (67). Erosion of the third MCP joint in a patient with RA. Longitudinal gray-scale US image of the third MCP joint shows cortical interruption (arrow) on the dorsal aspect of the third metacarpal head. That is consistent with an erosion in the bare area.

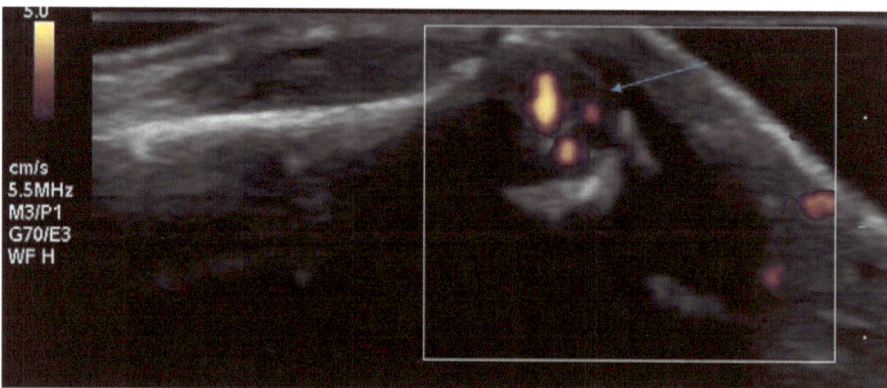

Fig. (68). Longitudinal power Doppler US image of the dorsal aspect of the third MCP joint shows PD signals (arrow) in the erosion of the third metacarpal head.

Fourth MCPs

Erosions of the fourth PIP joints (Fig. **69**).

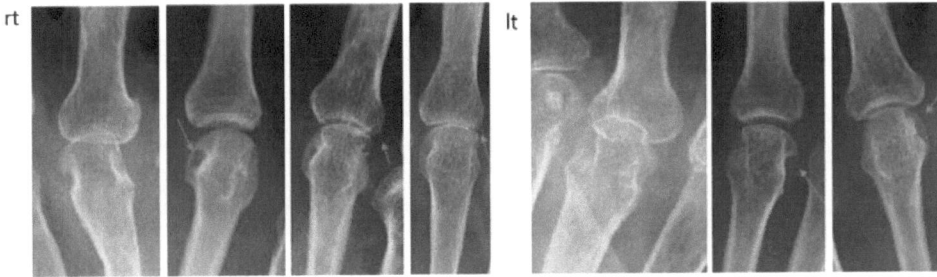

Fig. (69). Erosions of the 4th MCP joints.

Fifth MCPs

Erosions of the fifth MCP joints (Fig. **70**).

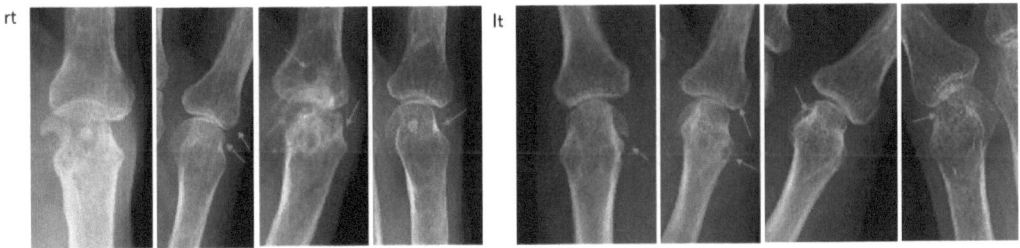

Fig. (70). Erosions of the 5th MCP joints.

DIPs

Arthritis and erosions of DIP joints are less common and less severe. Although involvement of the DIP joints is rare, it can occur in RA (Fig. **71**). However, the sole arthritis of the DIP joints is unusual in RA.

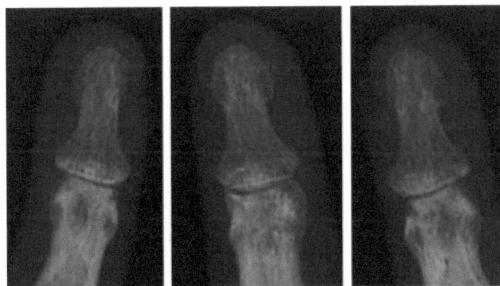

Fig. (71). Rarely, erosions of the DIP joints may be seen in patients with RA.

CMCs

Erosions of the CMC joints in RA (Fig. **72**).

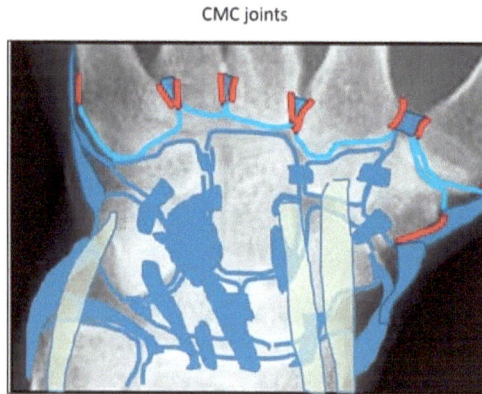

Fig. (72). A schema of the sites of erosions of the CMC joints in RA.

First CMCs

Erosions of the first CMC joints in RA (Figs. **73** and **74**).

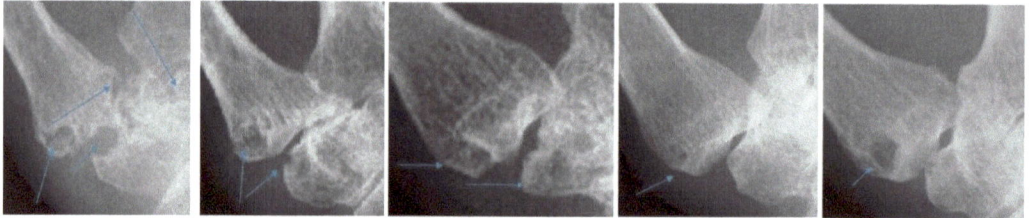

Fig. (73). Erosions of the right 1st CMC joints in patients with RA.

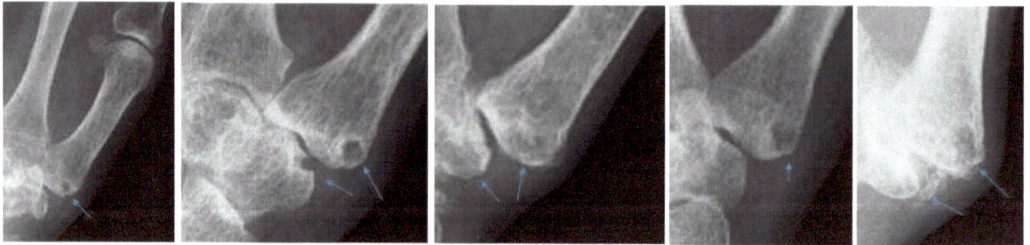

Fig. (74). Erosions of the left 1st CMC joints in patients with RA.

Second CMCs

Erosions of the second CMC joints in RA (Fig. **75**).

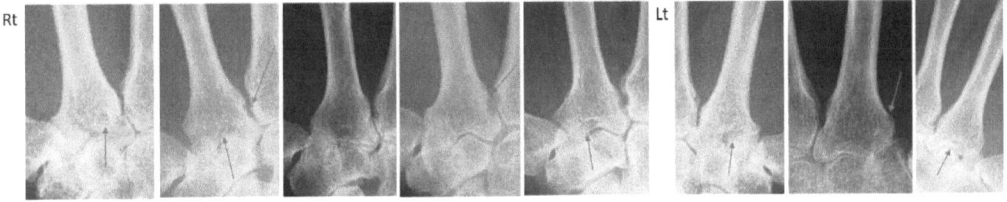

Fig. (75). Erosions of the 2nd CMC joints in patients with RA.

Third CMCs

Erosions of the fourth CMC joints in RA (Fig. **76**).

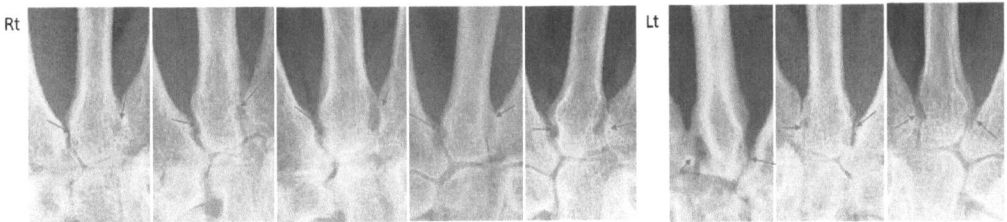

Fig. (76). Erosions of the 3rd CMC joints in patients with RA.

Fourth CMCs

Erosions of the fourth CMC joints in RA (Fig. **77**).

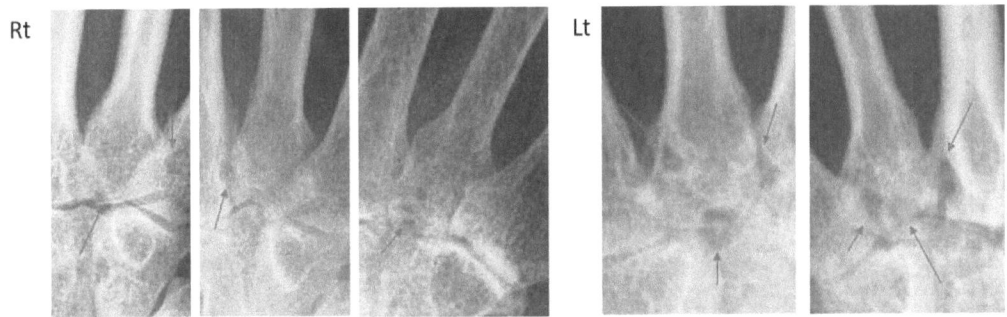

Fig. (77). Erosions of the 4th CMC joints in patients with RA.

Fifth CMCs

Erosions of the fifth CMC joints in RA (Fig. **78**).

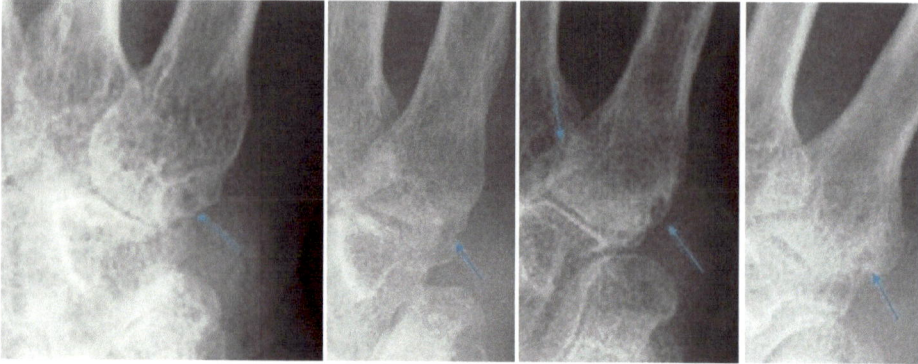

Fig. (78). Erosions of the 5th CMC joints in patients with RA.

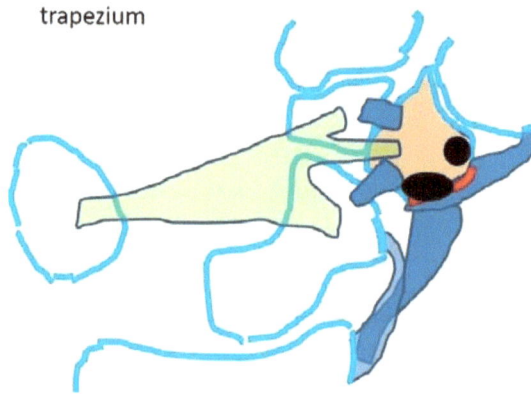

Fig. (79). A schema of the sites of erosions in the trapezium.

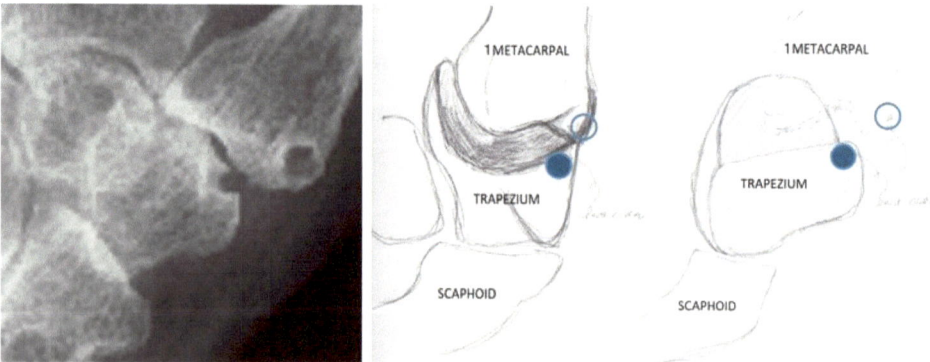

Fig. (80). A typical site of erosion of the trapezium in RA.

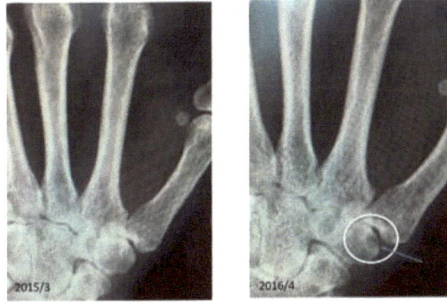

Fig. (81). Appearance of a novel erosion of the trapezium in a patient with RA.

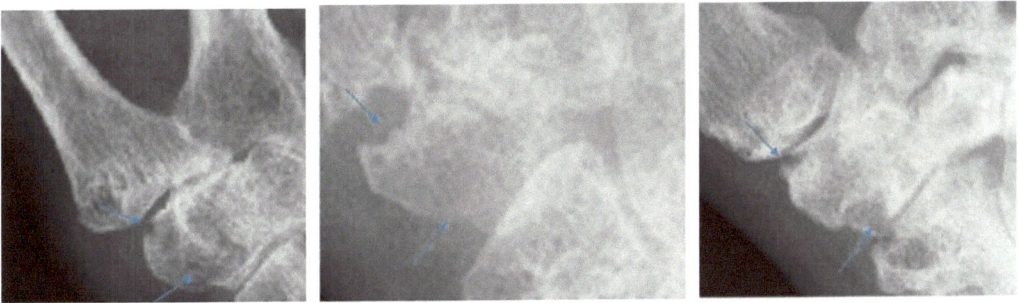

Fig. (82). Erosions of the right trapezium in RA.

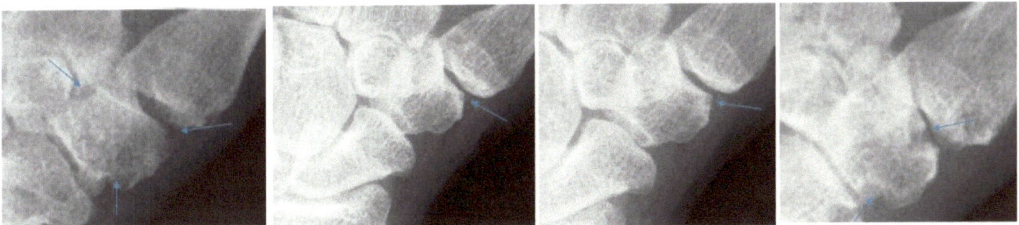

Fig. (83). Erosions of the left trapezium in RA.

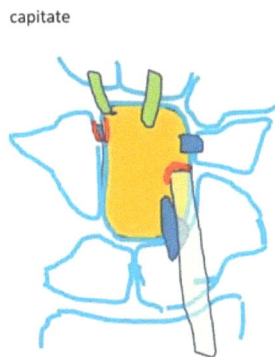

Fig. (84). A schema of the sites of erosions of the capitate.

Wrists

In the carpal bones, some sites of erosions are specific for RA. However, normal notches are also found. It is important to distinguish between these two conditions.

Trapezium

The sites of erosions in the trapezium (Figs. **79 - 82**).

Capitate

The sites of erosions in the capitate (Fig. **84**).

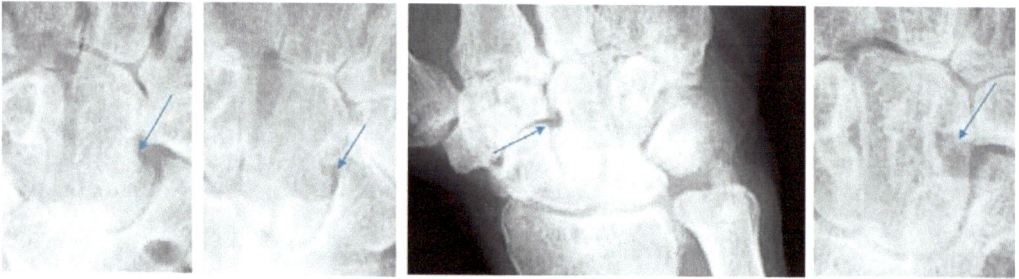

Fig. (85). Erosions of the capitate in patients with RA.

Hamate

The sites of erosions in the hamate (Fig. **86**).

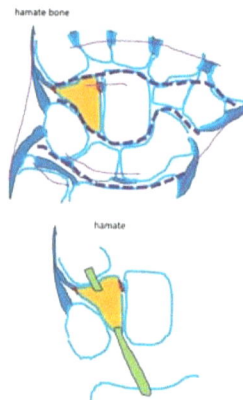

Fig. (86). A schema of the sites of erosions of the hamate bone.

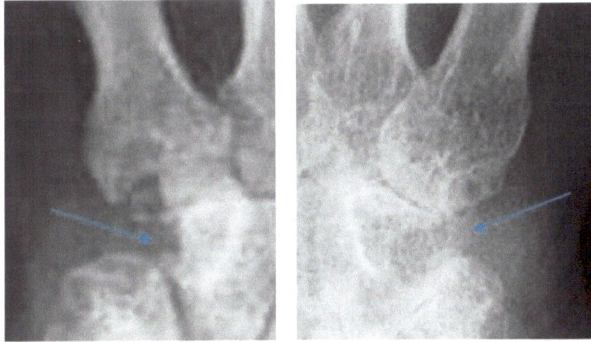

Fig. (87). Erosions of the hamate bone in patients with RA.

Scaphoid

The sites of erosions in the scaphoid (Figs. **88 - 92**).

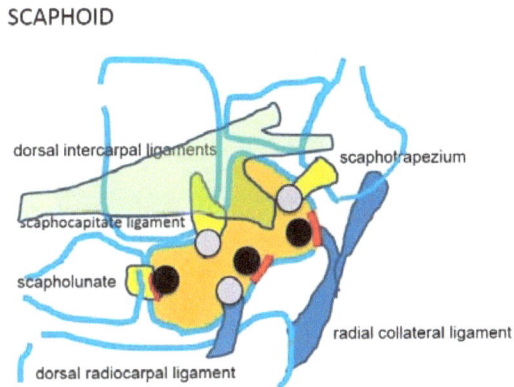

Fig. (88). A schema of the sites of erosions of the scaphoid.

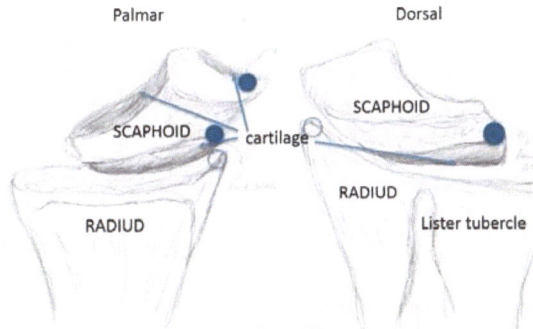

Fig. (89). A schema of the sites of erosions of the scaphoid.

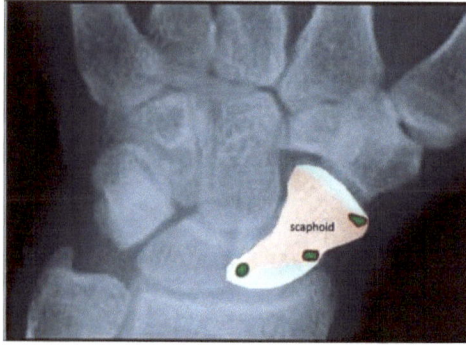

Fig. (90). The sites of erosions of the scaphoid in PA view of the left wrist.

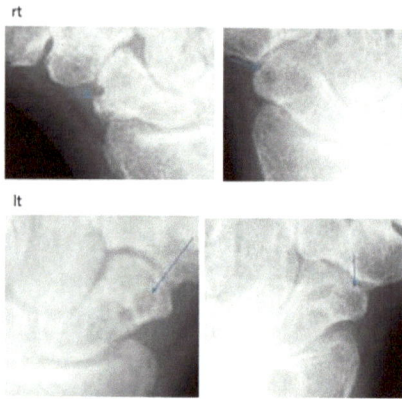

Fig. (91). Erosions at the radial collateral ligament attachment in patients with RA. PA views of the wrist show abnormalities of the scaphoid. Radiographs of the wrists show erosions of the lateral midportion of the scaphoid bone (arrows). Those are characteristic for RA.

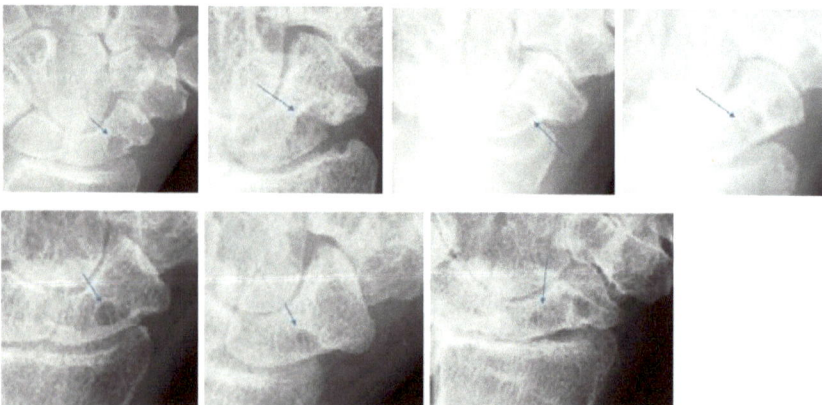

Fig. (92). Erosions at the scaphoid waist in patients with RA.

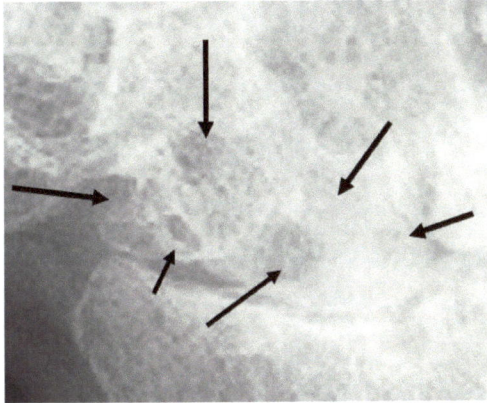

Fig. (93). Multiple erosions of the scaphoid in a patient with RA.

Lunate

The sites of erosions in the lunate (Figs. **94** and **95**).

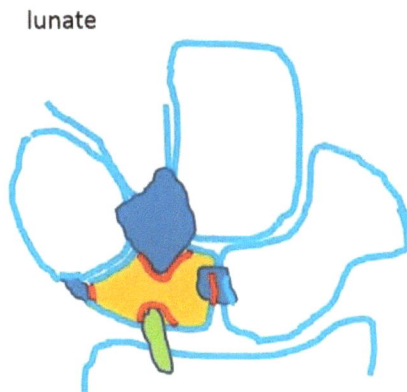

Fig. (94). A schema of the sites of erosions of the lunate.

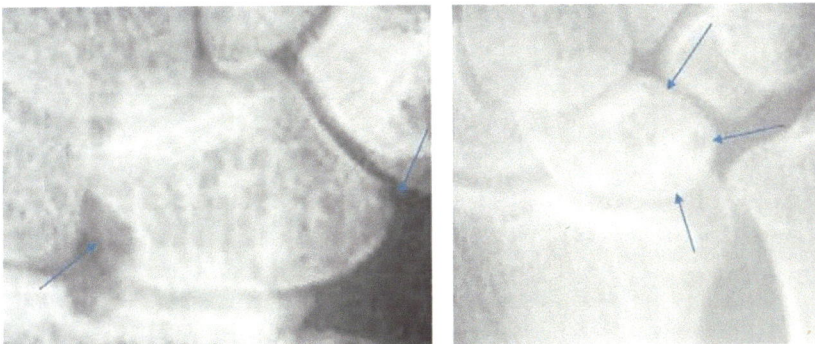

Fig. (95). Erosions of the right lunate in patients with RA.

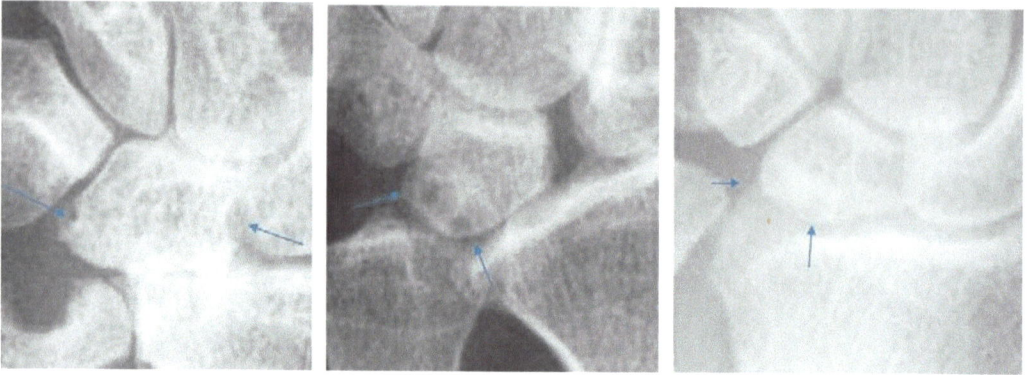

Fig. (96). Erosions of the left lunates in patients with RA.

Triquetrum

The sites of erosions in the triquetrum (Figs. **97 - 100**).

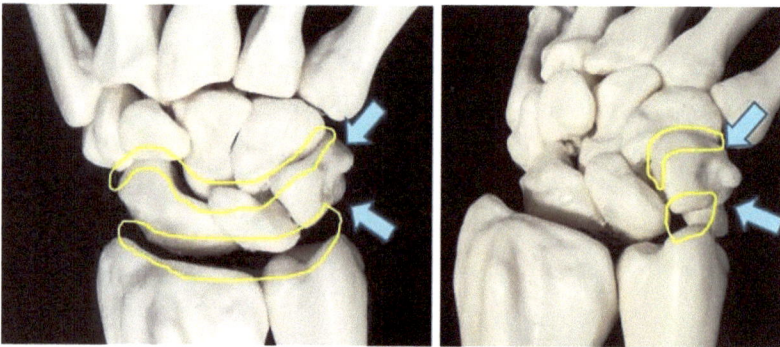

Fig. (97). Typical sites of erosions of the triquetrum in RA.

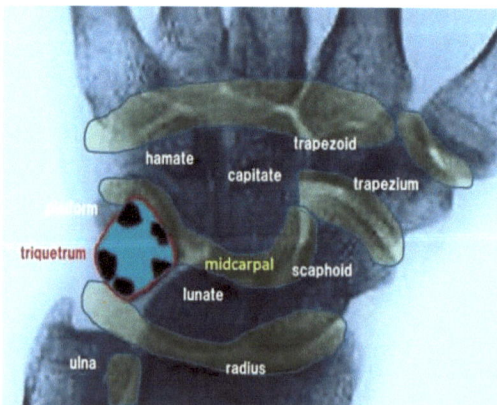

Fig. (98). The sites of erosions of the triquetrum in PA view of the left wrist.

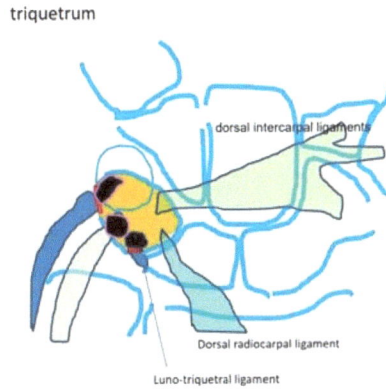

Fig. (99). A schema of the sites of erosions of the triquetrum.

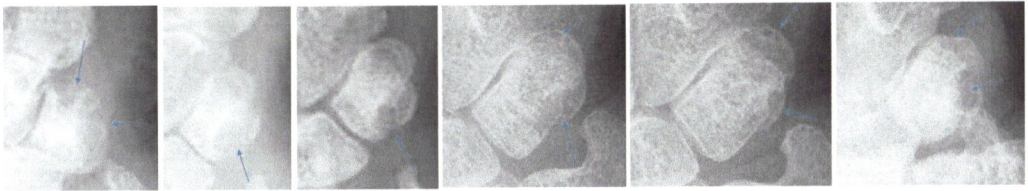

Fig. (100). Erosions of the right triquetrum in patients with RA.

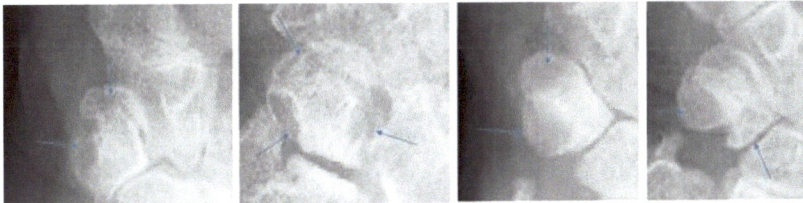

Fig. (101). Erosions of the left triquetrum in patients with RA.

Pisiform

The sites of erosions in the trapezium (Figs. **102 - 104**).

EROSIONS OF ULNAR STYLOID PROCESS AND RADIAL STYLOID PROCESS

Radius

1. Erosions of the styloid process of the radius (Fig. **106**)
2. Erosions near the styloid process of the radius in the RC joint (Fig. **107**)
3. Erosions at the center of the radius in the RA joints (Fig. **108**)
4. Erosions between the center and the ulnar side of the radius in RC joint (Fig. **109**)

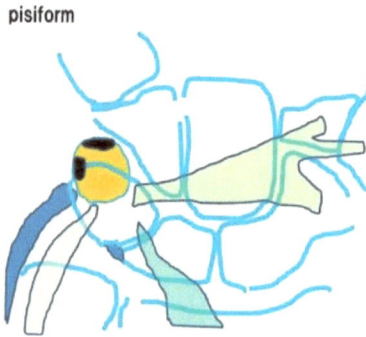

Fig. (102). A schema of the sites of erosions of the pisiform.

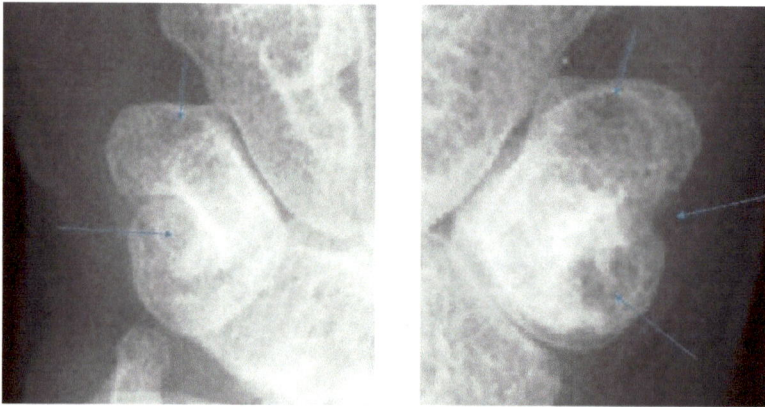

Fig. (103). Erosions of the pisiform in patients with RA.

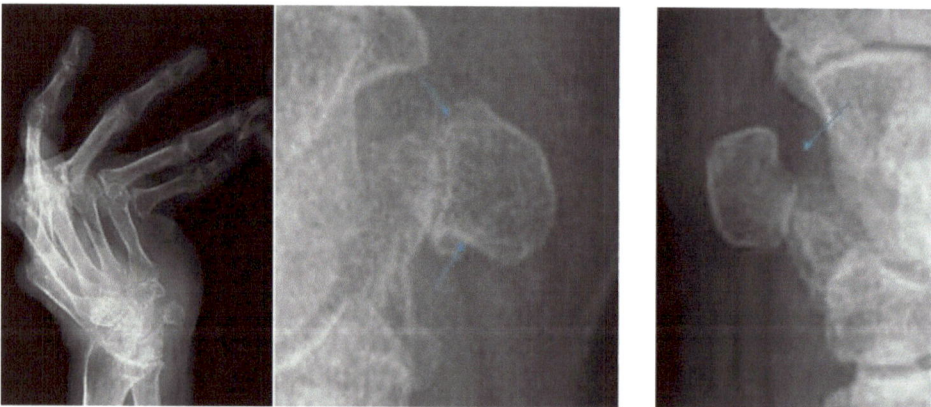

Fig. (104). Ball-catch views of the hand show erosions of the pisiform in patients with RA.

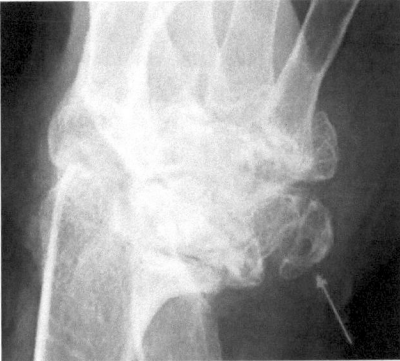

Fig. (105). Ball-catch view of the left hand shows erosions of the pisiform in a patient with advanced RA.

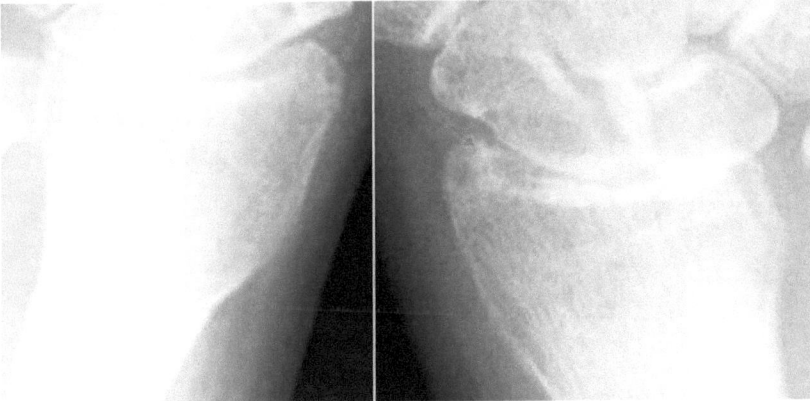

Fig. (106). PA views of the wrist show erosions at the styloid process of the radius in patients with RA.

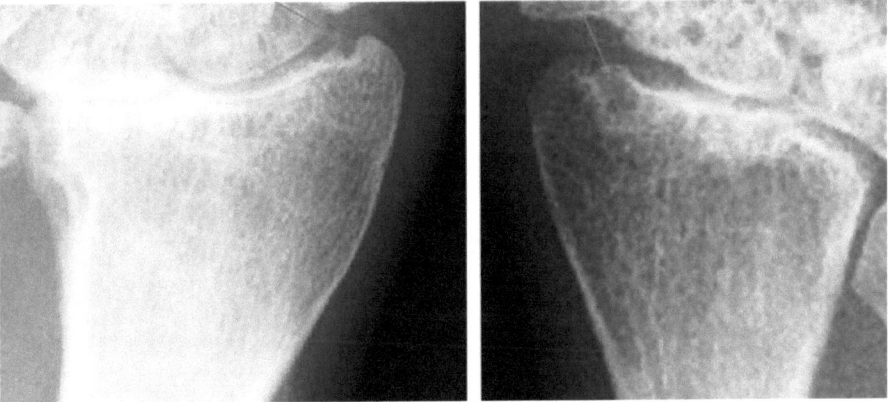

Fig. (107). PA views of the wrist show erosions near the styloid process of the radius of the RC joint in patients with RA.

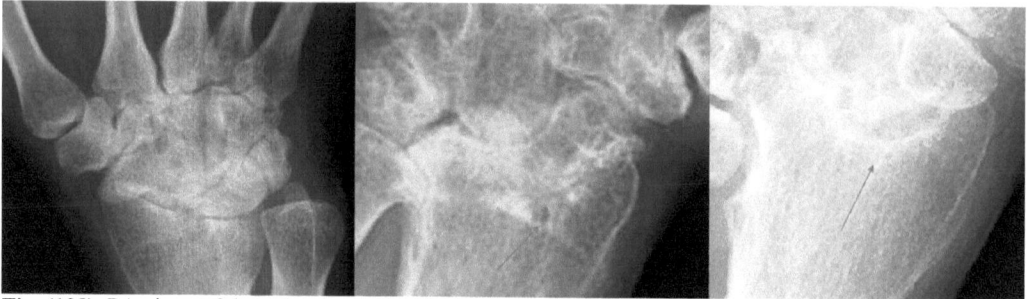

Fig. (108). PA views of the wrist show erosions at the center of the radius of the RC joint in patients with RA.

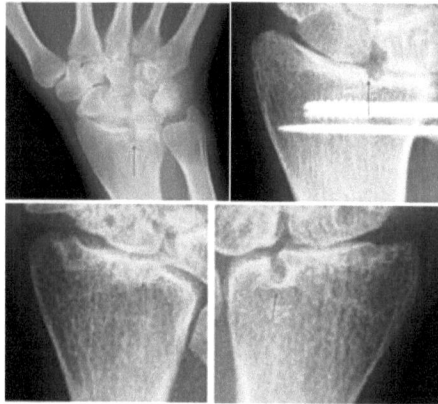

Fig. (109). Erosions between the center and the ulnar side of the radius in RC joint.

Distal Radioulnar Joints

The erosions of the distal radioulnar joints (Fig. **110**).

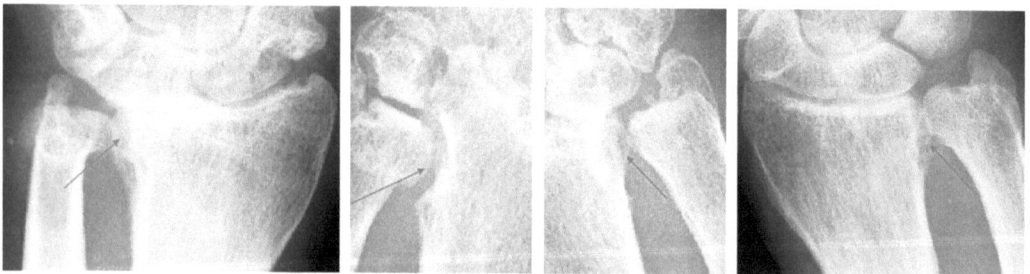

Fig. (110). Erosions of the distal radioulnar joint.

Ulna

The sites of erosions in the ulna (Figs. **111**).

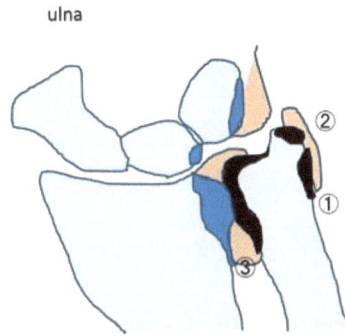

Fig. (111). A schema of the sites of erosions of the ulna.

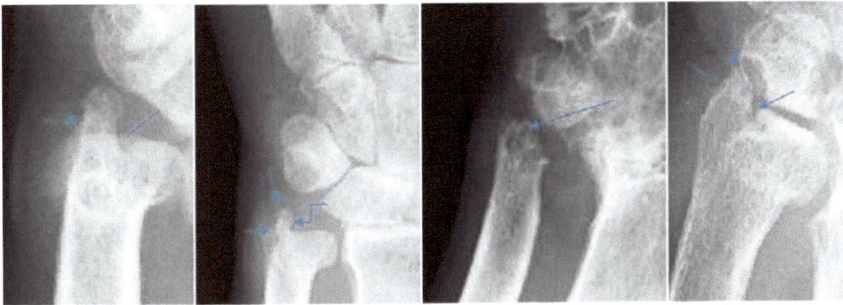

Fig. (112). Erosions of the ulna.

Elbows

Erosions on Olecranon

The erosions of the olecranon (Fig. **113**).

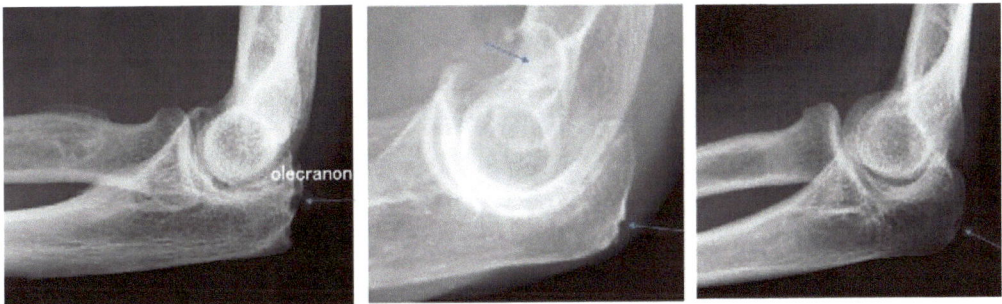

Fig. (113). Erosions on the olecranon of the elbow joint in patients with RA.

Erosions of Humeroradial Joints

There may be erosions at the head of the radius and the capitulum of the humerus in the humeroradial joint in RA (Fig. **114**).

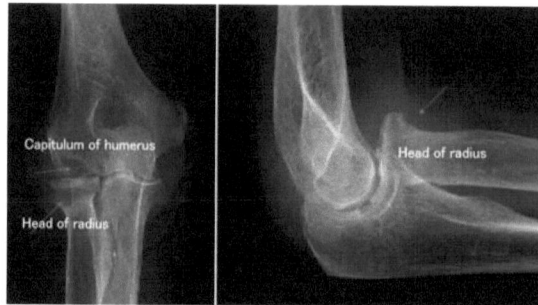

Fig. (114). Erosions of the head of the radius and the capitulum of the humerus of the elbow in a patient with RA.

Erisions of Humeroulnar Joints

The erosions of the humeroulnar joints (Fig. **115**).

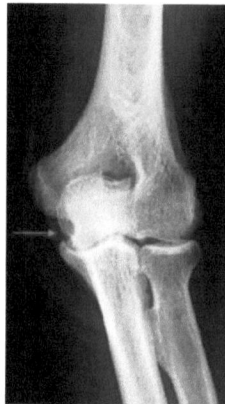

Fig. (115). An erosion of the humeroulnar joint in a patient with RA.

Erosions of Proximal Radioulnar Joints

The erosions of the proximal radioulnar joints (Fig. **116**).

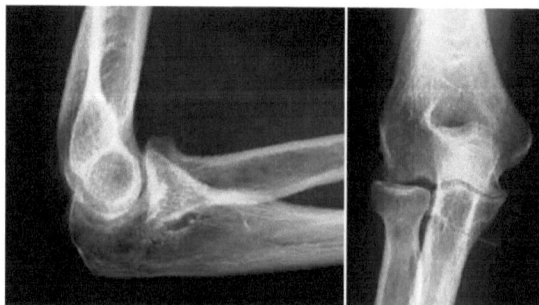

Fig. (116). An erosion of the proximal radioulnar joint in a patient with RA.

Shoulders

Erosions of Head of Humerus

The erosions of the head of humerus (Figs. **117 - 119**).

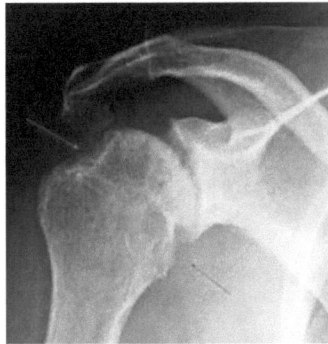

Fig. (117). AP view of the shoulder shows erosions of the head of the right humerus in a patient with RA.

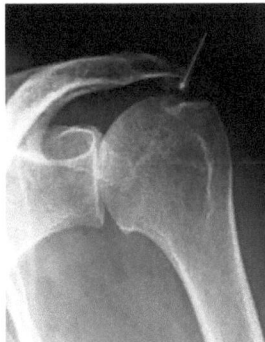

Fig. (118). AP view of the shoulder shows an erosion of the head of the left humerus in a patient with RA.

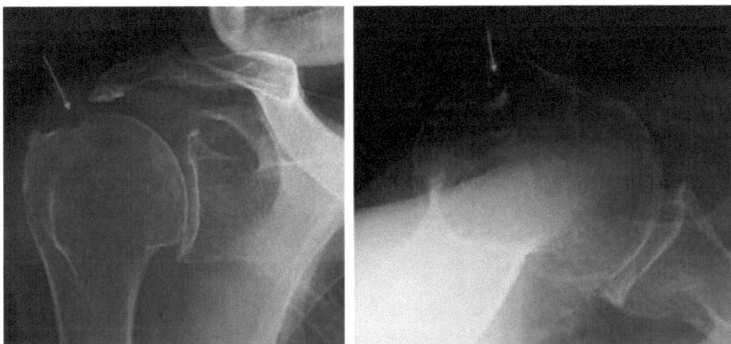

Fig. (119). AP view and axillary view of the shoulder show an erosion of the head of the right humerus in a patient with RA.

Erosions on Glenoids of Shoulders

Erosions on the glenoids of the shoulders in RA (Figs. **120 - 122**).

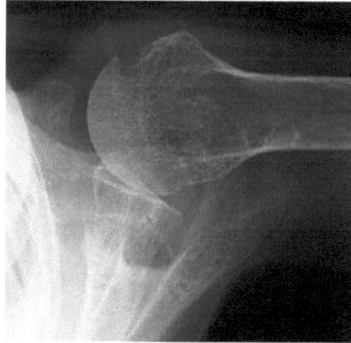

Fig. (120). Axillary view of the shoulder shows an erosion of the glenoid in a patient with RA.

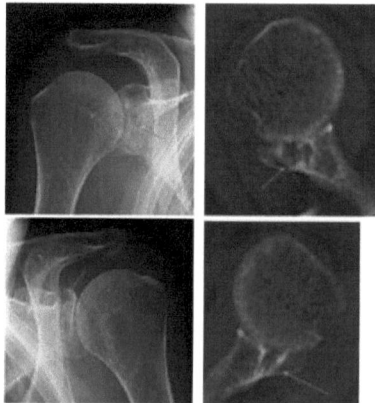

Fig. (121). AP views of the shoulders and CT images show erosions of the glenoids in a patient with RA.

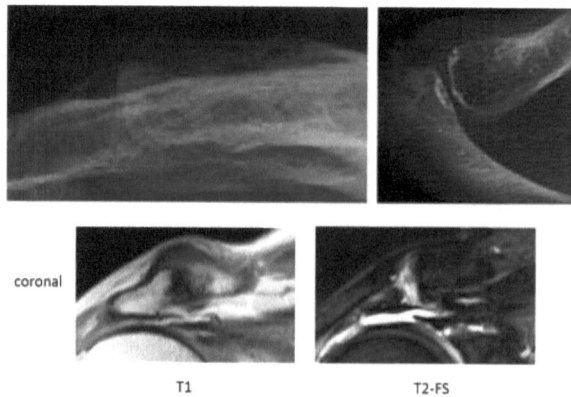

coronal   T1   T2-FS

Fig. (122). Eosions of the acromioclavicular (AC) joint. Plain radiograph, CT image, and MR images (T1 and T2-FS) show erosive lesions at the right AC joint in a patient with RA.

Hips

Erosion of Femoral Head

Erosions of the femoral head in RA (Fig. **123**).

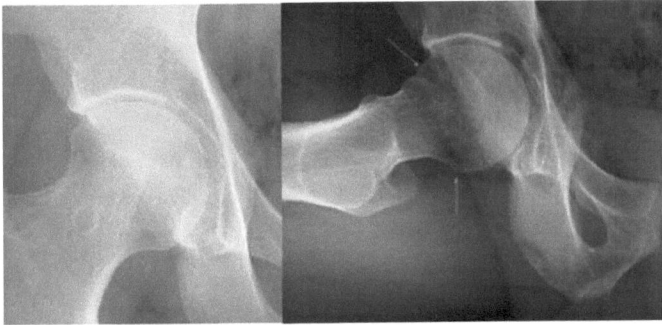

Fig. (123). Erosions of the femoral head of the right hip in a patient with RA.

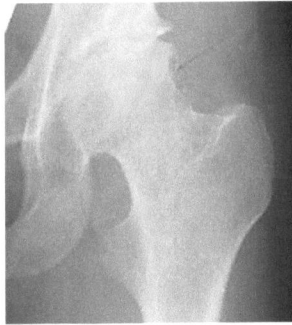

Fig. (124). An erosion of the femoral head of the left hip in a patient with RA.

Knees

Erosions of the knees in RA (Figs. **125 - 134**).

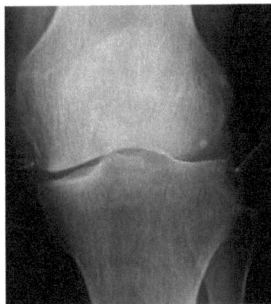

Fig. (125). AP view of the left knee shows typical erosion at the sites of bare areas in a patients with RA.

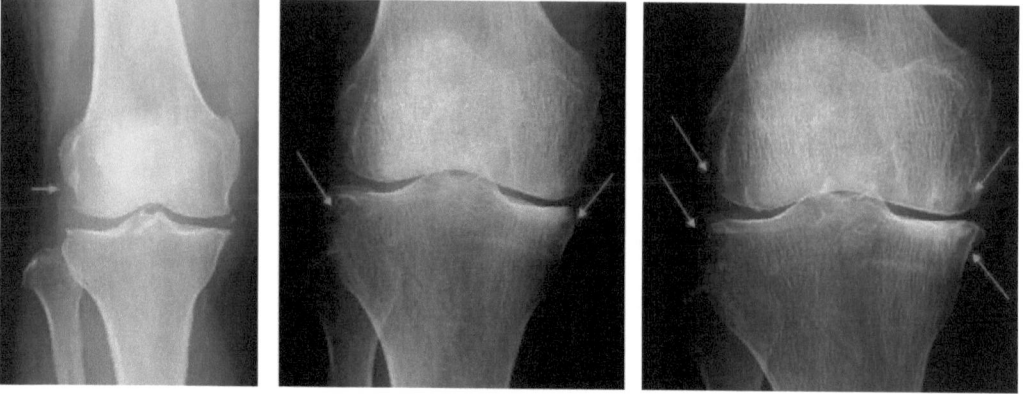

Fig. (126). Erosions of the right knees in patients with RA.

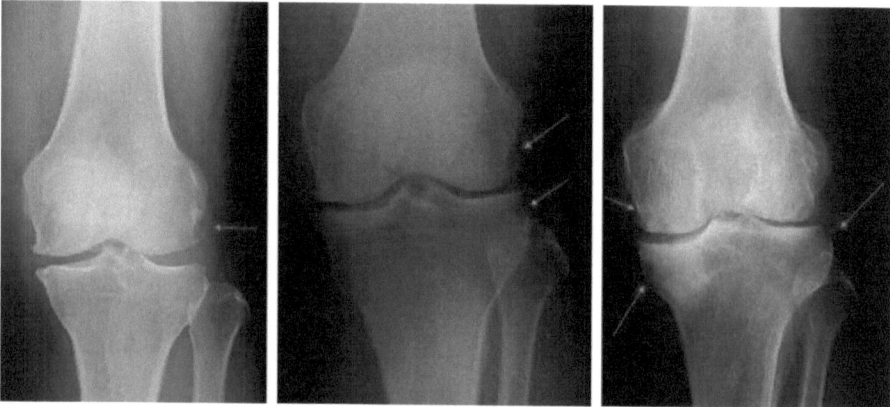

Fig. (127). Erosions of the left knees in patients with RA.

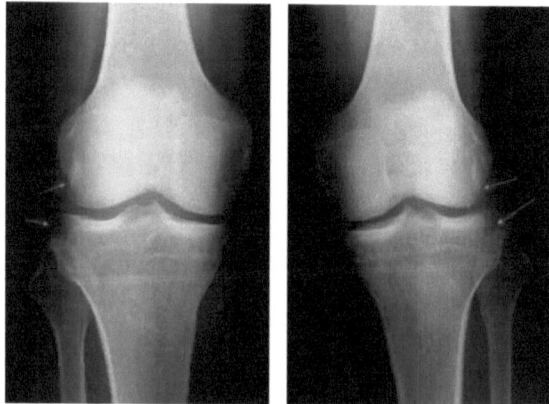

Fig. (128). AP views of the knees show erosions in a patient with RA.

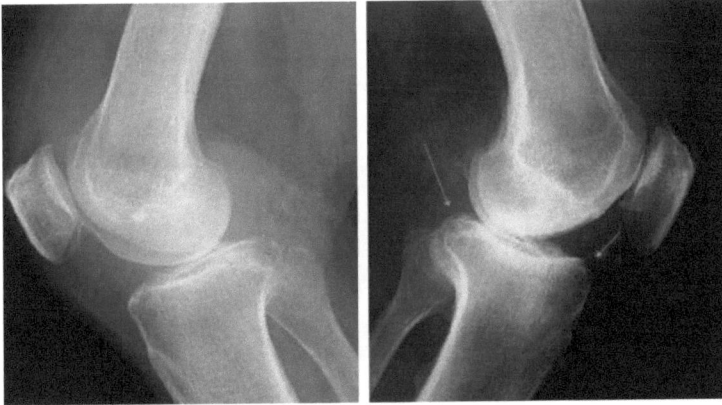

Fig. (129). Lateral views of the knees show erosions in patients with RA.

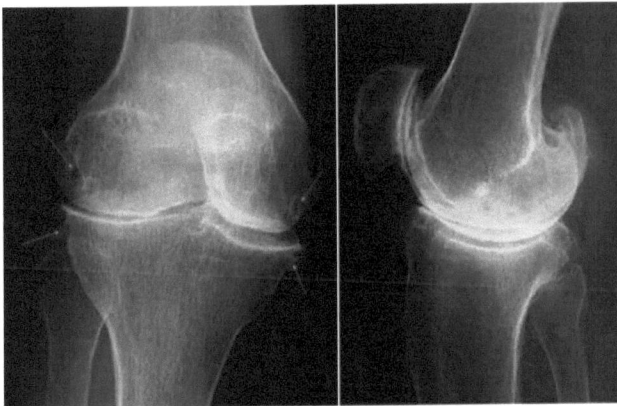

Fig. (130). AP view and lateral view of the right knee show advanced changes with erosions in a patient with RA.

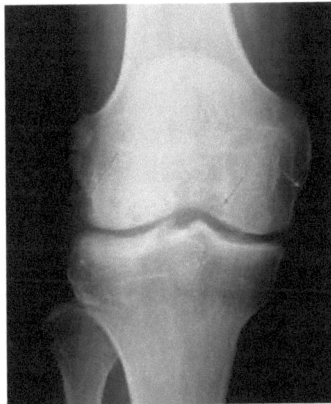

Fig. (131). AP veiw of the right knee shows multiple erosions in a patient with advanced RA.

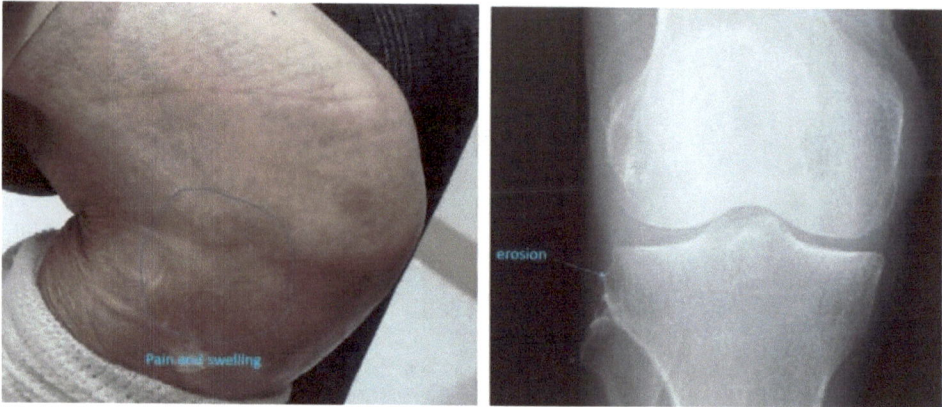

Fig. (132). Photograph of the right knee shows swelling of the soft tissue, and plain radiograph demonstrates an erosion of the right knee in a patient with RA.

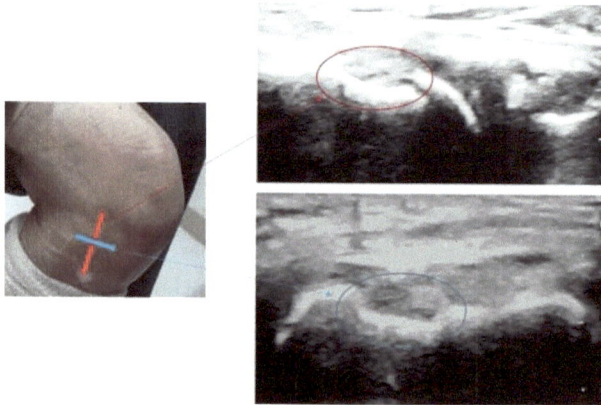

Fig. (133). Longitudinal and transverse gray-scale US images of the lateral side of the right knee show the large-sized erosion in the same patient with RA.

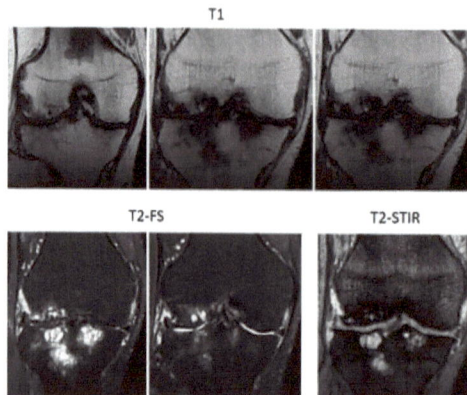

Fig. (134). MR images of the right knee including T1, T2-FS and T2-STIR show multiple erosions and bone edemas in the same patient with RA.

Ankles

Erosions of the ankles in RA (Fig. **135**).

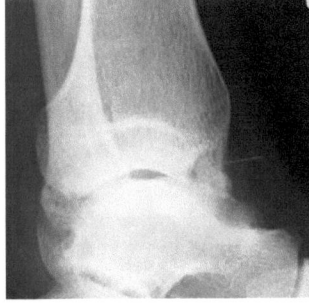

Fig. (135). Lateral view of the ankle shows an erosion of the tibia in a patient with RA.

Feet

Calcaneus

The sites of erosions of of the calcaneus in RA (Figs. **136 - 140**).

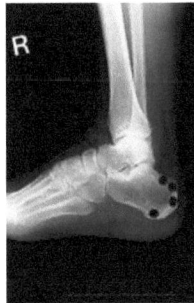

Fig. (136). The sites of erosions of the calcaneus in RA.

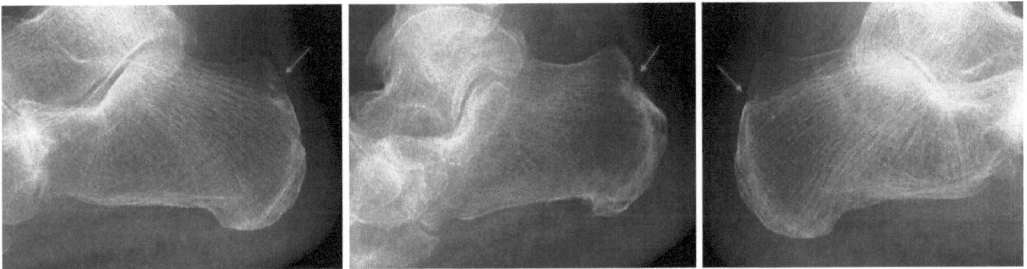

Fig. (137). Erosions of the posterior surface above the attachment of the Achilles tendon.

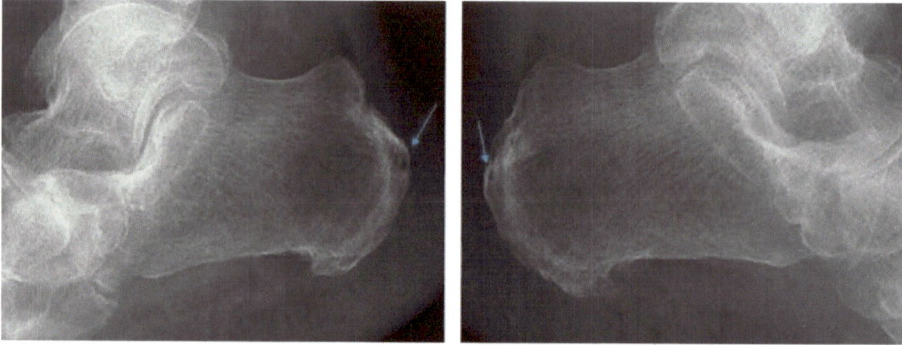

Fig. (138). Erosions of the posterior surface at the site of the attachment of the Achilles tendon.

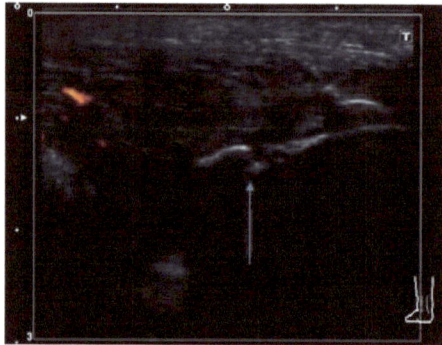

Fig. (139). Longitudinal power Doppler US image shows an erosion of the posterior surface at the site of the attachment of the Achilles tendon with a PD signal.

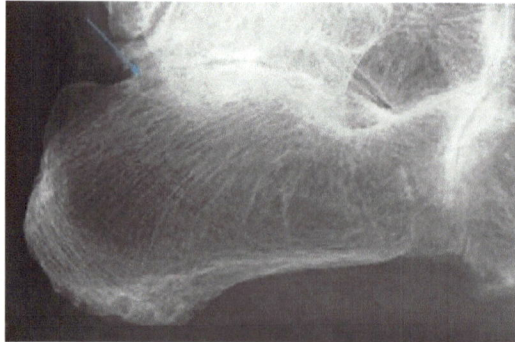

Fig. (140). An erosion at the superior surface of the calcaneus in a patient with RA.

Mid-foot

The erosions of the mid-feet in RA (Figs. **141 - 145**).

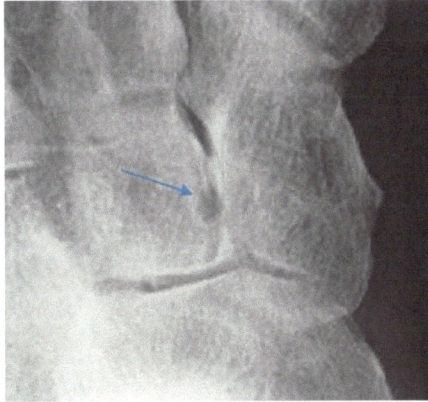

Fig. (141). An erosion between the lateral and the intermediate cuneiform in the left mid-foot.

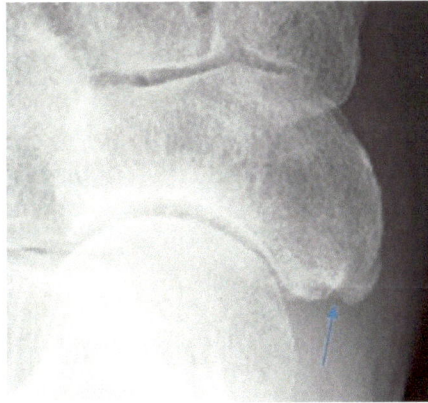

Fig. (142). An erosion of the talonavicular joint in the left mid-foot.

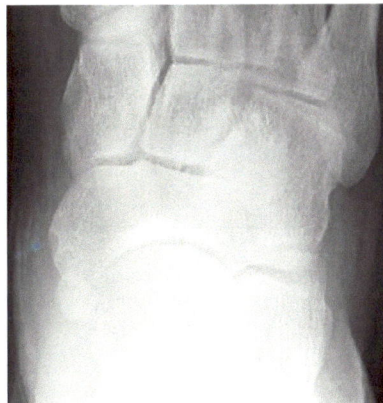

Fig. (143). An erosion of the right navicular.

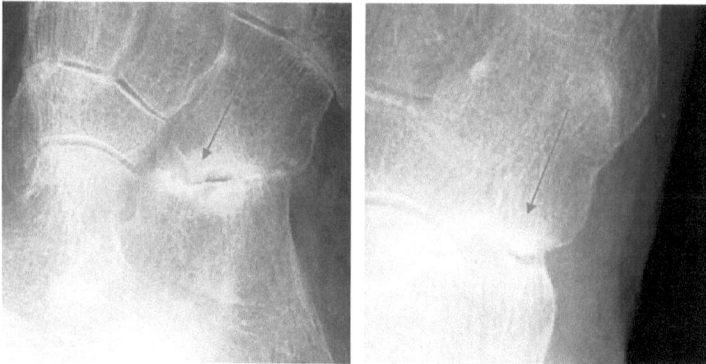

Fig. (144). Erosions of the calcaneocuboid joint in the left mid-foot.

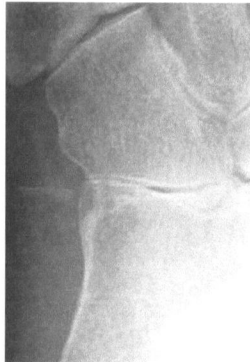

Fig. (145). An erosion of the calcaneocuboid joint in the left mid-foot.

TMTs

The erosions of of the TMT joints in RA (Figs. **146** and **147**).

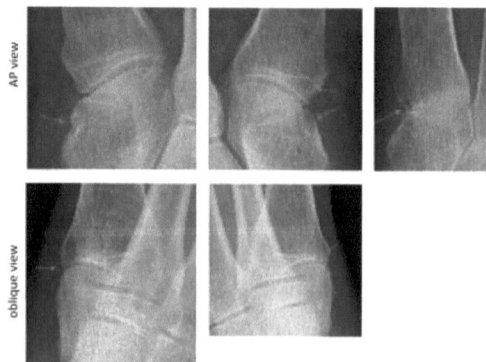

Fig. (146). AP views and oblique views of the foot show erosions of the first Tarsometatarsal (TMT) joints in patients with RA.

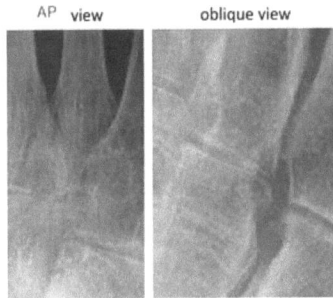

Fig. (147). AP view and oblique view of the foot show erosions of the third TMT joint in a patient with RA.

Toes

MTPs

The erosions of of the MTP joints in RA (Figs. **148 - 159**).

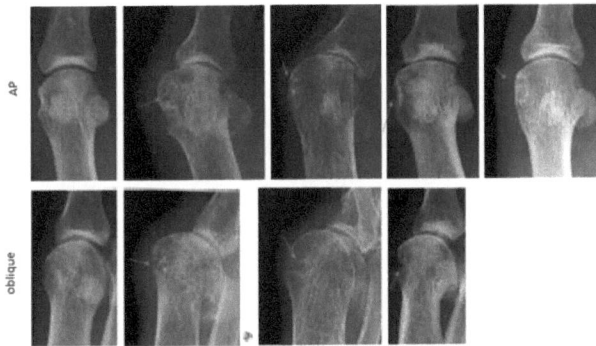

Fig. (148). AP views and oblique views of the right big toes show erosions of the first MTP joints in patients with RA.

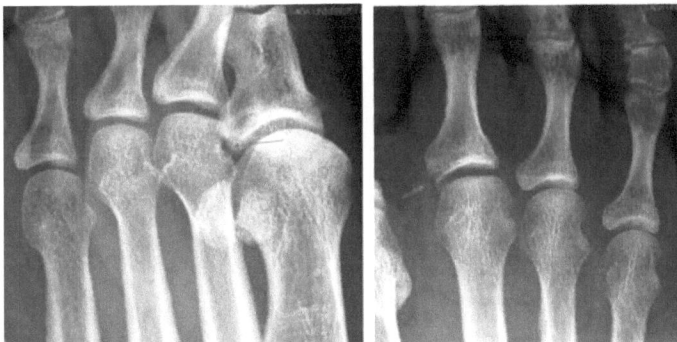

Fig. (149). AP views of the foot demonstrate erosions of the second MTP joints in a patient with RA. Left panel shows an erosion of the second metatarsal head. Right panel also shows an erosion of the base of the second proximal phalanx.

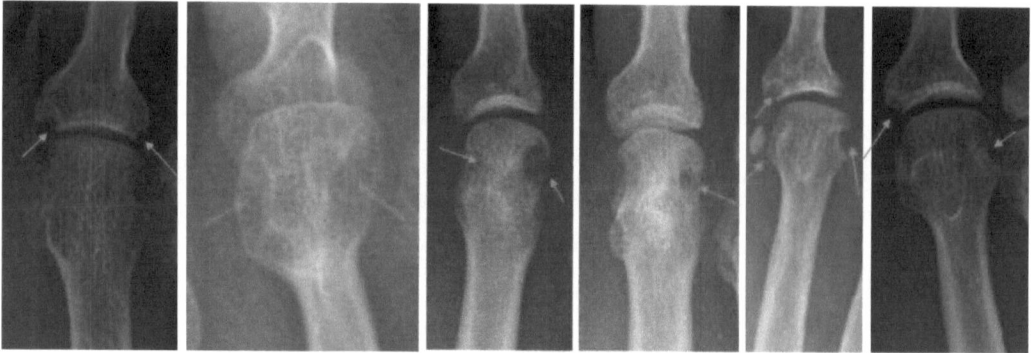

Fig. (150). AP views of the foot show erosions of the 2nd MTP joints in patients with RA.

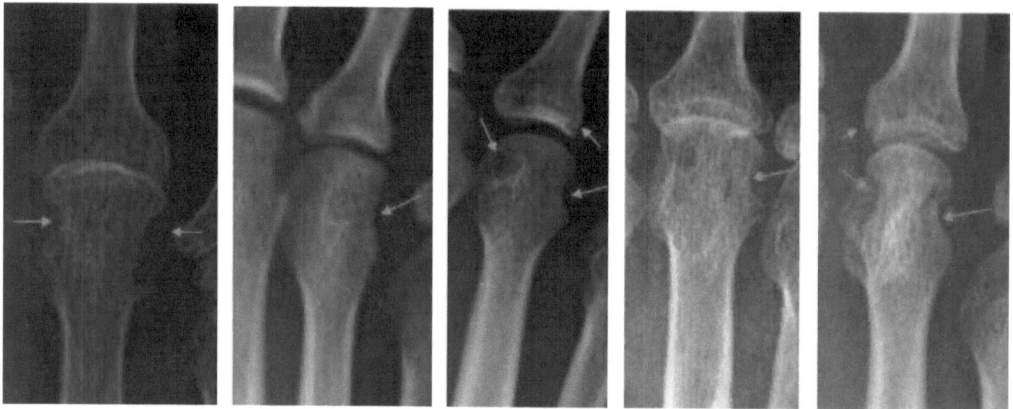

Fig. (151). AP views of the right foot show erosions of the 3rd MTP joints in patients with RA.

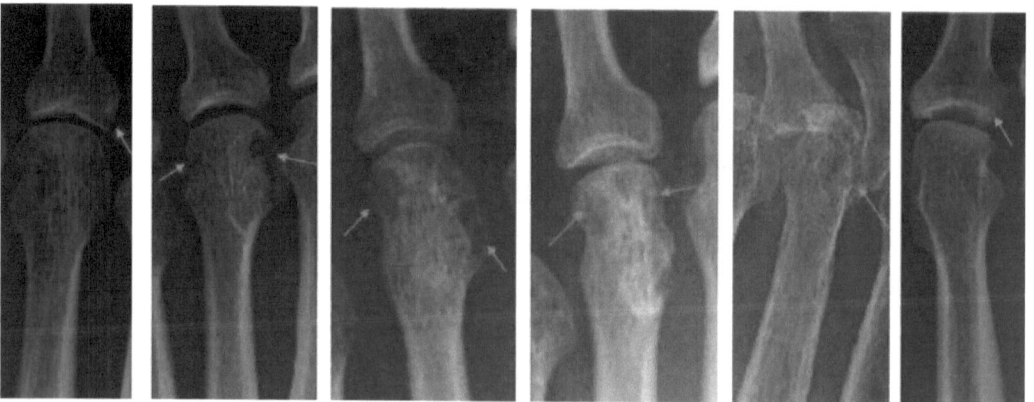

Fig. (152). AP views of the left foot show erosions of the 3rd MTP joints in patients with RA.

Rt   Lt

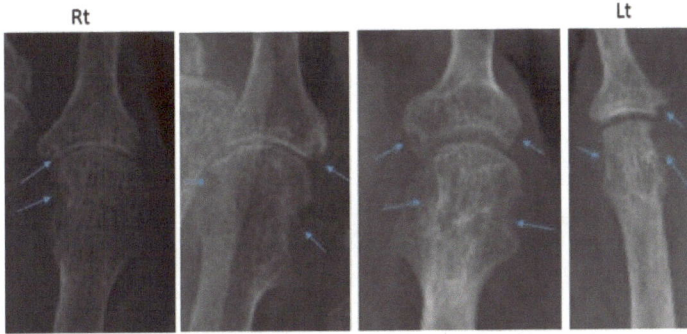

Fig. (153). AP views of the foot show erosions of the 4th MTP joints in patients with RA.

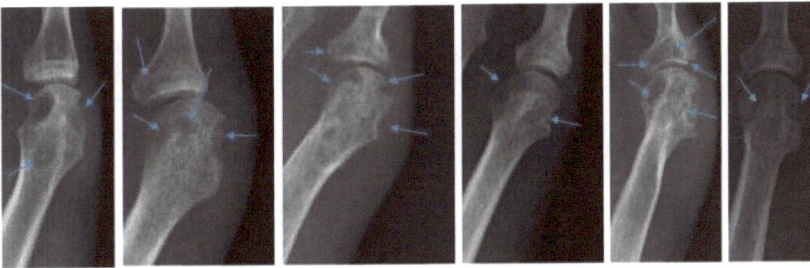

Fig. (154). AP views of the right foot show erosions of the fifth MTP joints in patients with RA.

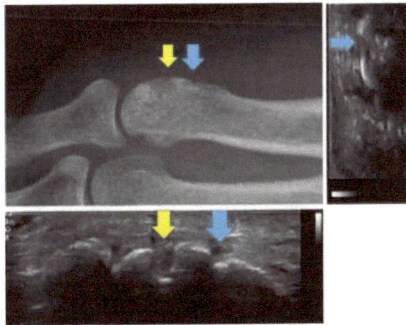

Fig. (155). AP view of the right fifth MTP joint shows two erosions (yellow and blue arrows) of the metatarsal head. They are confirmed by longitudinal and transverse gray-scale US images.

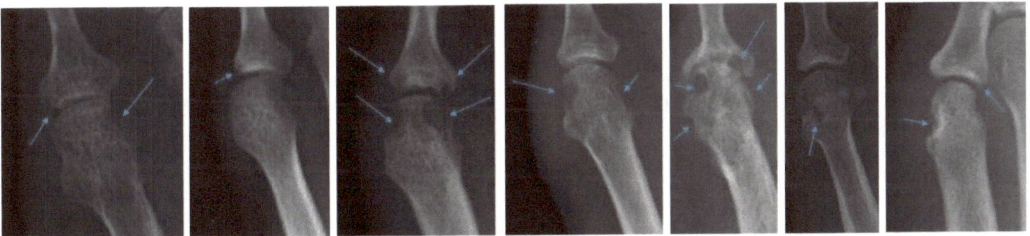

Fig. (156). AP views of the left foot show erosions of the left fifth MTP joints in patients with RA.

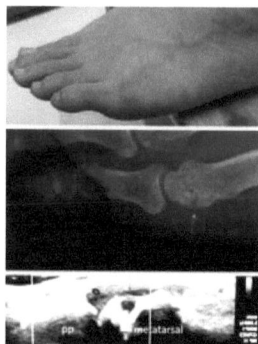

Fig. (157). Upper panel; photograph of swelling of the left fifth MTP joint in a patient with RA. Middle panel; AP view of the left fifth MTP joint shows an erosion of the metatarsal head. Lower panal; longitudinal power Doppler US image shows the erosion. pp: proximal phalanx.

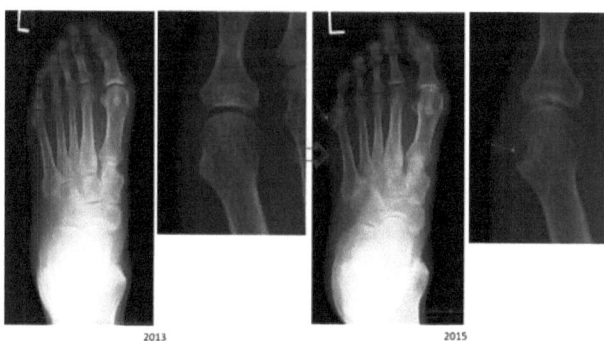

Fig. (158). AP views of the left foot demonstrate emergence of an erosion of the fifth MTP joint in a patient with RA.

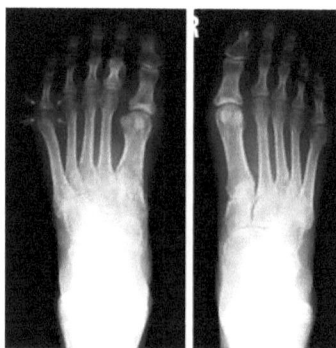

Fig. (159). AP views of the bilateral feet demonstrate typical marginal erosions at the fifth MTP joints in a patient with RA.

First IPs

The erosions of of the first IP joints in RA (Fig. **160**).

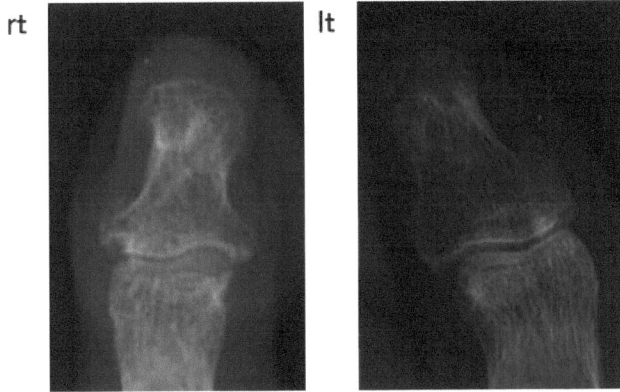

Fig. (160). AP views of the foot show erosions of the first IP joints in patients with RA.

Sternoclavicular Joints

The erosions of of the sternoclavicular joints in RA (Figs. **161** and **162**)

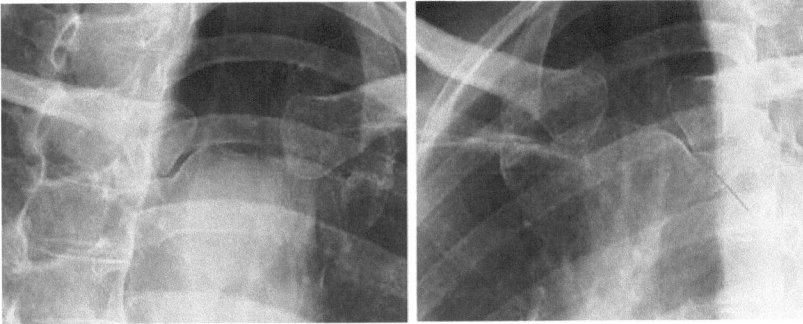

Fig. (161). Plain radiograph shows erosion of the sternoclavicular joint in a patient with RA.

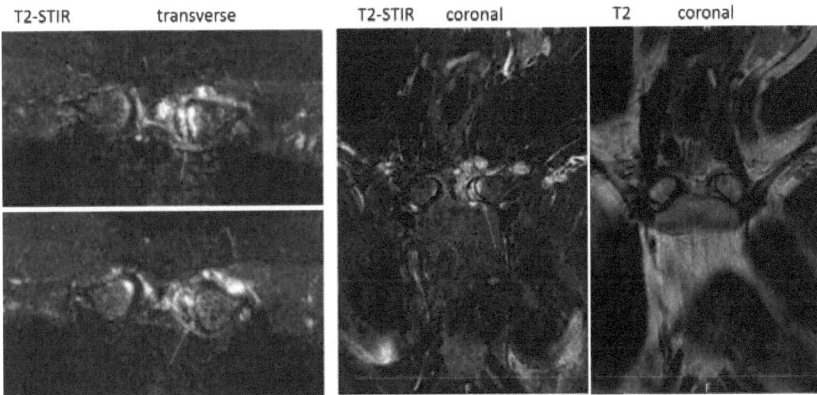

Fig. (162). MR images show erosions of the sternoclavicular joints in a patient with RA.

Pubic Symphysis

Erosions of the pubic symphysis in RA (Fig. **163**).

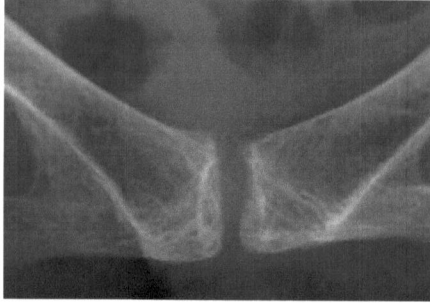

Fig. (163). An erosion of the pubic symphysis in a patient with RA.

BONE CYSTS

RC Joints

Bone cysts of the RC joints in RA (Figs. **165** and **166**).

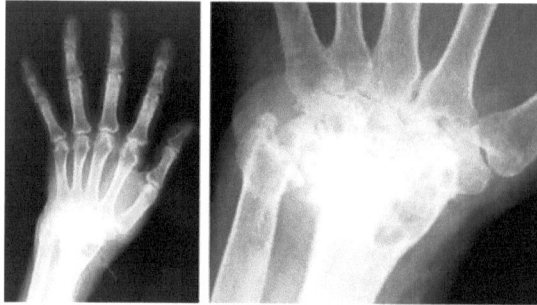

Fig. (165). Bone cysts of the left radius in a patient with RA.

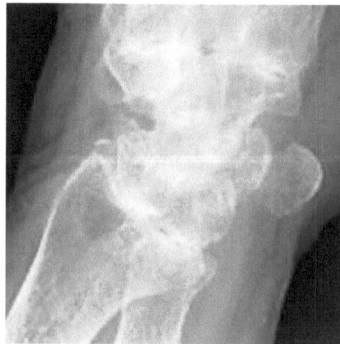

Fig. (166). Bone cysts of the left radius in a patient with RA.

Hips

Bone cysts of the hips in RA (Fig. **167**).

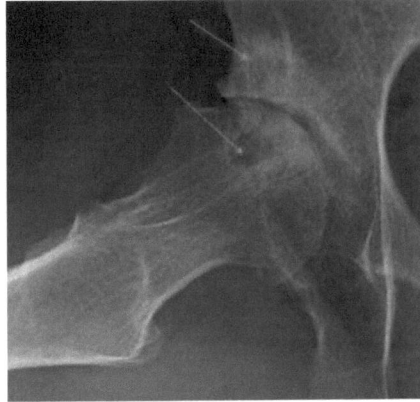

Fig. (167). Bone cysts of the right hip in a patient with RA.

Knees

Bone cysts of the knees in RA (Fig. **168**).

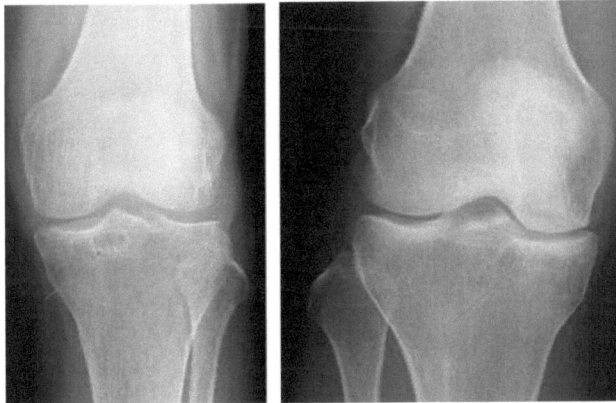

Fig. (168). AP views of the knee in patients with RA. Synovial bone cysts involve the tibial plateau, rheumatoid "geodes".

Mid-foot

Bone cysts of the mid-feet in RA (Fig. **169**).

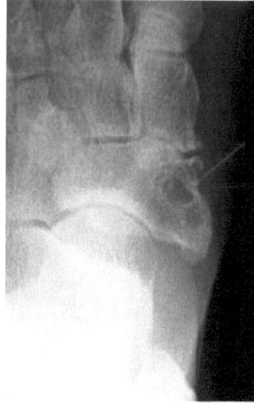

Fig. (169). Bone cyst formation in the navicular of a patient with RA.

MTP joints

Bone cysts of the MTP joints in RA (Fig. **170**).

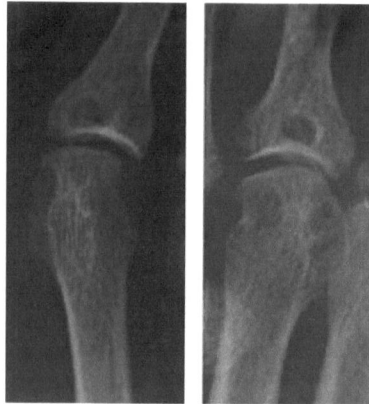

Fig. (170). AP view and oblique view of the foot show bone cyst formation in the second MTP joint of a patient with RA.

OSTEOPHYTE FORMATION

Proliferation of Bones at Joints

In RA, there may be osteophyte formation at the joints because patients with RA may have OA simultaneously and/or have the secondary OA changes due to RA and other reasons (Figs. **171 - 184**).

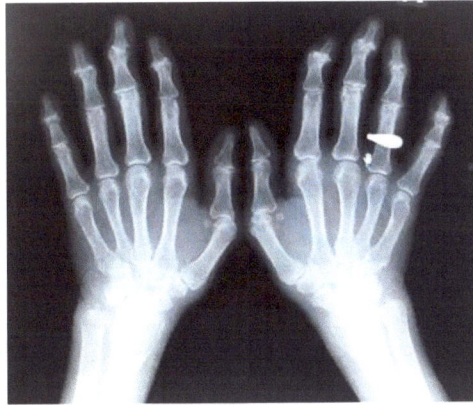

Fig. (171). PA view of the hands demonstrates osteophytes at the DIP joints that suggest OA, and marginal erosions that indicate RA. The patient has both OA and RA at the same time.

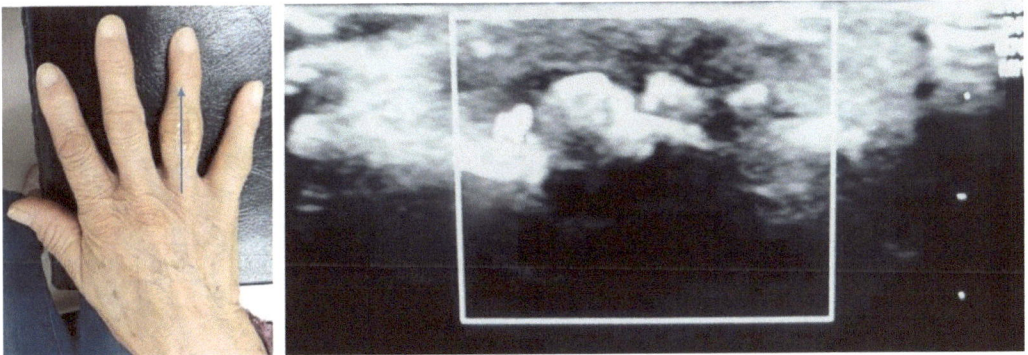

Fig. (172). Photograph of the right hand of the same patient (□□□! □□□□□□□□□□□□) shows swelling of the fourth PIP Joint. Longitudinal power Doppler US image of the dorsal aspect of the fourth PIP joint shows osteophytes related to OA. There is the small amount of Doppler signal that may be consistent with mild synovitis due to OA.

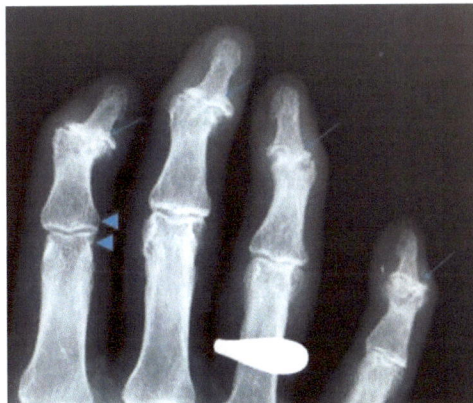

Fig. (173). PA view of the right hand show typical osteophytes of OA at all the DIP joints. In the PIP joints, there are also erosions.

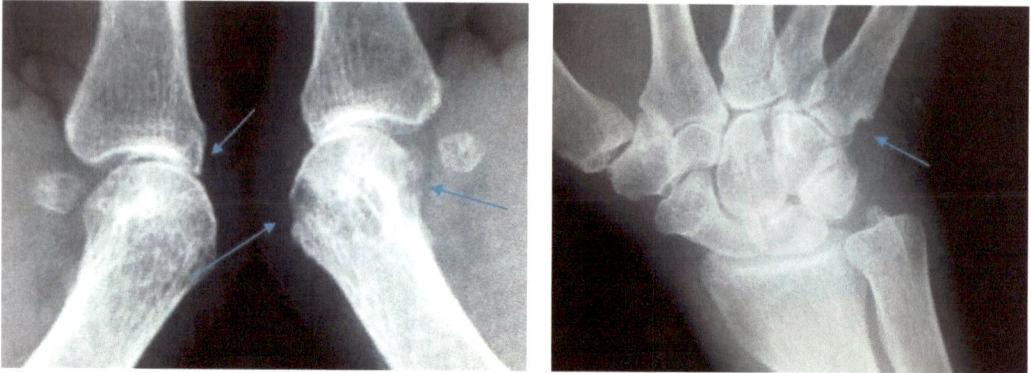

Fig. (174). PA views of the hands show typical erosions of RA at the first MCP joints and the right fifth CMC joint.

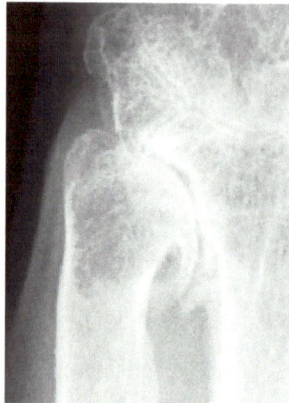

Fig. (175). PA view of the left wrist shows an osteophyte of the ulna in distal radioulnar joint that is compatible the secondary OA change due to RA.

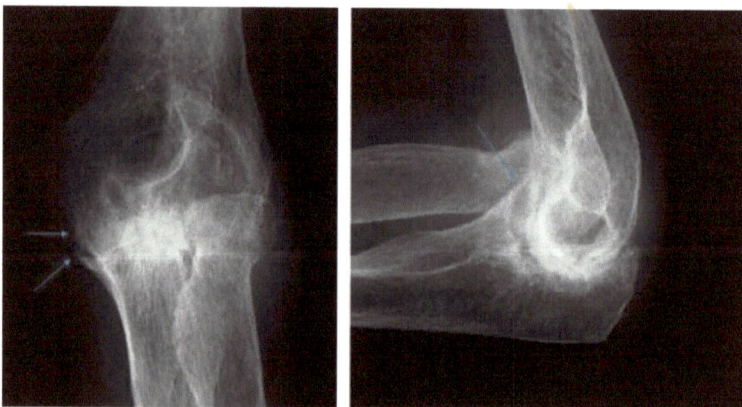

Fig. (176). AP view and lateral view of the right elbow show the secondary osteophytosis due to RA.

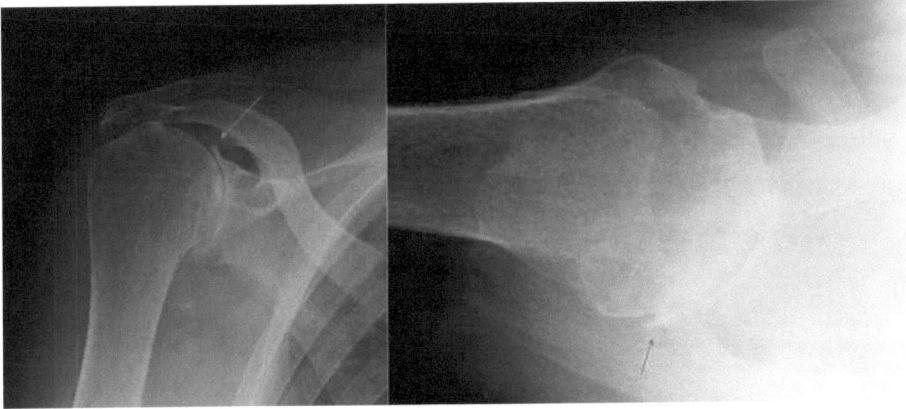

Fig. (177). AP view and axillary view of the right shoulder show an osteophyte of the secondary OA change due to RA.

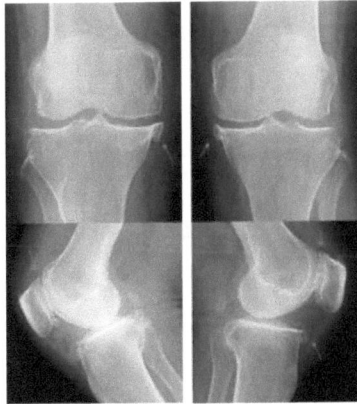

Fig. (178). AP views and axillary views of the knees show osteophytes of the secondary OA change due to RA.

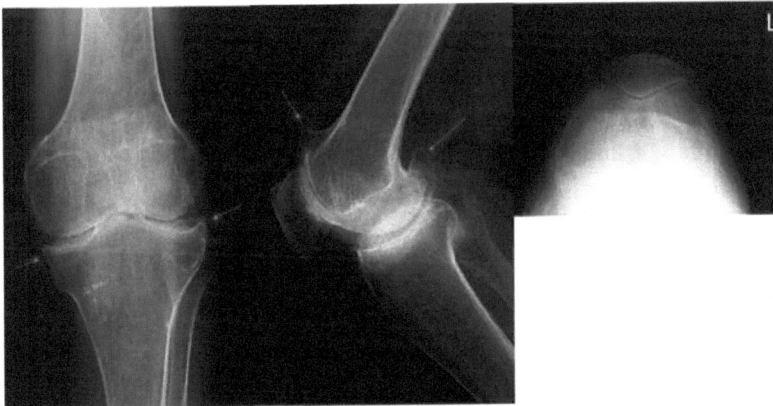

Fig. (179). Marked osteophyte formations of the secondary OA change due to RA in the right knee. There is also joint space narrowing (JSN) of the medial, lateral, and patellofemoral compartments.

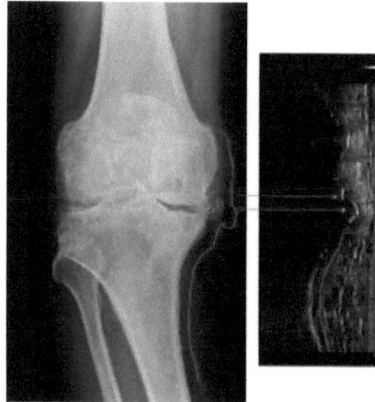

Fig. (180). Osteophyte of the secondary OA change due to RA in the right knee. Especially, medial side has strong changes. Outlines of medial side of the bone are very similar in plain radiograph and longitudinal gray-scale US image.

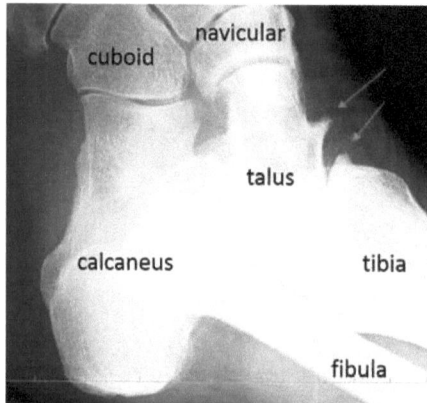

Fig. (181). Osteophytes of the left tibiotalar joint (ankle joint) in a patient with RA.

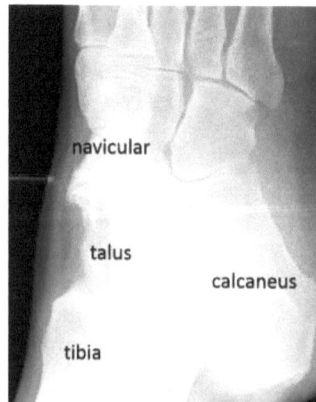

Fig. (182). Osteophytes of the talonavicular joint in a patient with RA.

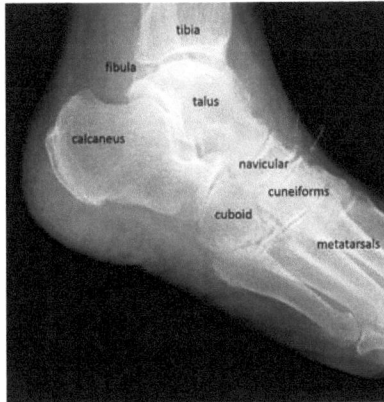

Fig. (183). Osteophytes of the cuneonavicular joint in a patient with RA.

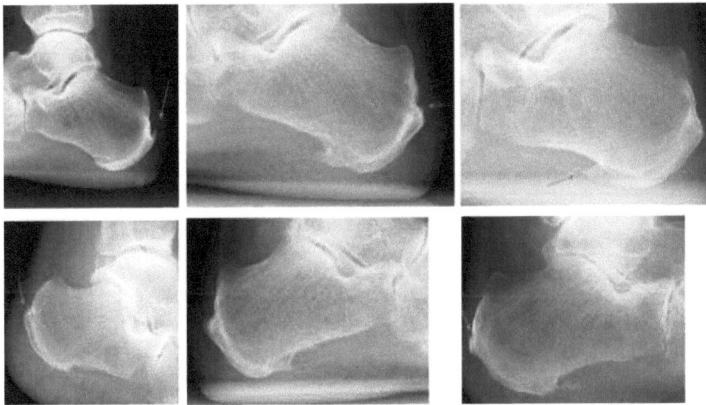

Fig. (184). Lateral views of the foot show the entheseal bony spur at Achilles insertion and at the plantar fascia in patients with RA.

CONSENT FOR PUBLICATION

Not applicable.

CONFLICT OF INTEREST

The author (editor) declares no conflict of interest, financial or otherwise.

ACKNOWLEDGEMENTS

The authors thank Ms. K. Eguchi and A. Ibe for secretarial assistance.

REFERENCES

[1]   Koarada S, Tada Y, Eds. Fundamental Rheumatological Knowledge of Arthritis Images of the Hand and Case Studies for General Physicians (Medical Procedures, Testing and Technology). New York: Nova Science Pub Inc 2013; pp. 1-222.

CHAPTER 4

C: Capsula Articularis, Intra Articular: Joint Spaces and Calcifications

Syuichi Koarada* and **Yukiko Takeyama**

Division of Rheumatology, Faculty of Medicine, Saga University, Saga, Japan

Abstract: Category C is the capsula articularis, intra articular. It includes the changes of joint paces and calcifications. In this category, joint space narrowing (JSN) and ankylosis are important in rheumatoid arthritis (RA). Also, joint effusion and synovitis are detectable by US and MRI.

Keywords: Ankylosis, Joint effusion, Joint Space Narrowing (JSN), Rheumatoid arthritis, Synovitis.

In normal persons, joint space consists of the cartilages between the bones. However, in patients with RA, the cartilages are damaged and the joint space becomes narrow. Also, the joint space narrowing is uniform.

US images of the normal joints of the hand (Figs. **1**, **2**).

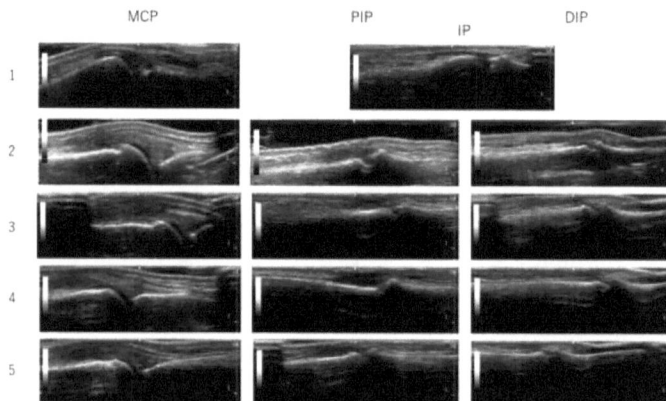

Fig. (1). Longitudinal gray-scale US images show normal joints of the hand.

* **Corresponding author Syuichi Koarada:** Division of Rheumatology, Faculty of Medicine, Saga University, Saga, Japan; Tel: 81-952-31-6511; E-mail: koarada@cc.saga-u.ac.jp

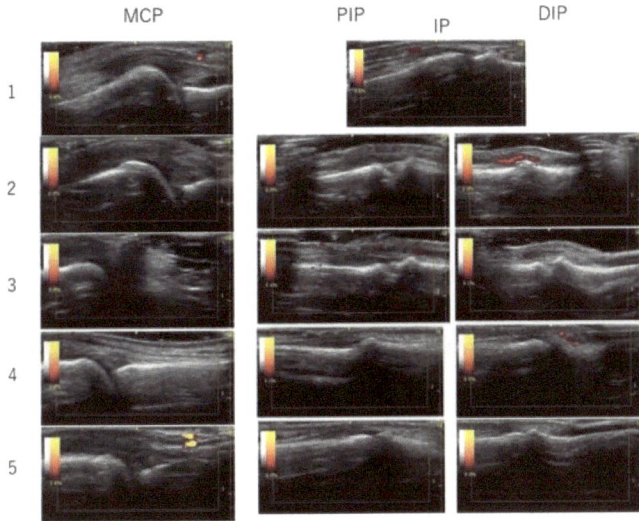

Fig. (2). Longitudinal power Doppler US images show normal joints of the hand.

JOINT SPACE NARROWING (JSN)

Joint space narrowing (JSN) in RA (Figs. **3**, **4**).

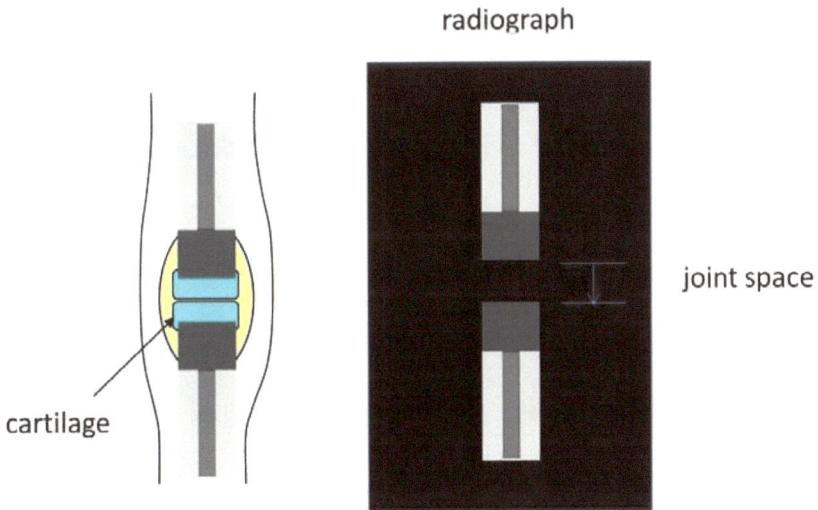

Fig. (3). A simplified schema of joint space. In normal persons, joint space consists of the cartilages between bones.

Fingers and Thumbs

IP Joints

JSN of the 1st IP joints in RA (Fig. **5**).

radiograph

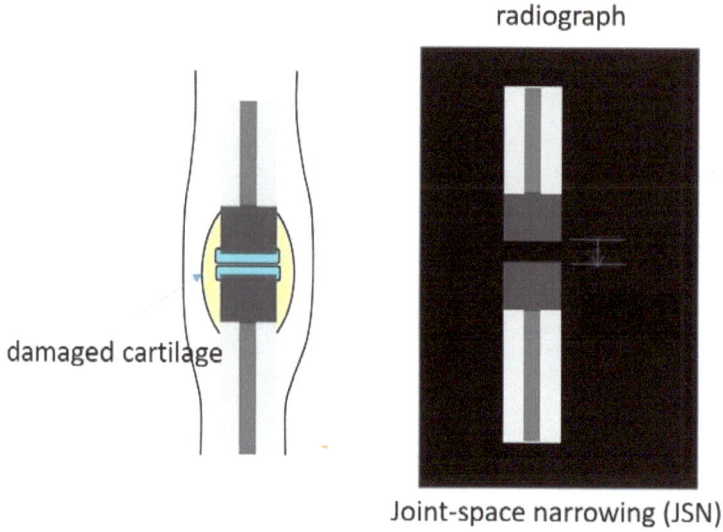

damaged cartilage

Joint-space narrowing (JSN)

Fig. (4). A simplified schema of joint space narrowing (JSN) in RA. When the cartilages are damaged, the joint space becomes narrow. Especially, in RA, joint space narrowing is uniform.

Rt 1th IP   Lt 1th IP

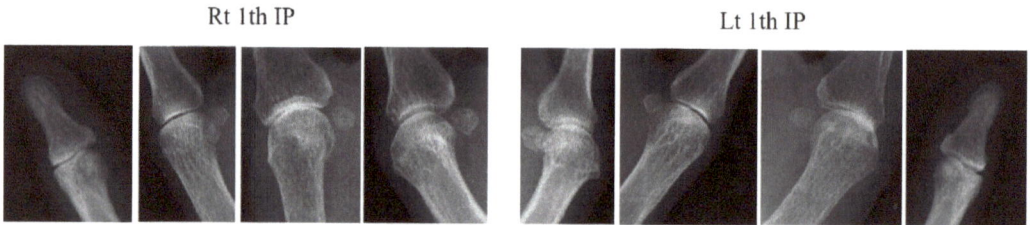

Fig. (5). Joint space narrowing of the 1st IP joints.

PIP Joints

JSN of the 2nd PIP joints in RA (Figs. **6**, **7**).

Rt 2nd PIP

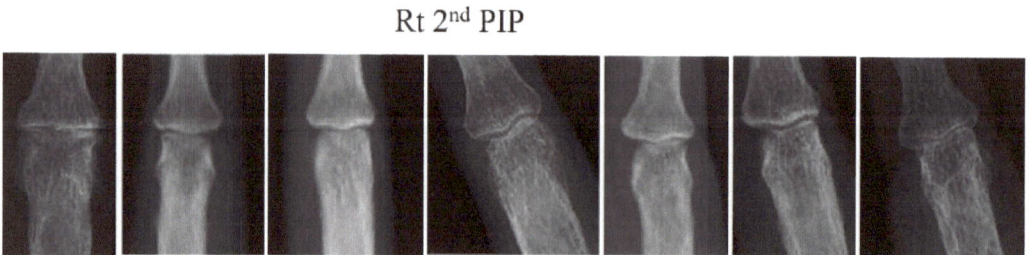

Fig. (6). Joint space narrowing of the right 2nd PIP joints.

Lt 2nd PIP

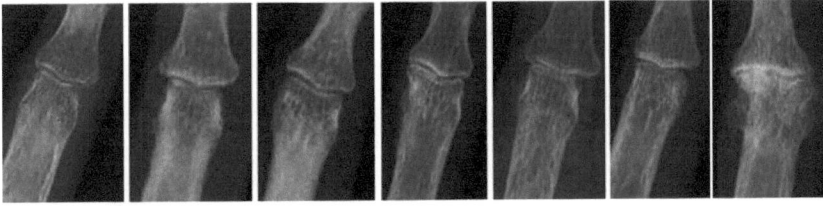

Fig. (7). Joint space narrowing of the left 2nd PIP joints.

JSN of the 3rd PIP joints in RA (Figs. **8, 9**).

Rt 3rd PIP

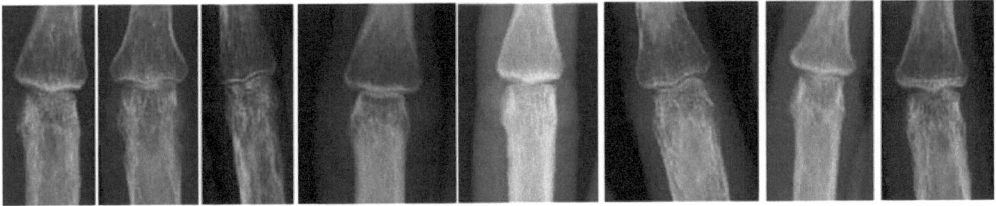

Fig. (8). Joint space narrowing of the right 3rd PIP joints.

Lt 3rd PIP

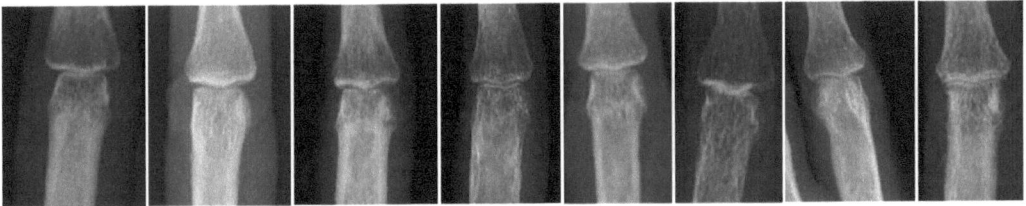

Fig. (9). Joint space narrowing of the left 3rd PIP joints.

JSN of the 4th PIP joints in RA (Figs. **10, 11**).

Rt 4th PIP

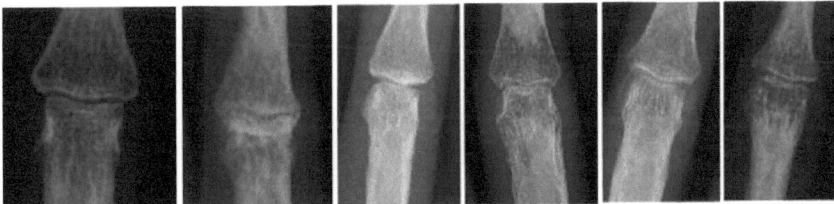

Fig. (10). Joint space narrowing of the right 4th PIP joints.

Lt 4th PIP

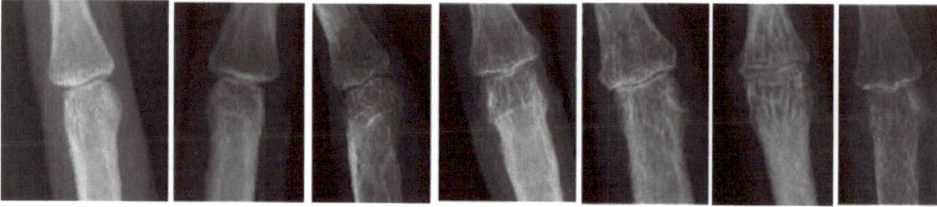

Fig. (11). Joint space narrowing of the left 4th PIP joints.

JSN of the 5th PIP joints in RA (Figs. **12**, **13**).

Rt 5th PIP

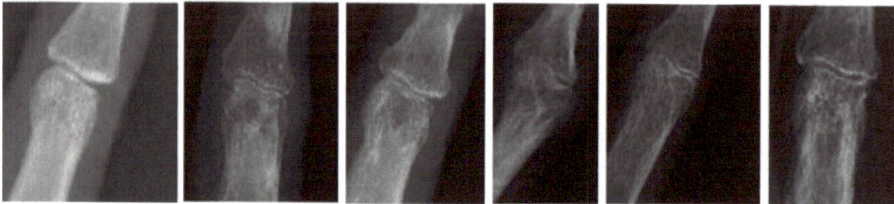

Fig. (12). Joint space narrowing of the right 5th PIP joints.

Lt 5th PIP

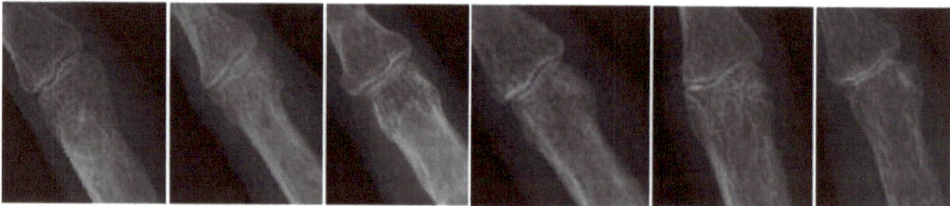

Fig. (13). Joint space narrowing of the left 5th PIP joints.

PIP joint US imaging (Fig. **14**).

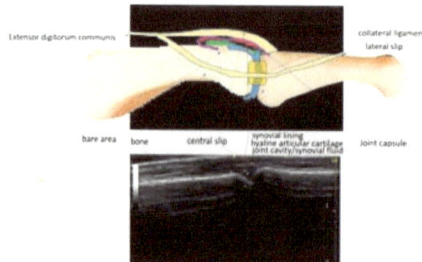

Fig. (14). Normal structure of the PIP joint and its US imaging.

MCP Joints

JSN of the 1st MCP joints in RA (Figs. **15, 16**).

Rt 1st MCP

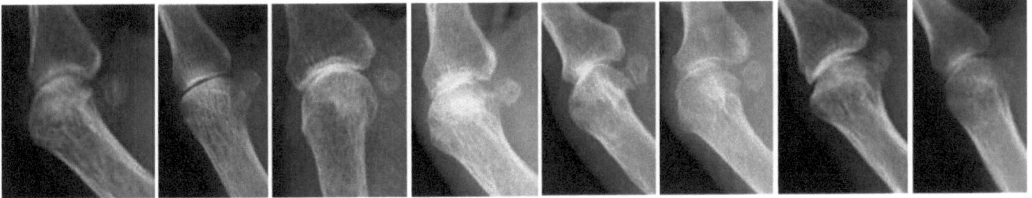

Fig. (15). Joint space narrowing of the right 1st MCP joints.

Lt 1st MCP

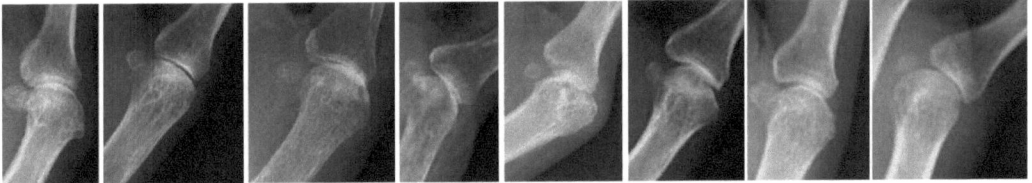

Fig. (16). Joint space narrowing of the left 1st MCP joints.

JSN of the 2nd MCP joints in RA (Figs. **17, 18**).

Rt 2nd MCP

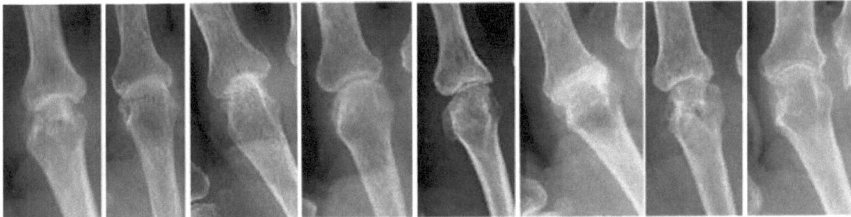

Fig. (17). Joint space narrowing of the right 2nd MCP joints.

Lt 2nd MCP

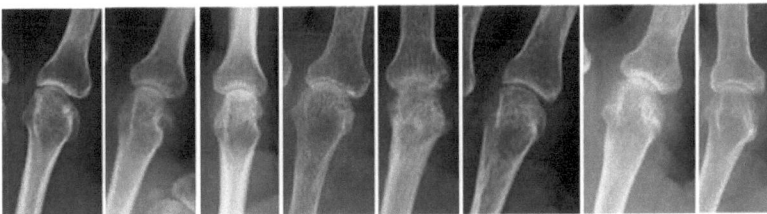

Fig. (18). Joint space narrowing of the left 2nd MCP joints.

JSN of the 3rd MCP joints in RA (Figs. **19, 20**).

Rt 3rd MCP

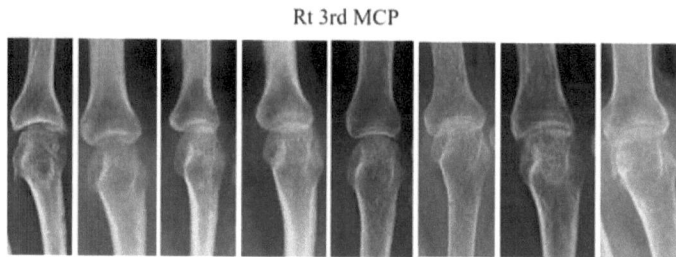

Fig. (19). Joint space narrowing of the right 3rd MCP joints.

Lt 3rd MCP

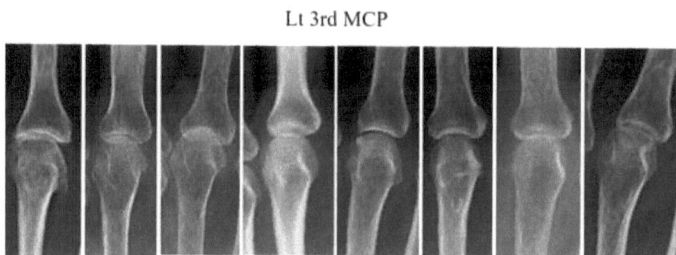

Fig. (20). Joint space narrowing of the left 3rd MCP joints.

JSN of the 4th MCP joints in RA (Figs. **21, 22**).

Rt 4th MCP

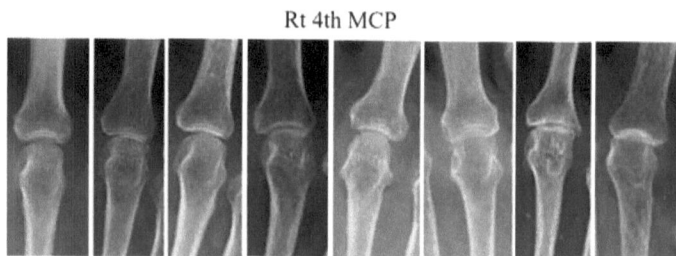

Fig. (21). Joint space narrowing of the right 4th MCP joints.

Lt 4th MCP

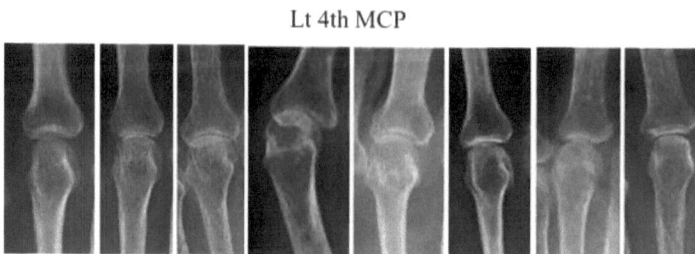

Fig. (22). Joint space narrowing of the left 4th MCP joints.

JSN of the 5th MCP joints in RA (Figs. **23, 24**).

Rt 5th MCP

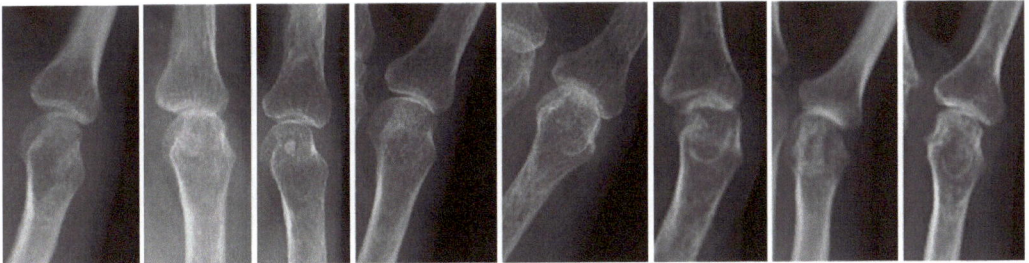

Fig. (23). Joint space narrowing of the right 5th MCP joints.

Lt 5th MCP

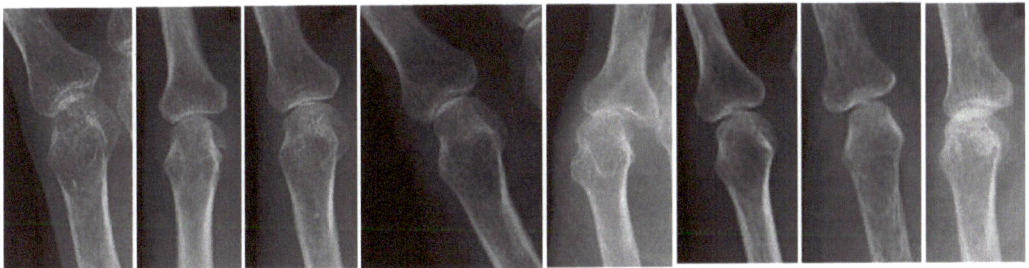

Fig. (24). Joint space narrowing of the left 5th MCP joints.

MCP joint US imaging (Figs. **25, 26**).

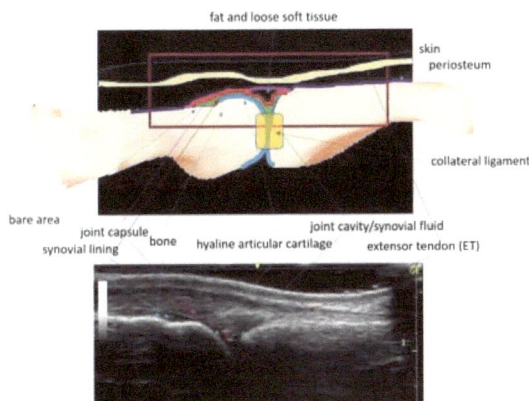

Fig. (25). Normal structure of the MCP joint and its US imaging.

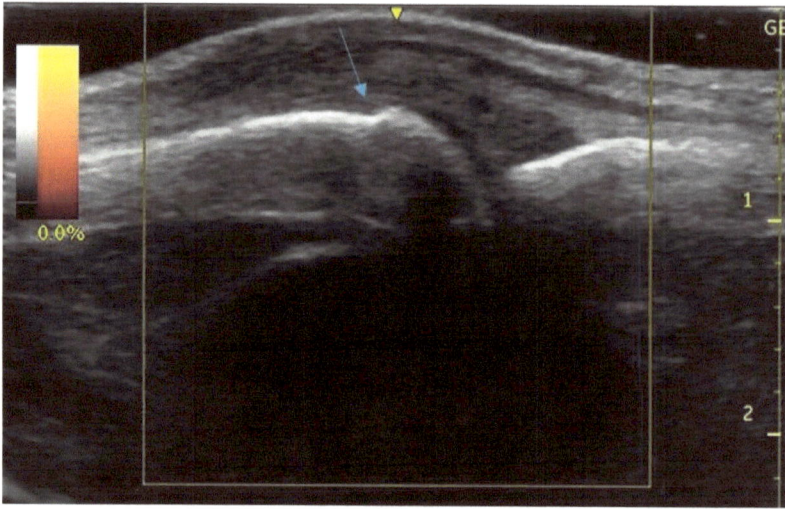

Fig. (26). Longitudinal US images of the dorsal aspect of the second MCP joint in a normal person. Doppler US image shows none of Doppler signals. Also, normal smooth indentation (arrow) is a pseudo-erosion on the dorsal aspect of the second metacarpal head. Sometimes it may be mistaken for an erosion.

MCP joint MR imaging (Fig. **27**).

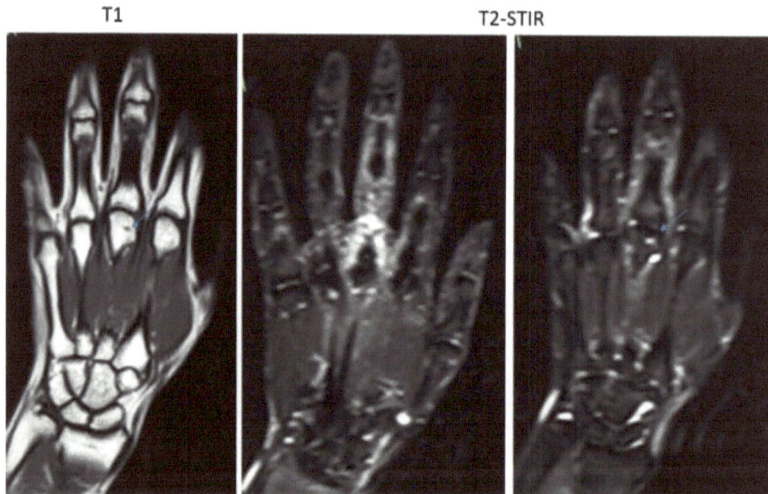

Fig. (27). Left panel: Coronal T1-weighted MR image shows small erosion (arrow). Middle panel: Coronal T2-short inversion time inversion-recovery (STIR) MR image shows marked synovitis at the third MCP joint. Right panel: Another image of coronal T2-STIR shows high intensity area of the third metacarpal head (arrow).

DIP Joints

DIP joint US imaging (Fig. **28**).

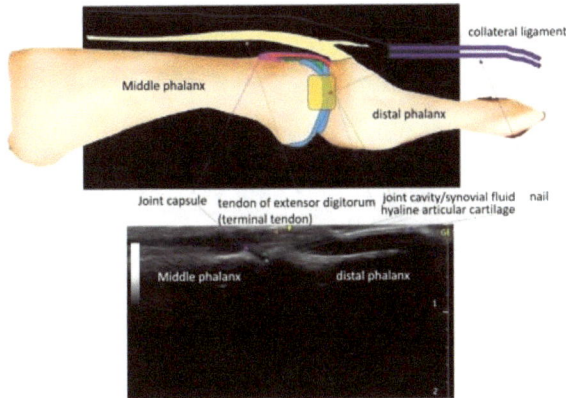

Fig. (28). Normal structure of the DIP joint and its US imaging.

Wrists

JSN of the wrists in RA (Figs. **29**, **30**).

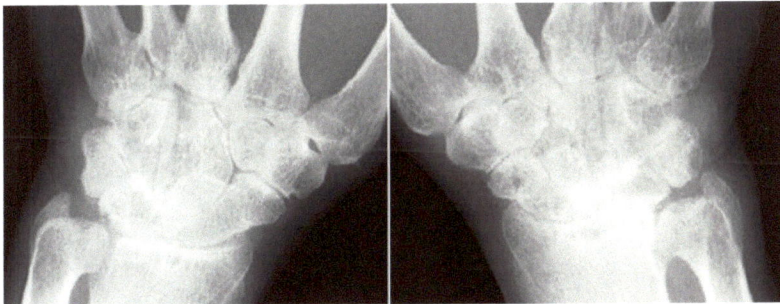

Fig. (29). Severe joint space narrowing of the wrists in a patient with RA.

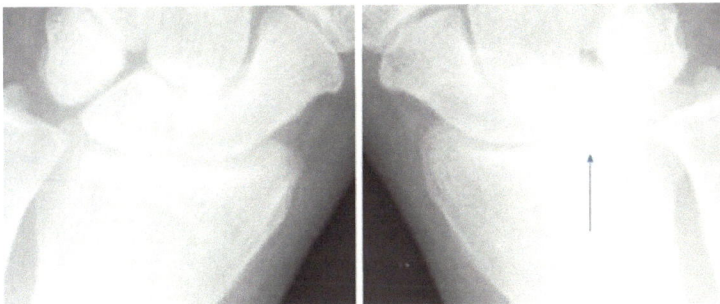

Fig. (30). Moderate joint space narrowing of the right radiocarpal joint in a patient with RA.

Elbows

JSN of the elbows in RA (Figs. **31**, **32**).

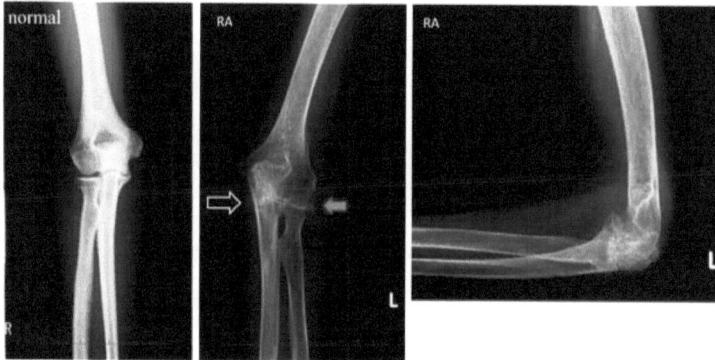

Fig. (31). Joint space narrowing of the elbows.

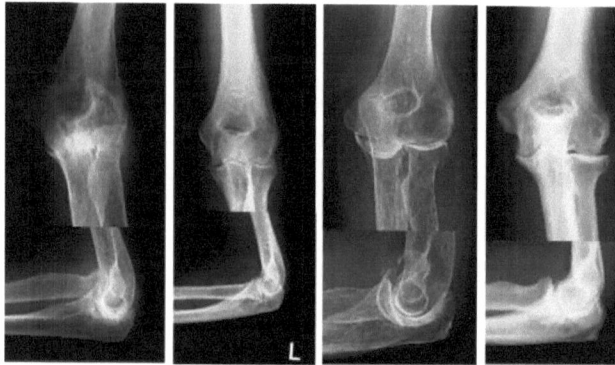

Fig. (32). Various patterns of joint space narrowing of the elbows.

Shoulders

JSN of the shoulders in RA (Figs. **33**, **34**).

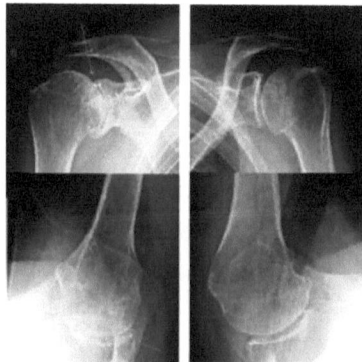

Fig. (33). Joint space narrowing of the right shoulder in a patient with RA.

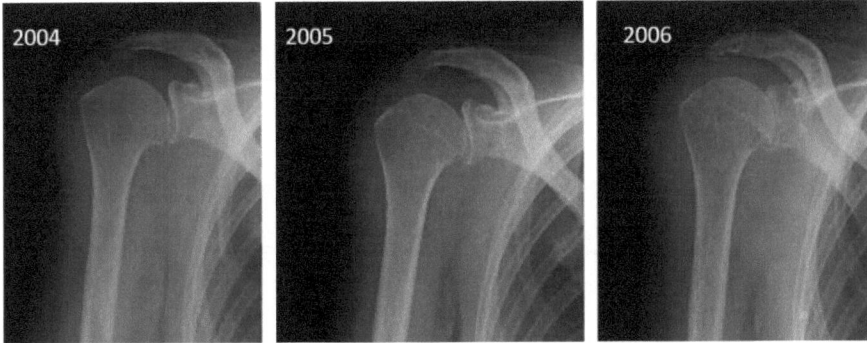

Fig. (34). From left to right progressive changes over a 2-year period of joint space narrowing at the right shoulder in a patient with RA.

Hips

JSN of the hips in RA (Fig. **35**).

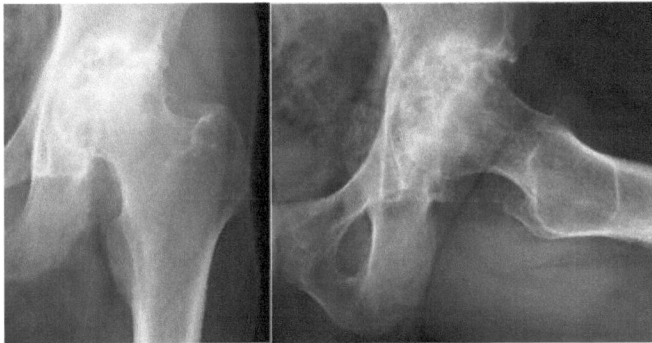

Fig. (35). Joint space narrowing of the left hip in a patient with RA.

Knees

JSN of the knees in RA (Figs. **36-39**).

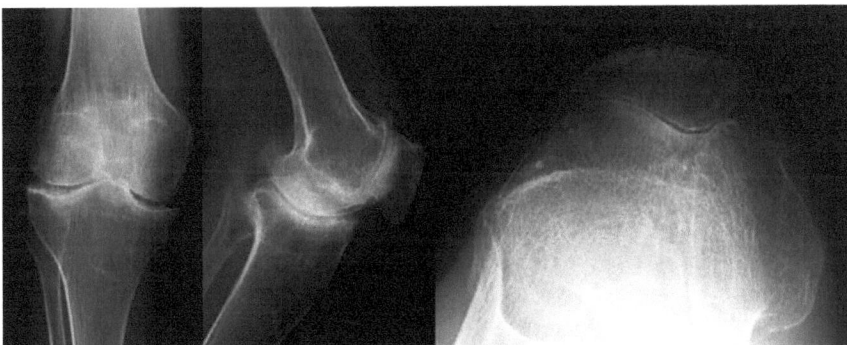

Fig. (36). Joint space narrowing with severe OA changes of the right knee in a patient with RA.

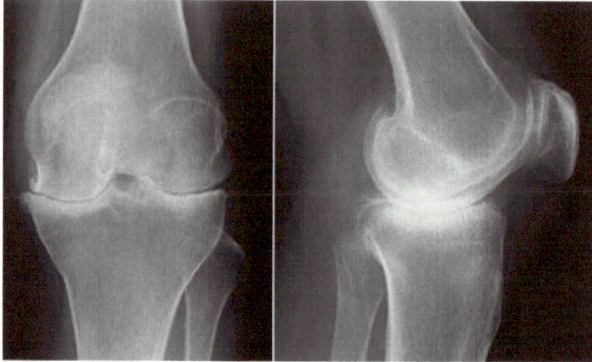

Fig. (37). Joint space narrowing with mild OA changes of the left knee in a patient with RA. AP view of the left knee shows symmetric reduction of both the medial and the lateral femorotibial joint spaces.

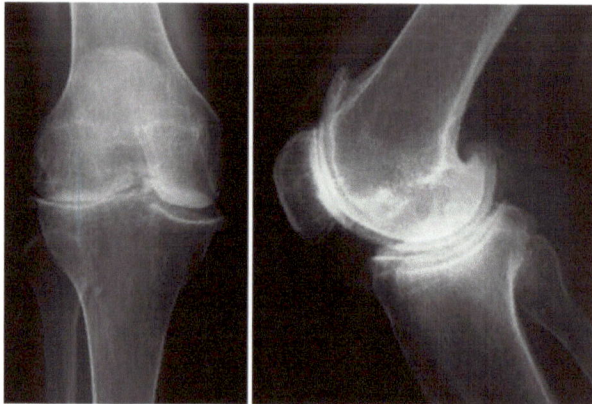

Fig. (38). Joint space narrowing of the lateral side of the right knee in a patient with RA.

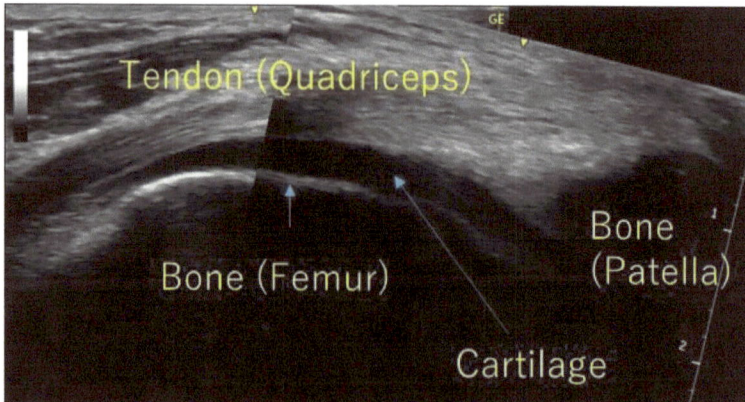

Fig. (39). Longitudinal US image of the knee shows the normal cartilage of the joint.

Ankles

JSN of the ankles in RA (Fig. **40**).

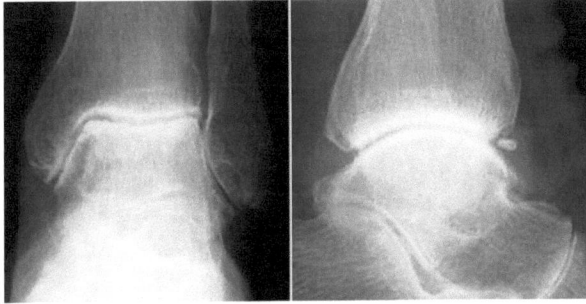

Fig. (40). Joint space narrowing of the left ankle in a patient with RA.

ANKYLOSIS

Ankylosis of the joints in RA (Figs. **41-46**).

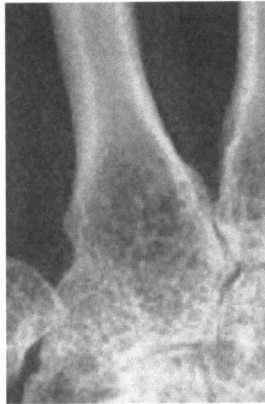

Fig. (41). Ankylosis of the trapezoid and the second metacarpal bone at the right 2nd CMC joint in a patient with RA.

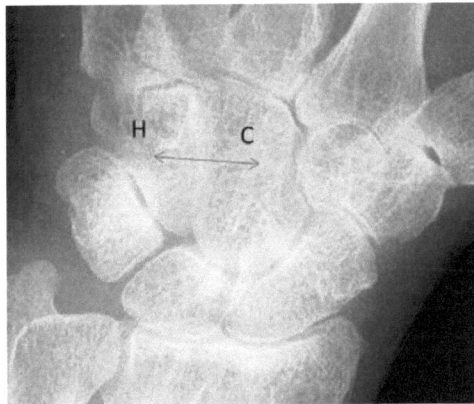

Fig. (42). PA view of the left wrist shows ankylosis between the capitate and the hamate.

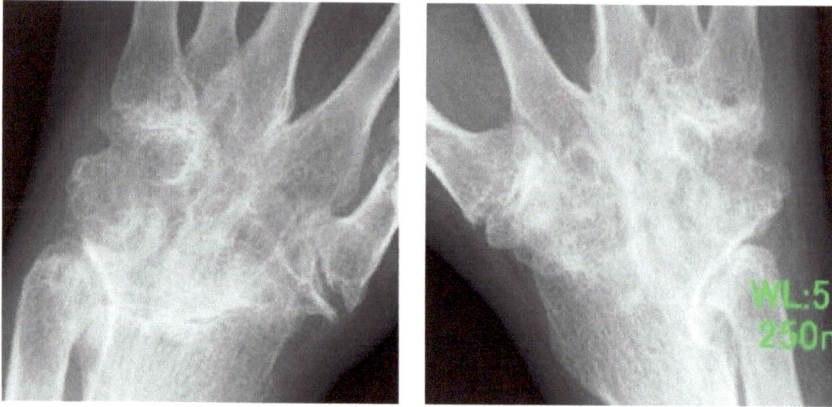

Fig. (43). PA views of the wrists show marked ankylosis of most of the carpal bones and the radius in a patient with RA.

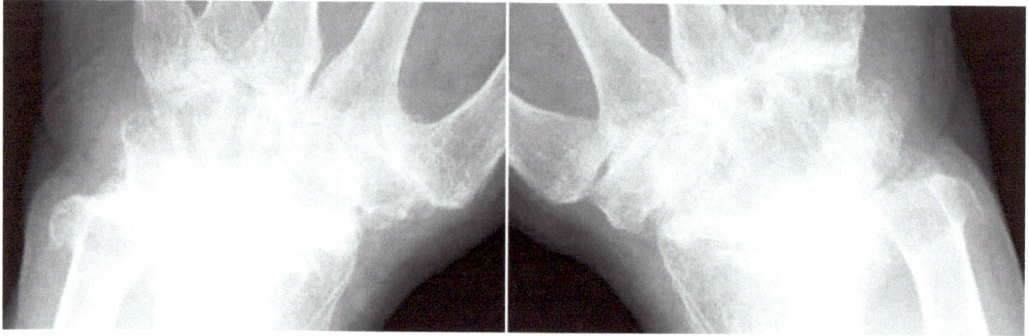

Fig. (44). PA views of the wrists show partial collapse of fused carpal bones in a patient with RA.

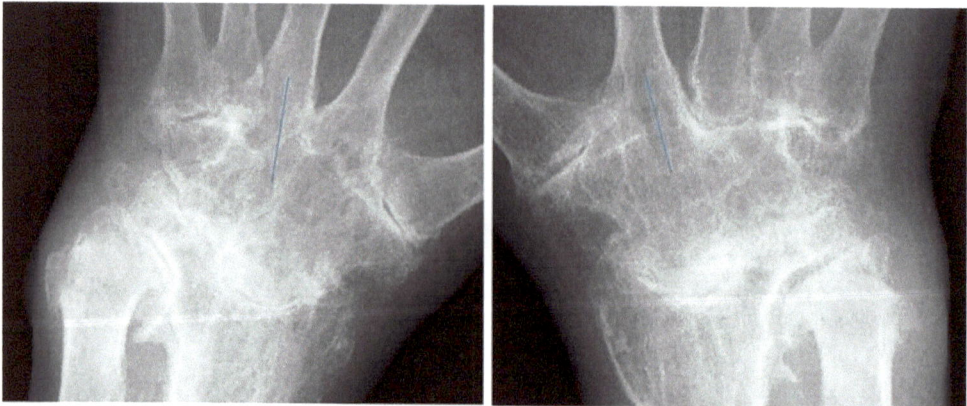

Fig. (45). PA views of the wrists show marked ankylosis of most of the carpal bones and the metacarpal bones in a patient with RA.

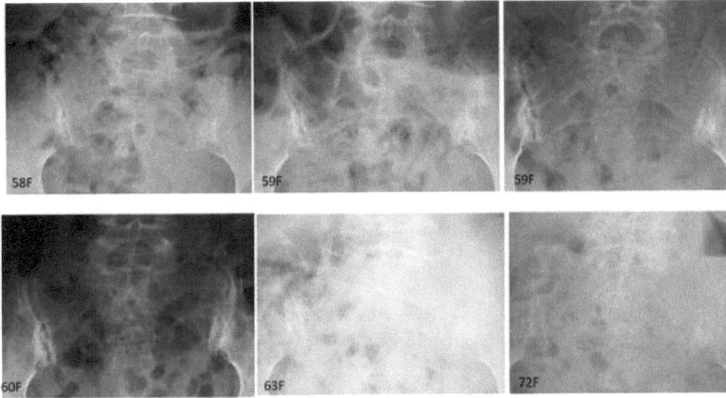

Fig. (46). AP views of the pelvis of a patient of RA shows ankylosis of the bilateral sacroiliac joints.

Joint Space Widening

JSW in RA (Figs. **47-50**).

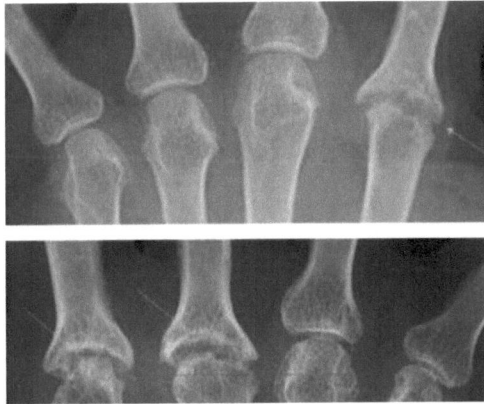

Fig. (47). The radiographs of the MCP joints show the joint space widening in a patient with RA. Occasionally, joint space may be widened by strong damage and destruction of the joints.

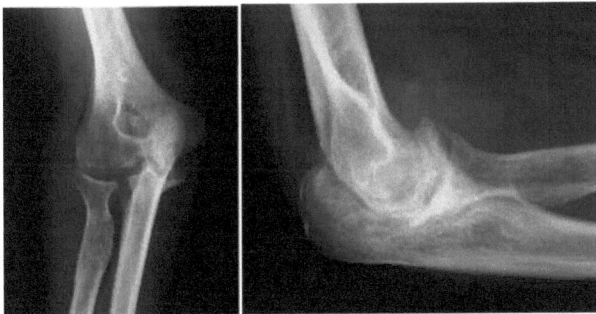

Fig. (48). The radiographs of the elbow show the joint space widening in a patient with RA.

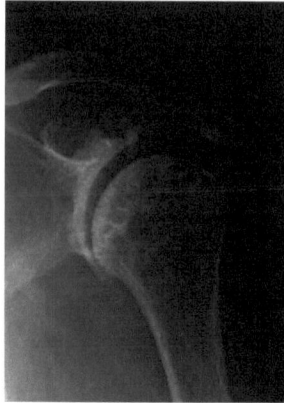

Fig. (49). AP view of the left shoulder shows the joint space widening in a patient with RA.

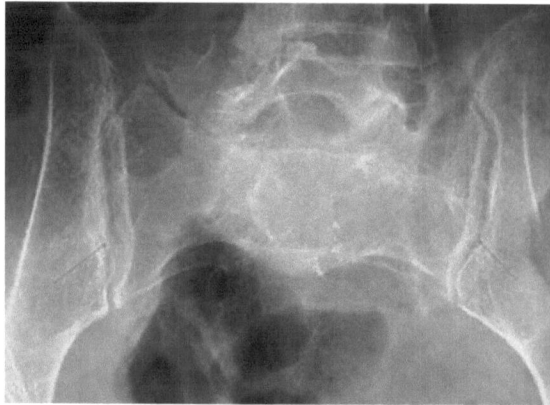

Fig. (50). Joint space widening of the sacroiliac joint in a patient with RA.

Calcification in Joints

Calcification of the shoulder joint in RA (Fig. **51**).

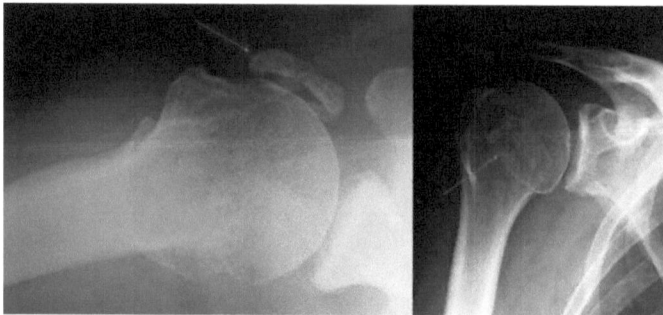

Fig. (51). Calcification of the shoulder joint in a patient with RA.

Joint Effusion

MCP Joint

Joint effusion of the MCP joints in RA (Fig. **52**).

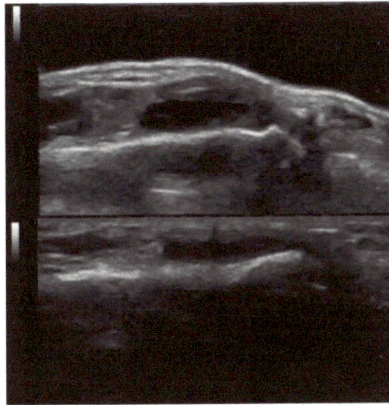

Fig. (52). Joint effusion in the 2nd MCP joint in a patient with RA. When the same joint is hardly pressed, effusion disappears, but proliferated synovium is not changed.

Elbows

Joint effusion of the elbows in RA (Fig. **53**).

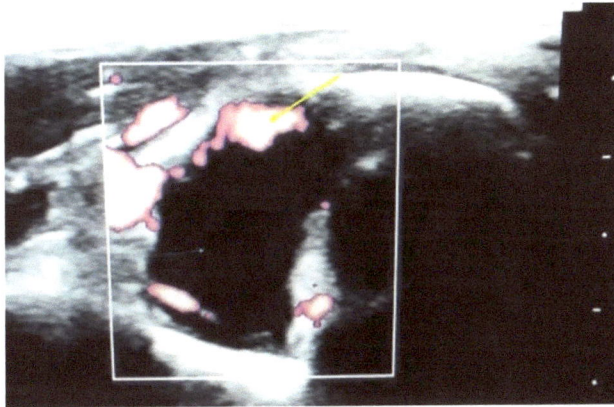

Fig. (53). Longitudinal power Doppler US image over the olecranon process and the posterior aspect of the distal humerus shows joint effusion without PD signals (blue arrow) and synovitis (yellow arrow) with PD signals of the elbow.

Knees

Joint effusion of the knees in RA (Figs. **54, 55**).

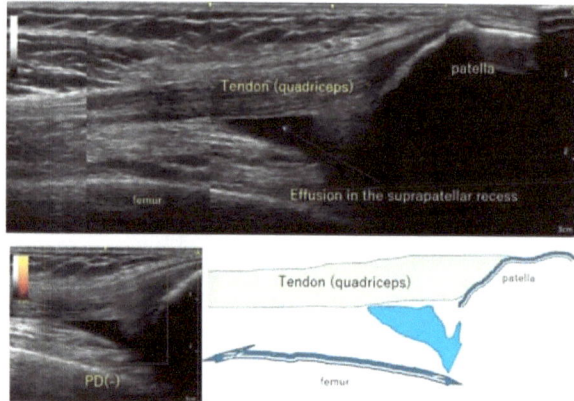

Fig. (54). Mild effusion in the suprapatella recess. There is no power Doppler signal at the knee in a patient with RA and SLE (rhupus).

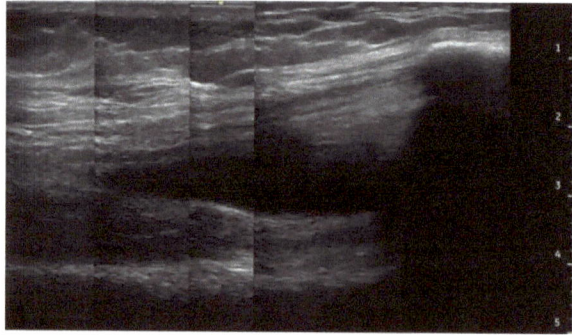

Fig. (55). Moderate effusion in the suprapatella recess in a patient with RA.

Synovitis

PIP joints

Synovitis of the PIP joints in RA (Figs. **56**, **57**).

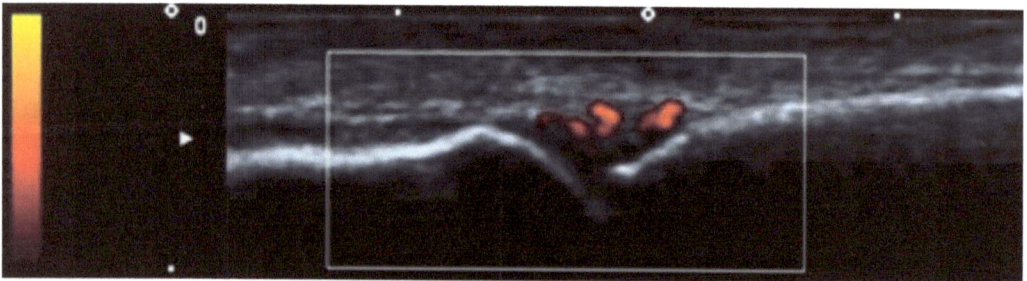

Fig. (56). Longitudial power Doppler US image of the PIP joint shows synovitis with PD signals in a patient with RA.

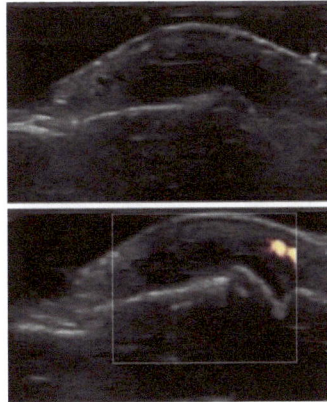

Fig. (57). Long-axis US images of the dorsal aspect of the first IP joint in a patient with RA. Power Doppler US image shows mild intra-articular synovial Doppler signal consistent with active synovitis.

MCP Joints

Synovitis of the MCP joints in RA (Figs. **58-65**).

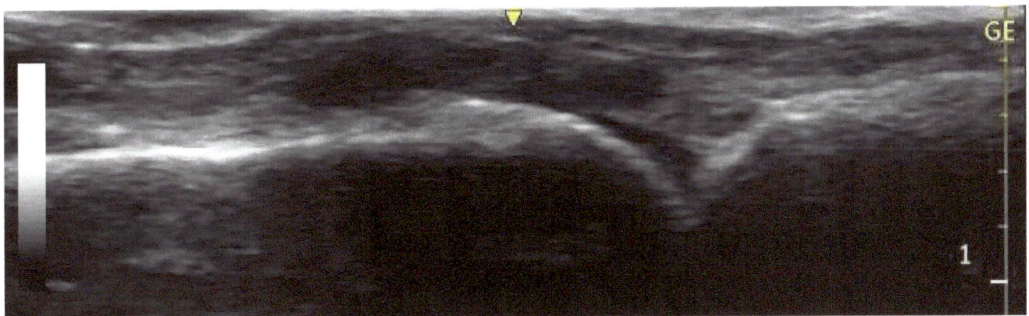

Fig. (58). Longitudinal gray-scale US image of the dorsal aspect of the third MCP joint in a patient with RA. The gray-scale US image shows the synovial proliferation.

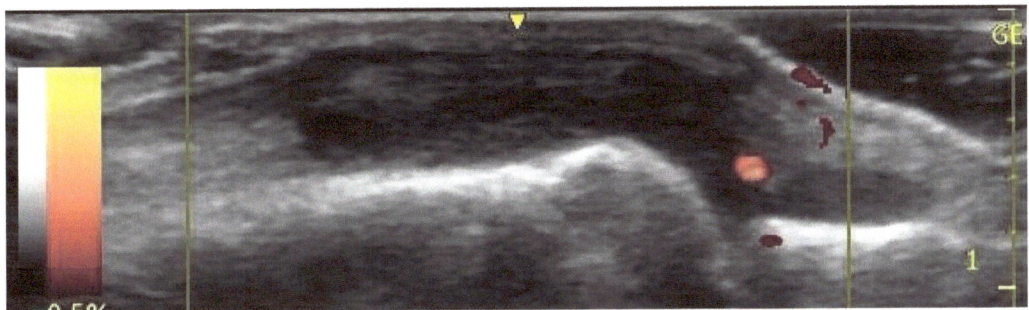

Fig. (59). Longitudinal power Doppler US image of the dorsal aspect of the third MCP joint in a patient with RA. Power Doppler US image shows mild intra-articular synovitis with PD signals.

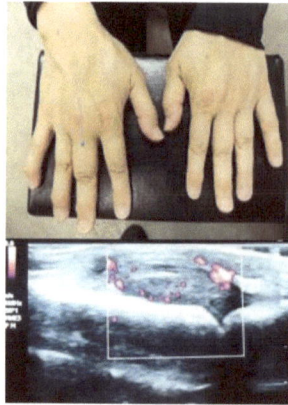

Fig. (60). Photograph of the hands shows swelling of the third MCP joint in a patient with RA. Longitudinal color Doppler US image of the dorsal aspect of the third MCP joint shows synovitis with PD signals.

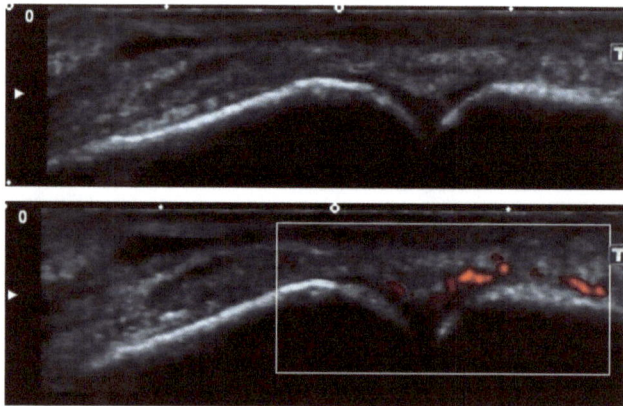

Fig. (61). Longitudinal gray-scale and power Doppler US images of the third MCP joint show synovitis with PD signals in a patient with RA and SLE.

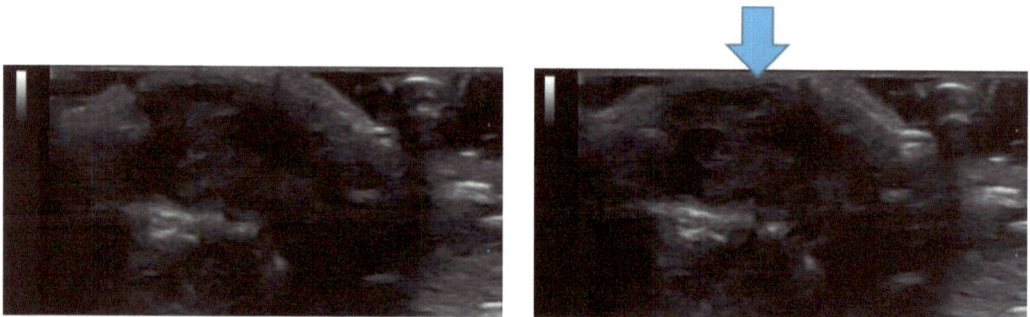

Fig. (62). Left panel; Longitudinal gray-scale US image of the dorsal aspect of the right third MCP joint shows strong synovial thickening in a patient with RA. Right panel; When the same joint is hardly pressed, it will not be changed. The synovitis consists of synovium but not joint effusion.

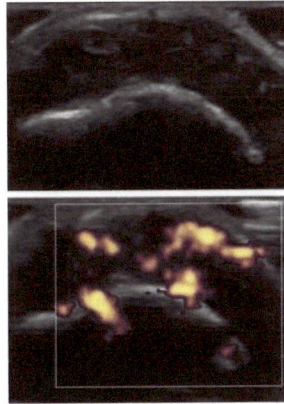

Fig. (63). Longitudinal US images of the dorsal aspect of the third MCP joint in a patient with RA. Upper panel: Gray-scale US image shows isoechoic synovial proliferation. Lower panel: Power Doppler US image shows markedly increased intra-articular PD signals consistent with active synovitis.

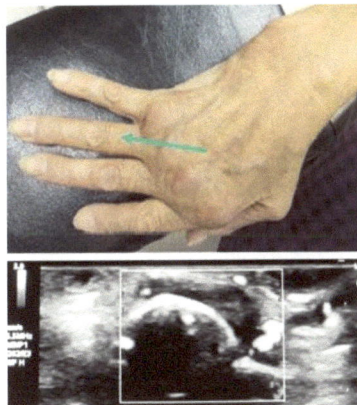

Fig. (64). Deformities of the fingers and synovitis in a patient with RA. Longitudinal US image of dorsal aspect of the fourth MCP joint shows synovitis with PD signals.

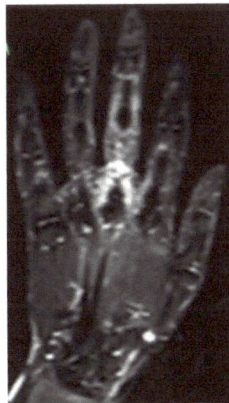

Fig. (65). MR image of the left hand in a patient with RA. T2-STIR image shows synovitis of the MCP joint.

Wrists

Synovitis of the wrists in RA (Figs. **66-85**).

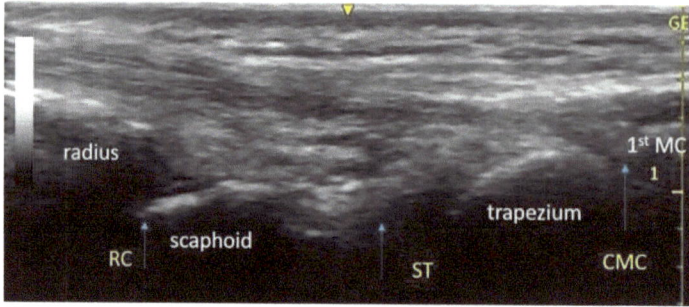

Fig. (66). Longitudinal gray-scale US image of radial side of the wrist in a normal person. CMC, First carpometacarpal joint; ST, scaphotrapezial joint; RC, radiocarpal joint.

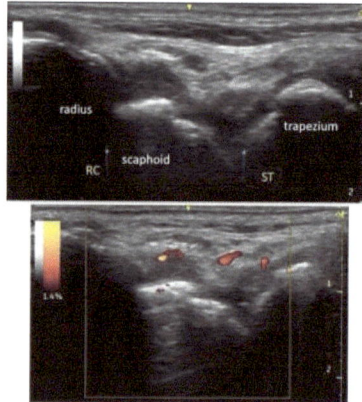

Fig. (67). Longitudinal gray-scale and power Doppler US images of radial side of the wrist show synovitis of the RC joint and the ST joint in a patient wirh RA. ST, scaphotrapezial joint; RC, radiocarpal joint.

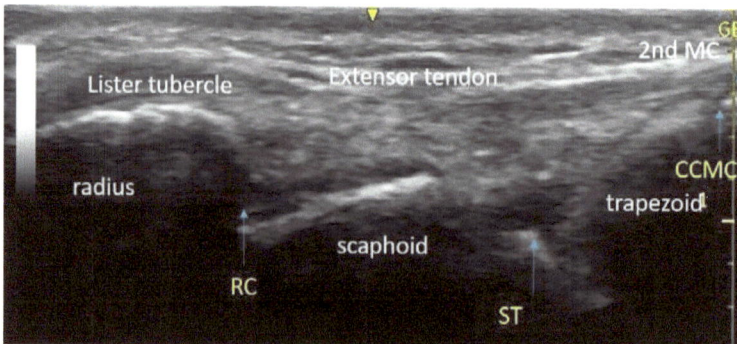

Fig. (68). Longitudinal gray-scale US image of dorsal aspect of Lister tubercle in a normal person. CCMC, common carpometacarpal joint; ST, scaphotrapezial joint; RC, radiocarpal joint.

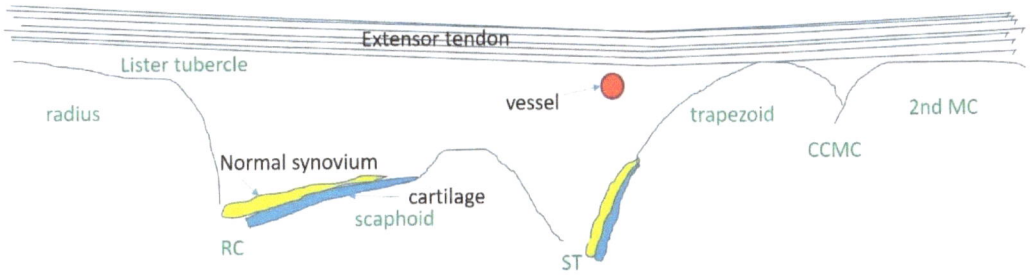

Fig. (69). A simplified schema of longitudinal image of dorsal aspect of Lister tubercle in normal persons.

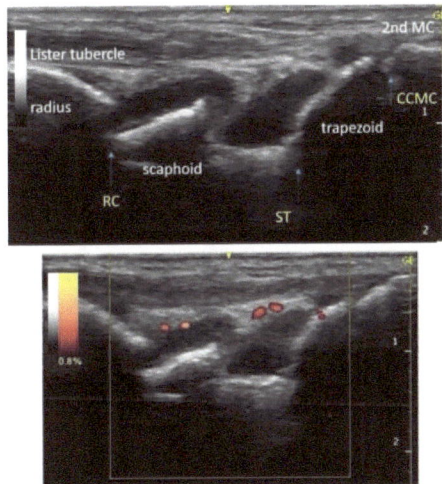

Fig. (70). Longitudinal gray-scale and power Doppler US images of dorsal aspect of Lister tubercle show synovitis of the RC joint and the ST joint in a patient wirh RA. ST, scaphotrapezial joint; RC, radiocarpal joint.

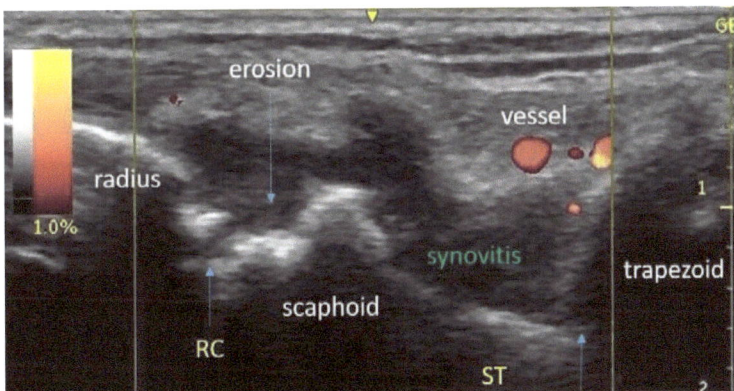

Fig. (71). Synovitis of the RC joint and the ST joint in a patient with RA.

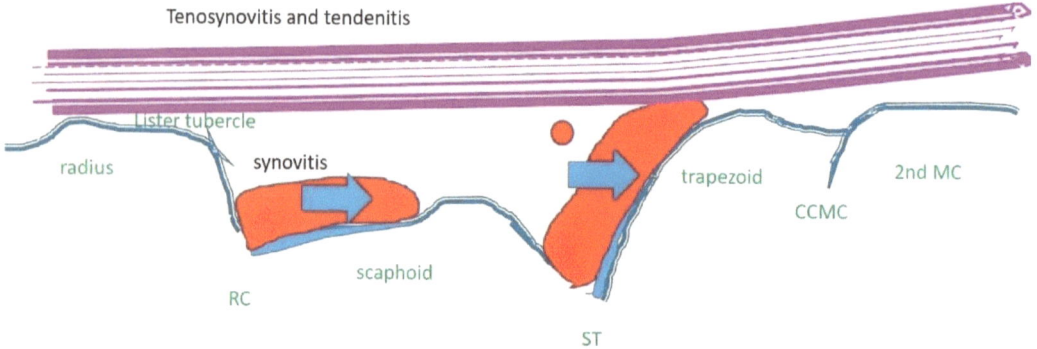

Fig. (72). A simplified schema of longitudinal image of dorsal aspect of Lister tubercle in RA. Synovitis of the RC joint and the ST joint with tenosynovitis of the extensor tendon may be observed. Usually, synovitis of the wrist will extend peripherally from the cleft between articulations. This pattern is different form the synovitis of the MCP joint and the PIP joint that extends proximally.

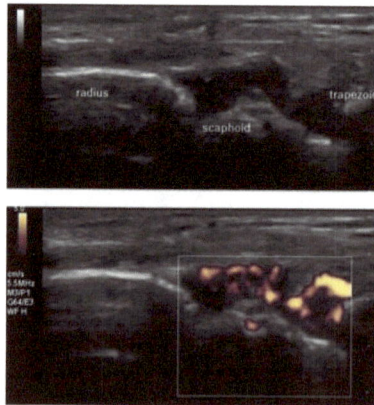

Fig. (73). Longitudinal gray-scale and power Doppler US images of dorsal aspect of the RC joint and the ST joint in a patient with RA. There are erosion and synovitis at the joints.

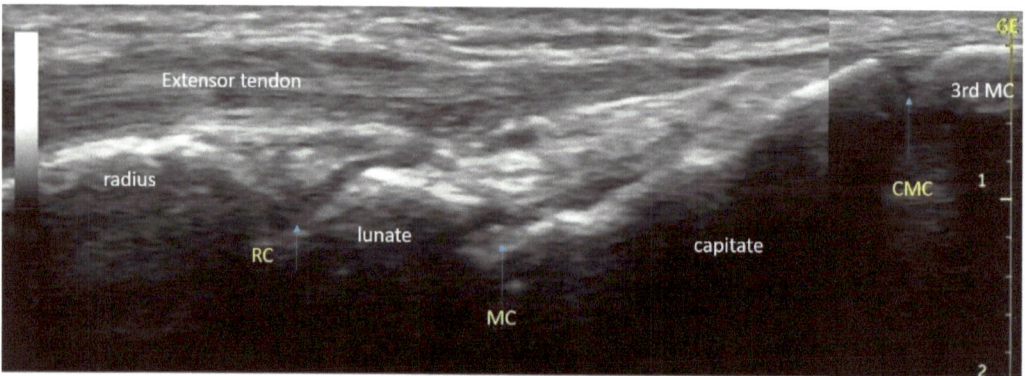

Fig. (74). Longitudinal gray-scale US image of dorsal aspect at the center of the wrist in a normal person. CMC, the third carpometacarpal joint; MC, midcarpal joint; RC, radiocarpal joint.

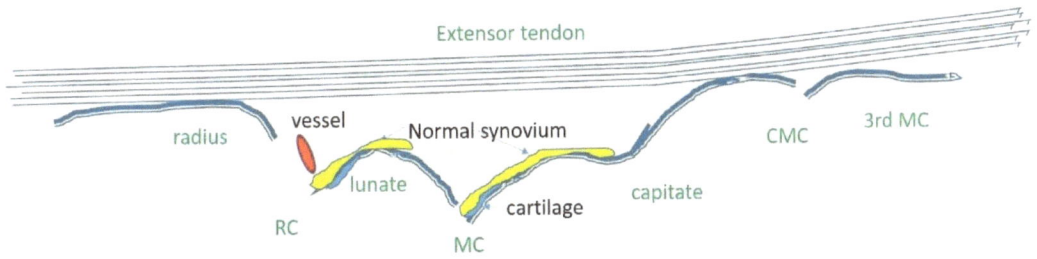

Fig. (75). A simplified schema of Longitudinal image of dorsal aspect at the center of the wrist in normal persons.

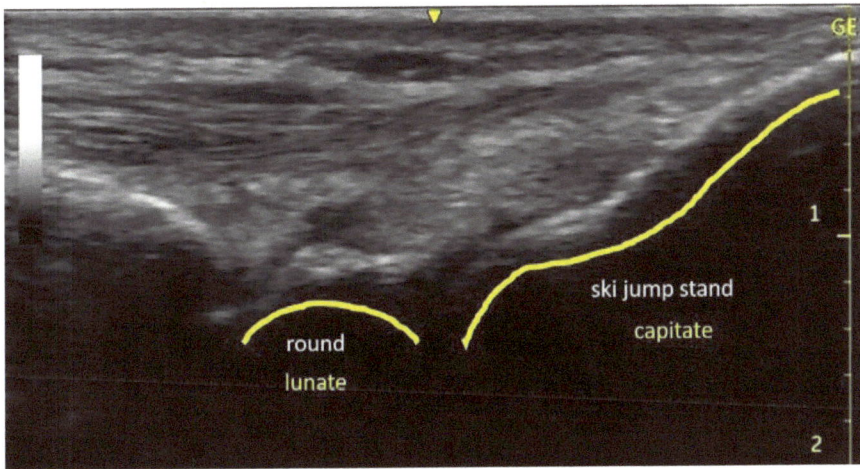

Fig. (76). The shape of the capitate likes a ski jump stand and the shape of the lunate is round as the moon in a normal person.

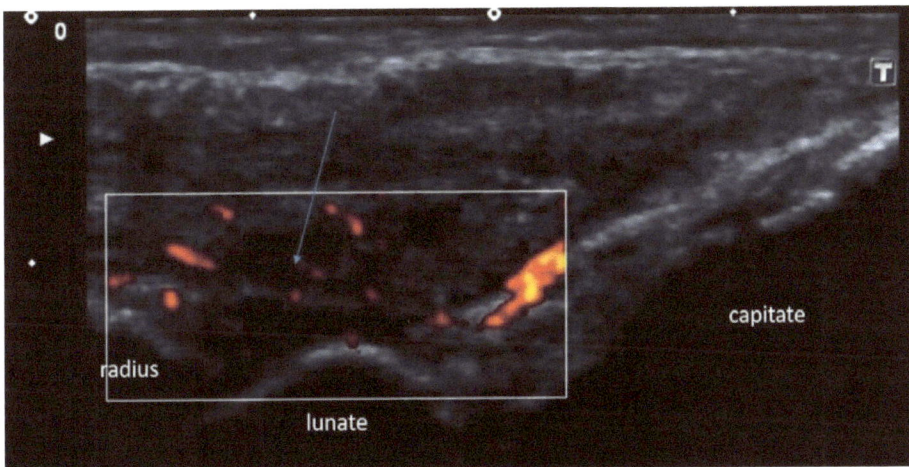

Fig. (77). Mild synovitis of the wrist in a patient with rhupus (RA and SLE).

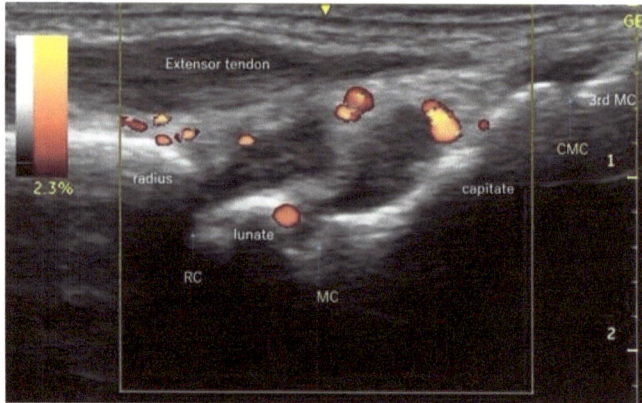

Fig. (78). Longitudinal gray-scale and power Doppler US images of dorsal aspect at the center of the wrist show synovitis of the RC joint and the MC joint in a patient wirh RA. CMC, the third carpometacarpal joint; MC, midcarpal joint; RC, radiocarpal joint.

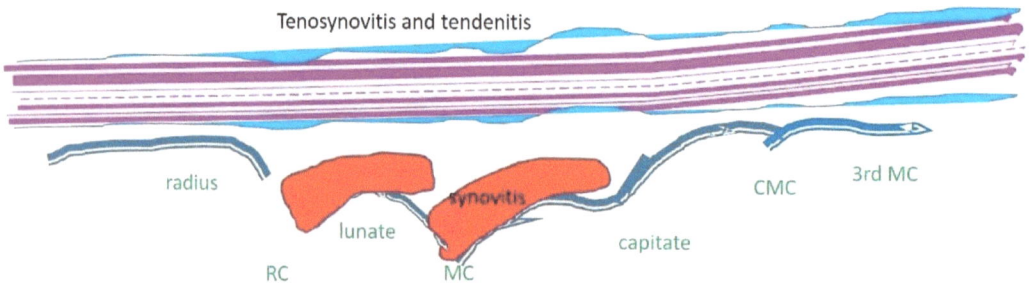

Fig. (79). A simplified schema of longotudinal image of dorsal aspect at the center of the wrist in RA. Synovitis of the RC joint and the ST joint with tenosynovitis of the extensor tendon occurs.

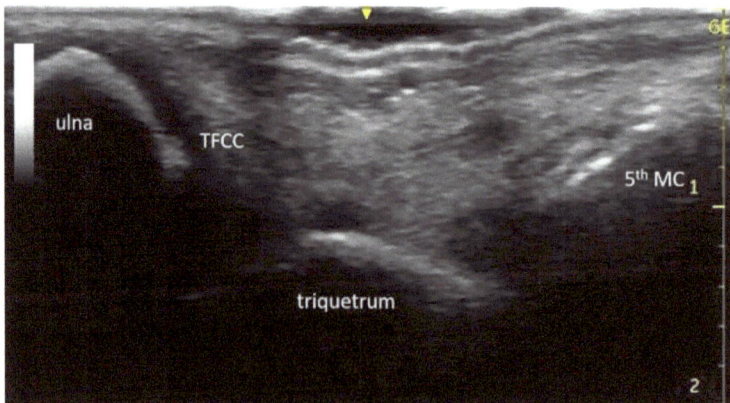

Fig. (80). Longitudinal gray-scale US image of dorsal aspect of the ulna in the wrist of a normal person. TFCC, triangular fibrocartilage complex.

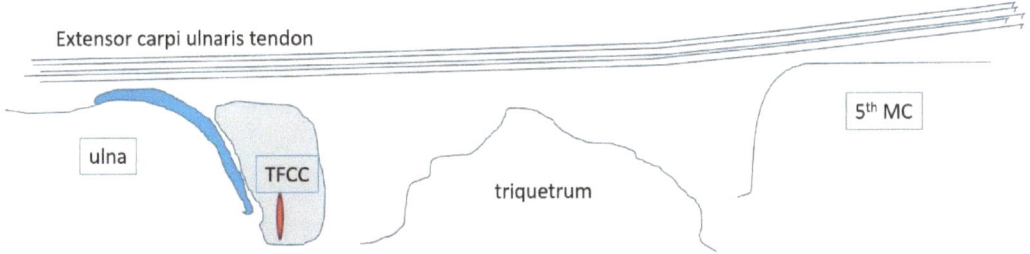

Fig. (81). A simplified schema of Longitudinal image of dorsal aspect of the ulna in the wrist.

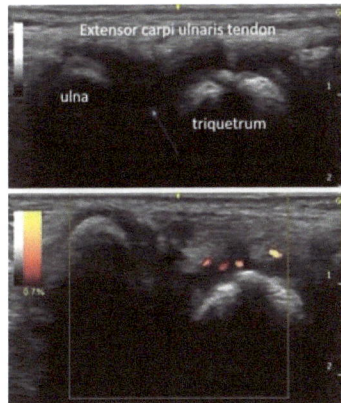

Fig. (82). Longitudinal gray-scale and power Doppler US images of dorsal aspect of the ulna in the wrist joint show synovitis. Hypo-echoic area with increased power Doppler is consistent with synovitis in a patient with RA.

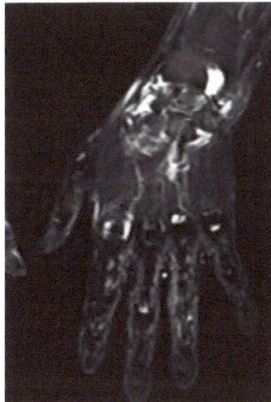

Fig. (83). MR image of the left hand in a patient with RA. T2-STIR image shows synovitis of the wrist.

FDG (^{18}F-fluorodeoxyglucose-positron emission tomography/computed tomograph) joint uptake reflectes inflammation in the affected joints in patients with RA [1 - 2]. FDG changes in inflamed joints are correlated with DAS28 joint scores [3].

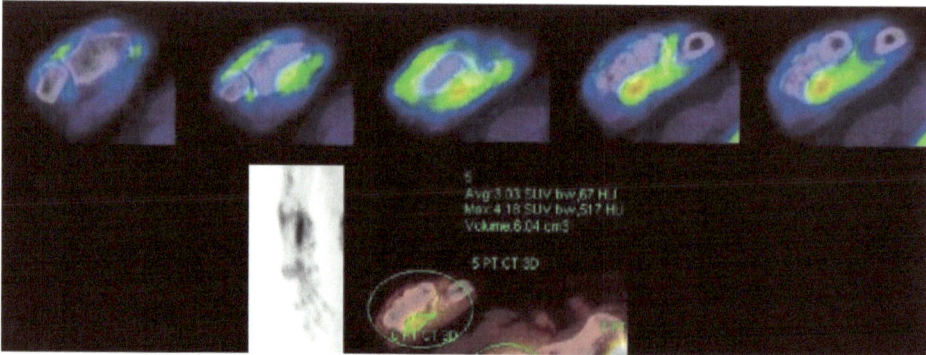

Fig. (84). FDG-PET/CT findings of the right wrist in a patient with rheumatoid arthritis (RA). Remarkable FDG uptake due to synovitis around the wrist.

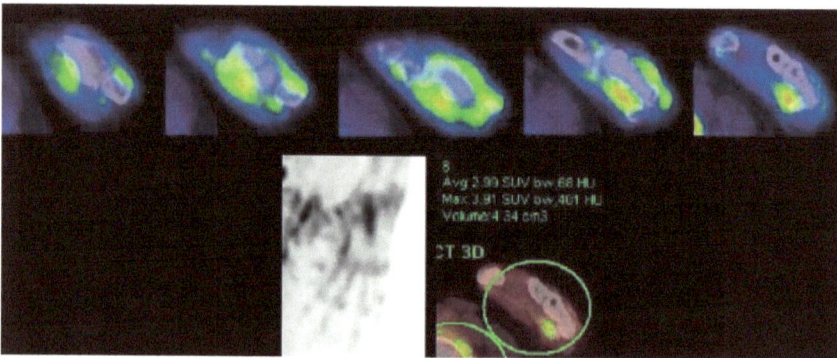

Fig. (85). FDG-PET/CT findings of the left wrist in a patient with rheumatoid arthritis (RA). Remarkable FDG uptake due to synovitis around the wrist.

Elbows

Synovitis of the elbows in RA (Figs. **86-93**).

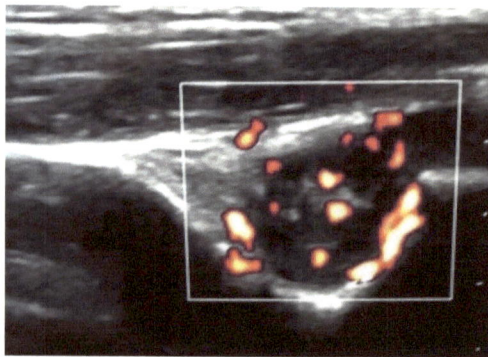

Fig. (86). Longitudinal power Doppler US image over the olecranon process and the posterior aspect of the distal humerus shows synovitis with PD signals of the elbow in a patient with RA.

Posterior

Lateral

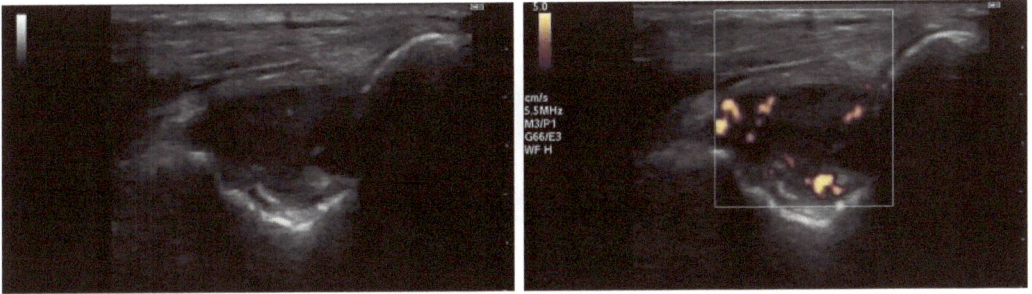

Fig. (87). Longitudinal gray-scale and power Doppler US images over the olecranon process and the posterior aspect of the distal humerus show synovitis with PD signals of the elbow in a patient with RA.

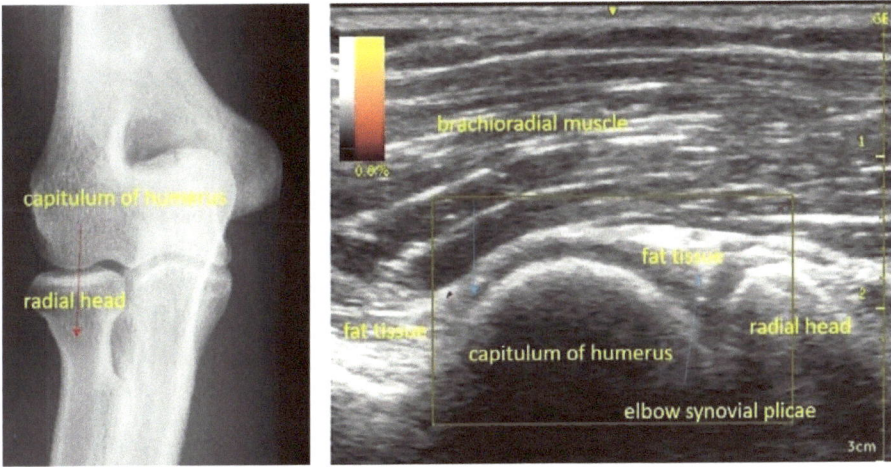

Fig. (88). Longitudinal gray-scale US image of lateral side of the elbow in a normal person.

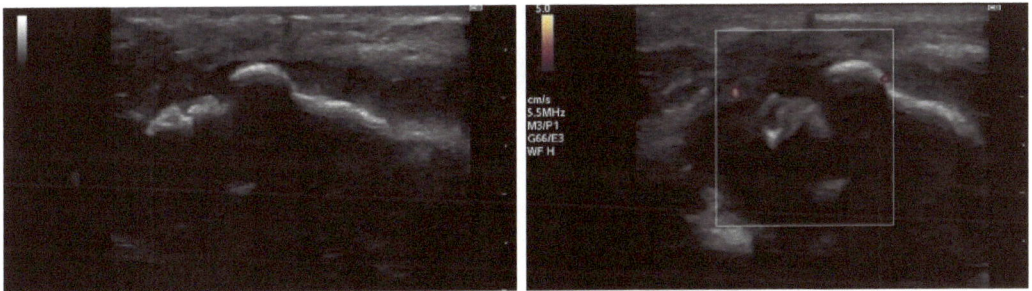

Fig. (89). Longitudinal gray-scale and power Doppler US images of lateral side of the elbow show mild synovitis with a PD signal and erosive lesions at the humeroradial joint. The radial head can be observed.

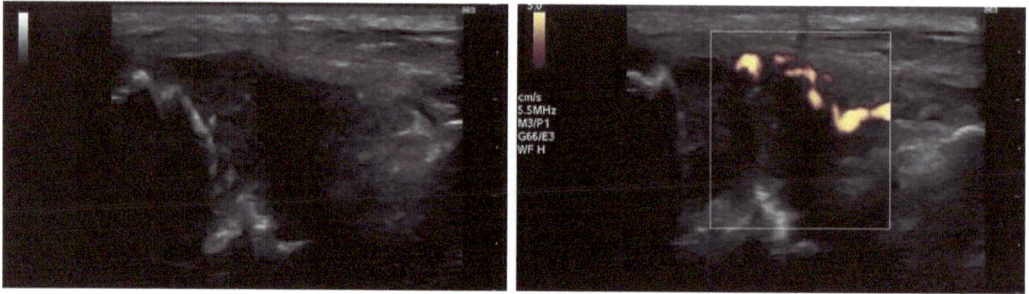

Fig. (90). Longitudinal gray-scale and power Doppler US images of lateral side of the elbow show synovitis with PD signals and erosive lesions at the humeroradial joint.

Medial

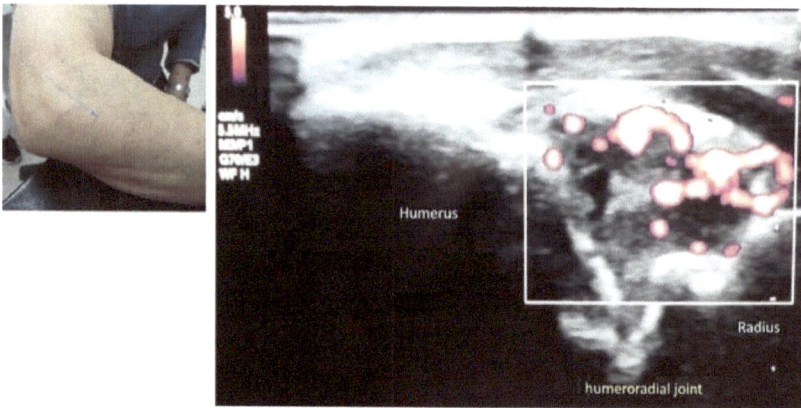

Fig. (91). Longitudinal power Doppler US image of lateral side of the elbow shows severe synovitis with PD signals and erosive lesions at the humeroradial joint.

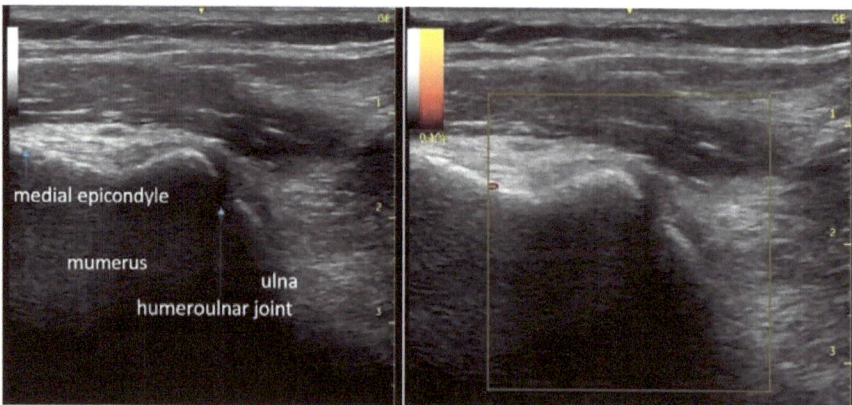

Fig. (92). Longitudinal gray-scale and power Doppler US images of medial side of the elbow in a normal person.

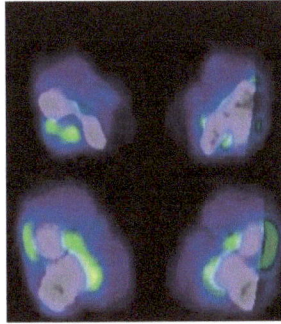

Fig. (93). FDG-PET/CT findings of the elbows in a patient with rheumatoid arthritis (RA). Remarkable FDG uptake due to synovitis around the elbows.

Shoulders

Synovitis of the shoulders in RA (Figs. **94, 95**).

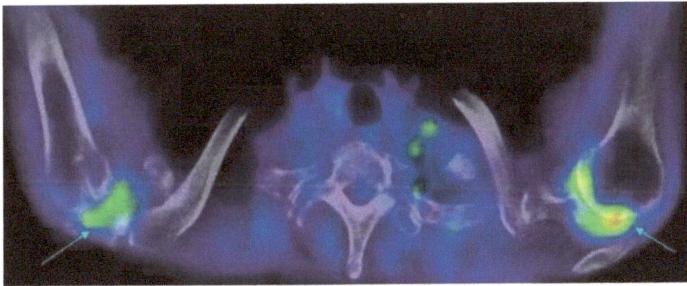

Fig. (94). Image of 18 F-fluorodeoxyglucose-positron emission tomography-computed tomography (FDG-PET/CT) shows arthritis of the shoulder joint in a patient with RA.

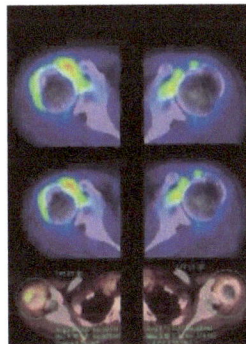

Fig. (95). FDG-PET/CT findings of the shoulders in a patient with rheumatoid arthritis (RA). Remarkable FDG uptake due to synovitis around the shoulders.

Hips

Synovitis of the knees in RA (Fig. **96**).

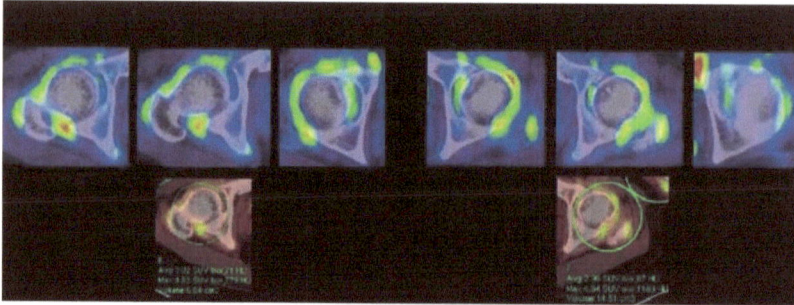

Fig. (96). FDG-PET/CT findings of the hips in a patient with rheumatoid arthritis (RA). Remarkable FDG uptake due to synovitis around the hips.

Knees

Synovitis of the knees in RA (Figs. **97-99**).

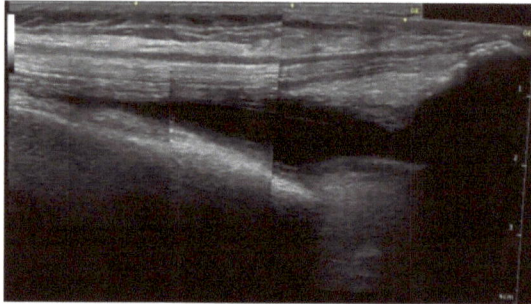

Fig. (97). Longitudinal gray-scale US image of the knee shows septic arthritis in a patient with RA.

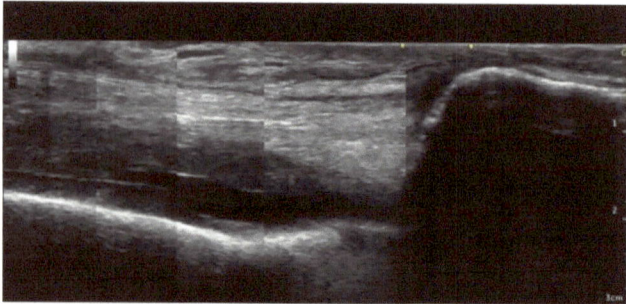

Fig. (98). Longitudinal gray-scale US image shows decreased joint effusion of septic arthritis after treatment in the same patient with RA (Fig. **97**).

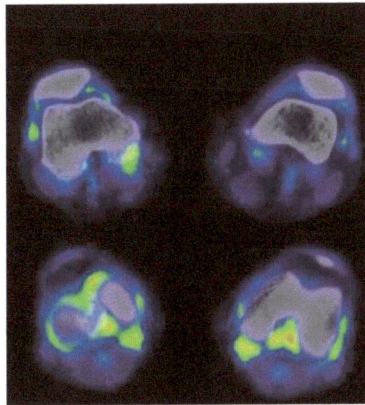

Fig. (99). FDG-PET/CT findings of the knees in a patient with rheumatoid arthritis (RA). Remarkable FDG uptake due to synovitis around the knees.

CONSENT FOR PUBLICATION

Not applicable.

CONFLICT OF INTEREST

The author (editor) declares no conflict of interest, financial or otherwise.

ACKNOWLEDGEMENTS

The authors thank Ms. K. Eguchi and A. Ibe for secretarial assistance.

REFERENCES

[1]   Okamura K, Yonemoto Y, Arisaka Y, *et al.* The assessment of biologic treatment in patients with rheumatoid arthritis using FDG-PET/CT. Rheumatology (Oxford) 2012; 51: 1484-91.

[2]   Yamashita H, Kubota K, Mimori A. Clinical value of whole-body PET/CT in patients with active rheumatic diseases. Arthritis Res Ther 2014; 16: 423.

[3]   Elzinga EH, van der Laken CJ, Comans EF, *et al.* 18F-FDG PET as a tool to predict the clinical outcome of infliximab treatment of rheumatoid arthritis: an explorative study. J Nucl Med 2011; 52: 77-80.

CHAPTER 5

D: Distribution

Syuichi Koarada[*] and **Akihito Maruyama**

Division of Rheumatology, Faculty of Medicine, Saga University, Saga, Japan

Abstract: Category D is the distribution of joint involvement. It includes the four "Distributions" in the body, the region, the joint and the time. These four categories provide important keys for the diagnosis of rheumatoid arthritis (RA) and differential diagnosis of various rheumatic diseases.

Keywords: Differential diagnosis, Distribution, Rheumatoid arthritis.

INTRODUCTION

Four components of "D": Distributions" include

1. Distribution in the body
2. Distribution in the region
3. Distribution in the joint
4. Distribution in the time

These four components of joint involvement provide important keys for the diagnosis of various rheumatic diseases. Especially, in RA, the pattern of the distributions is very specific for the disease.

Differential diagnosis of polyarthritis is important for the diagnosis of RA [1].

DISTRIBUTION IN BODY

In RA patients, any of synovial joints can be affected. However, especially, the MCP joints and the PIP joints are the most frequently involved and affected joints are bilateral and symmetrical [2, 3]. And, the atlantoaxial joint is involved in the spine.

A schema of the distribution of arthritis of RA in the whole body (Fig. **1**).

---

[*] **Corresponding author Syuichi Koarada:** Division of Rheumatology, Faculty of Medicine, Saga University, Saga, Japan; Tel: 81-952-31-6511; E-mail: koarada@cc.saga-u.ac.jp

Gallium and bone scintigraphy illustrates the distribution of arthritis and inflammation in patients with RA (Figs. **2 - 12**). The distribution of arthritis in primary and secondary SS (RA-based) (Fig. **13**).

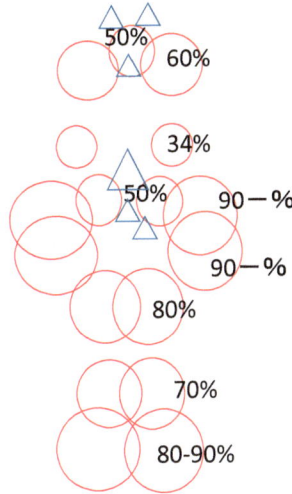

Fig. (1). A schema of the distribution of arthritis of RA in the whole body. The distribution of arthritis may be helpful in the evaluation of patients with RA. Peripheral small joints including the hands and the feet are mainly involved in RA [4].

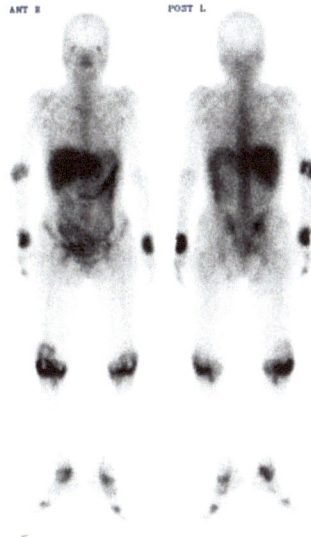

Fig. (2). Gallium scintigraphy illustrates the distribution of arthritis in the whole body in a patient with RA.

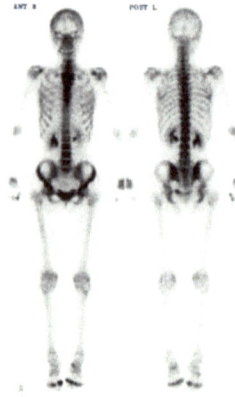

Fig. (3). Bone scan; The distribution of arthritis in RA. The affected joints are mainly smaller joints in the same patient with RA as seen in Fig. (2).

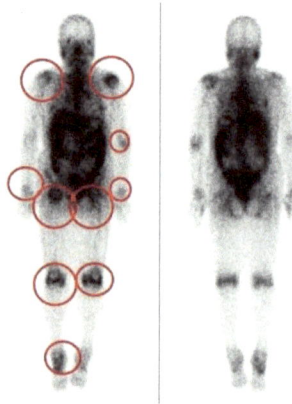

Fig. (4). Gallium scintigraphy; A schema of the distribution of arthritis in elderly onset rheumatoid arthritis (EORA). The affected joints are mainly larger joints.

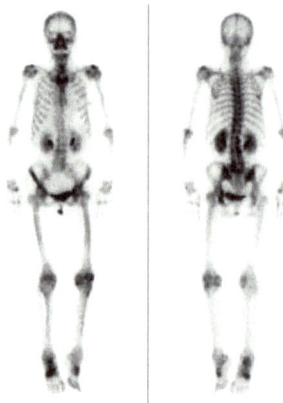

Fig. (5). Bone scan; The distribution of arthritis in elderly onset rheumatoid arthritis (EORA). The affected joints are mainly larger joints in the same patient with RA as seen in Fig. (4).

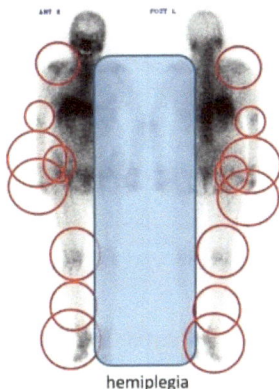

Fig. (6). A schema of the distribution of arthritis with a patient with RA who has hemiplegia. The affected joints are mainly in one side of the body.

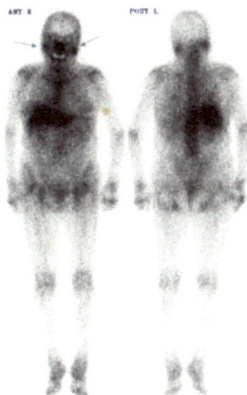

Fig. (7). Gallium scintigraph shows the distribution of arthritis in RA and parotitis of Sjögren's syndrome.

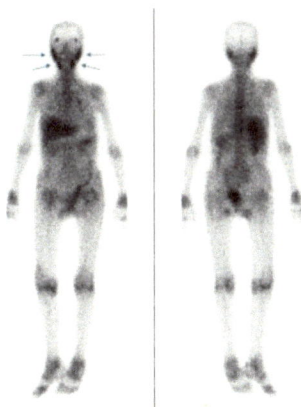

Fig. (8). Gallium scintigraphy shows the distribution of parotitis and submandibular sialoadenitis due to Sjögren's syndrome with polyarthritis.

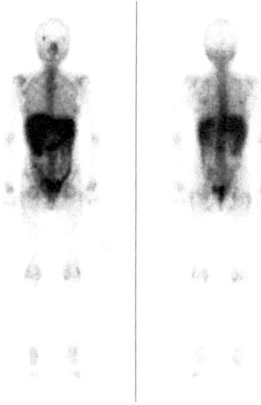

Fig. (9). Gallium scintigraphy shows the distribution of arthritis in rhupus (RA and SLE).

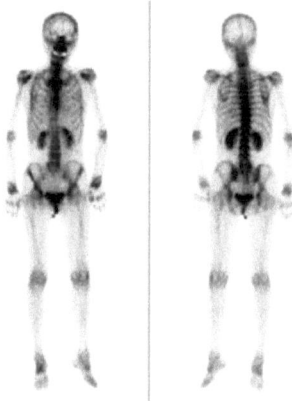

Fig. (10). Bone scan shows the arthritis distribution of large and small joints in rhupus (RA and SLE).

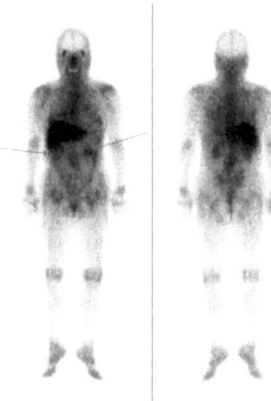

Fig. (11). Gallium scintigraph shows the distribution of arthritis and lupus nephritis in rhupus (RA and SLE).

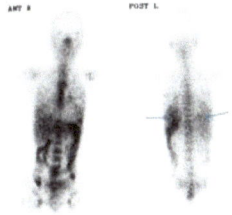

Fig. (12). Gallium scintigraph shows the interstitial pneumonitis and mild arthritis.

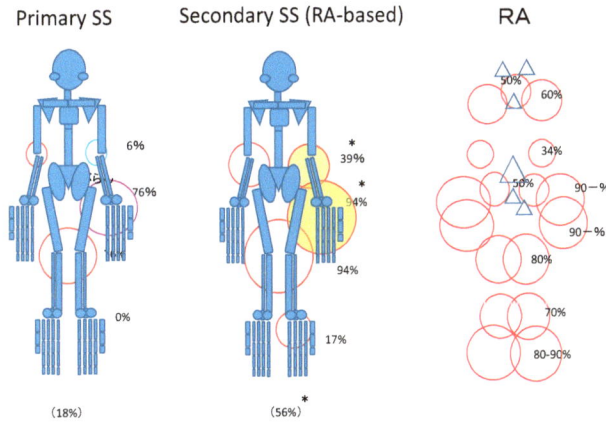

Fig. (13). The distribution of arthritis in primary and secondary SS (RA-based) [4].

DISTRIBUTION IN THE REGIONS IN RA

Hands

The distribution of radiologic changes within the joints, especially in the hands provides important information for appropriate diagnosis of RA and other rheumatic diseases. Usually, patients with RA have arthritis at the PIP joints, the MCP joints and the wrists but not the DIP joints (Figs. **14 - 30**).

Other rheumatic diseases have specific and/or non-specific distribution. For example, psoriatic arthritis may affect the DIP joints, the PIP joints and the MCP joints. Calcium pyrophosphate dehydrate deposition (CPPD) and gout may affect the MCP joints and the RC joints. The pattern of the distribution is useful to make differential diagnosis of various arthritis.

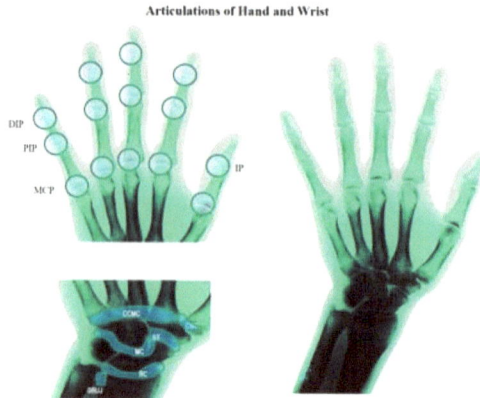

Fig. (14). Articulations of the hand and the wrist.

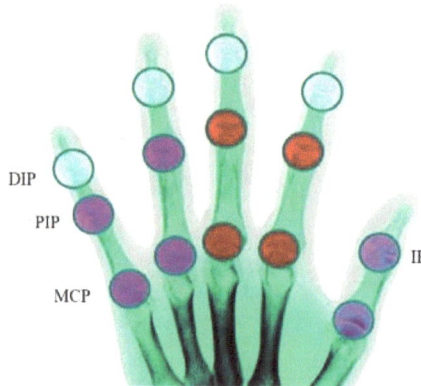

Fig. (15). The sites of the involvement with RA of the hand. Patients with RA have arthritis at the PIP, and MCP joints but not the DIP joints in the hand. (Red, generally [100-80%]; purple, frequently [80-60%], yellow, sometimes [60-40%]; blue, occasionally [40-20%]; green; rarely [20-0%]. The frequencies are in the cohort of our patients [SARAs cohort])

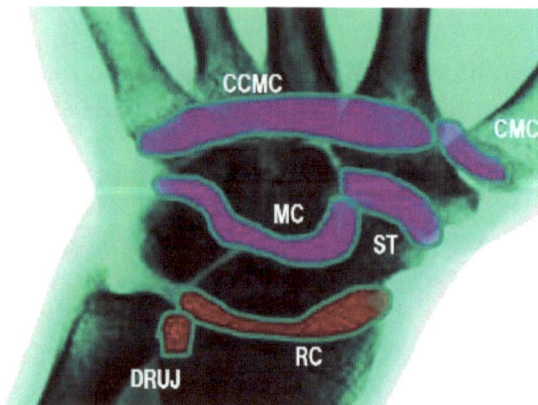

Fig. (16). The sites of the involvement with RA of the wrist.

Fig. (17). The erosive sites with early RA of the wrist.

Fig. (18). Erosions of the wrist in a patient with RA. An compartmental abnormalities of the wrist are seen.

Fig. (19). Erosions of the wrist in a patient with RA. Erosions of the radial side of the wrist are predominant .

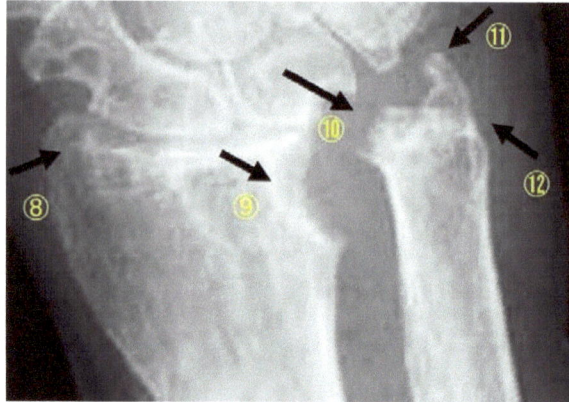

Fig. (20). Erosions of the distal end and the styloid process of the ulna in a patient with RA.

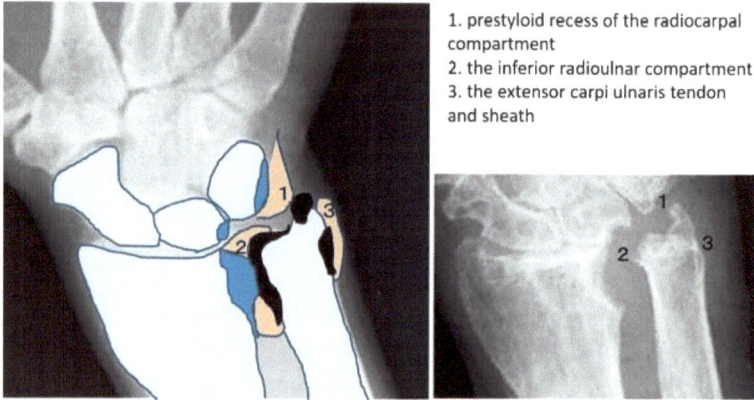

1. prestyloid recess of the radiocarpal compartment
2. the inferior radioulnar compartment
3. the extensor carpi ulnaris tendon and sheath

Fig. (21). The erosive sites of the distal end and the styloid process of the ulna in RA. There are three distinct areas in the distal portion of the ulna including the prestyloid recess of the radiocarpal compartment (1), the inferior radioulnar compartment (2), and the extensor carpi ulnaris tendon and sheath (3).

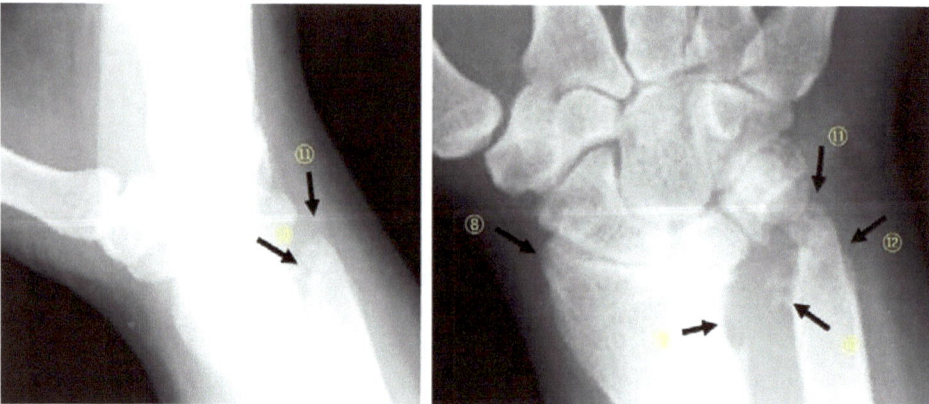

Fig. (22). Severe erosions of the distal end and the styloid process of the ulna.

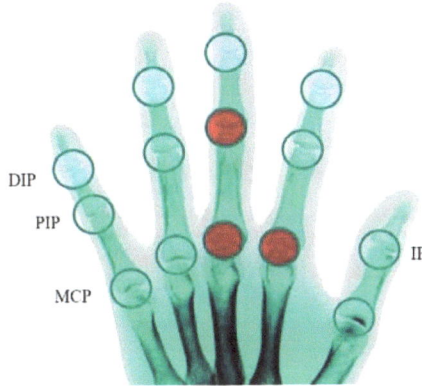

Fig. (23). The sites of the involvement with early RA of the hand.

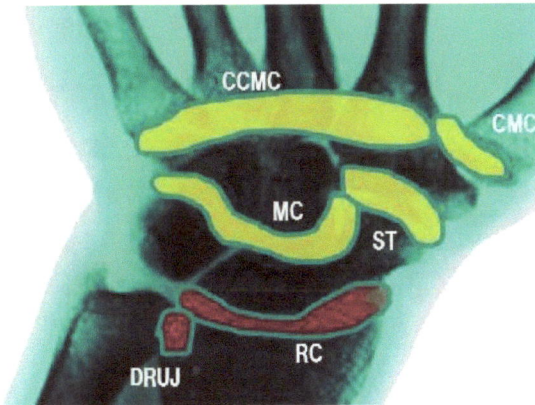

Fig. (24). The sites of the involvement with early RA of the wrist.

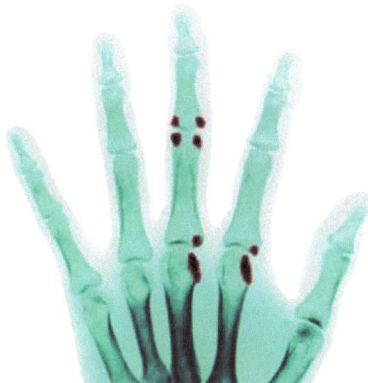

Fig. (25). The sites of erosions <u>with early RA of the hand</u>. Early erosions may occur on radial side of the bases of proximal phalanges and the heads of metacarpal bones at the second and third MCP joints. Also, erosions may appear on radial and ulnar sides of <u>the base of the middle phalange and the head of the proximal phalange at the third PIP joint</u>. The involvement of DIP joints is very rare.

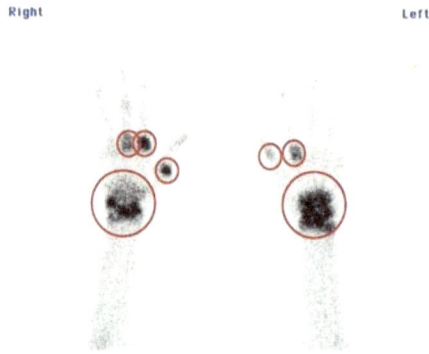

Fig. (26). Bone scan illustrates common sites of the involvement of arthritis of the hands in RA. Bone scan may help to evaluate the distribution of arthritis.

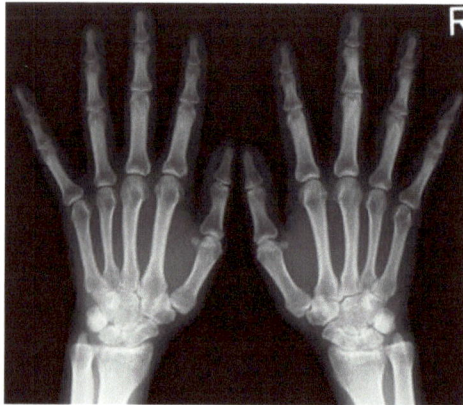

Fig. (27). Plain radiograph of the hands in a patient with RA shows periarticular osteoporosis at the PIP joints, the MCP joints and the carpal bones.

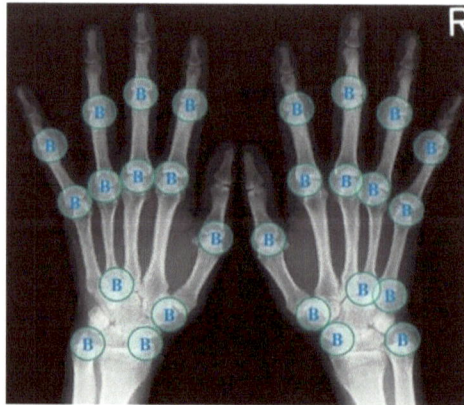

Fig. (28). The sites of arthritis of the hands and wrists in the same patient with RA (Fig. **27**).

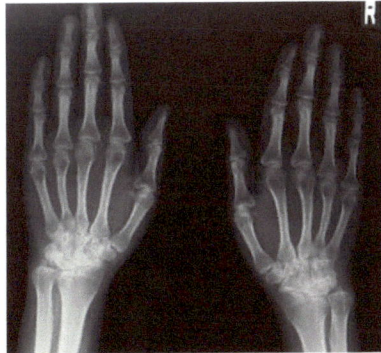

Fig. (29). Plain radiograph of the hands in a patient with advanced RA shows various characteristic changes of RA including A (mal-alighment), B (periarticular osteoporosis and erosions) and C (joint space narrowing) at the PIP joints, the MCP joints and the carpal bones.

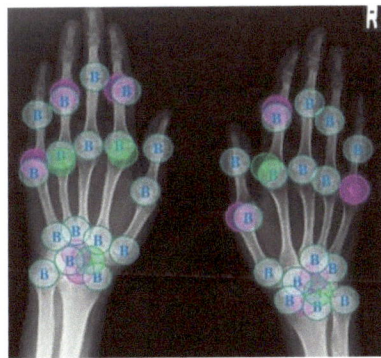

Fig. (30). The distribution of the sites of the involvement in the hands and the wrists suggests the diagnosis of advanced RA.

Shoulders

The sites of the involvement with RA of the shoulder (Fig. **31**).

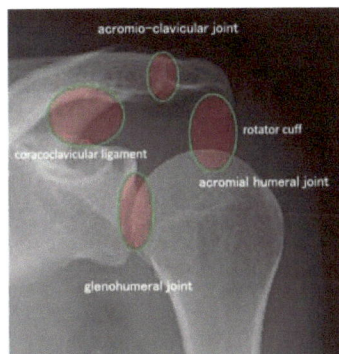

Fig. (31). The sites of the involvement with RA of the shoulder.

Pelvis

The sites of the involvement with RA of the pelvis (Fig. **32**).

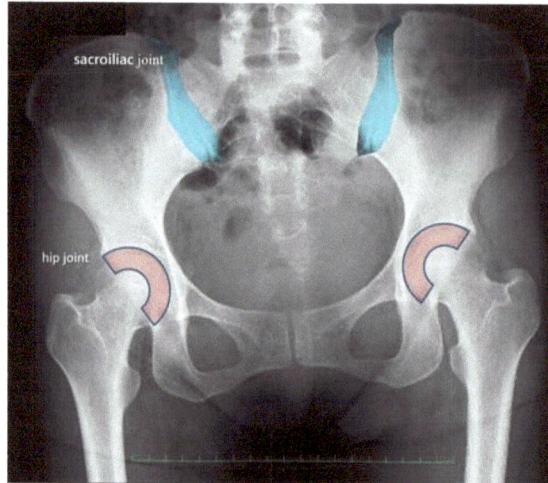

Fig. (32). The sites of the involvement with RA of the pelvis.

Knees

The sites of the involvement with RA of the knees (Fig. **33**).

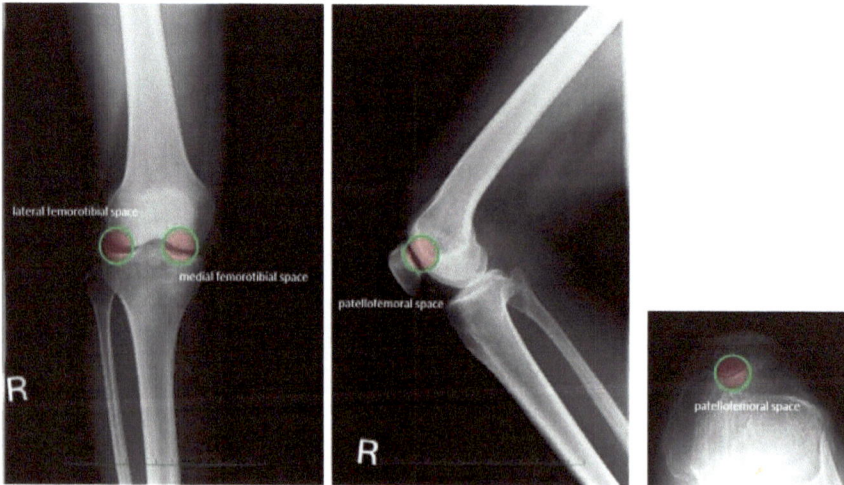

Fig. (33). The sites of the involvement with RA of the knee.

Feet

The sites of the involvement with RA of the feet (Figs. **34 - 37**).

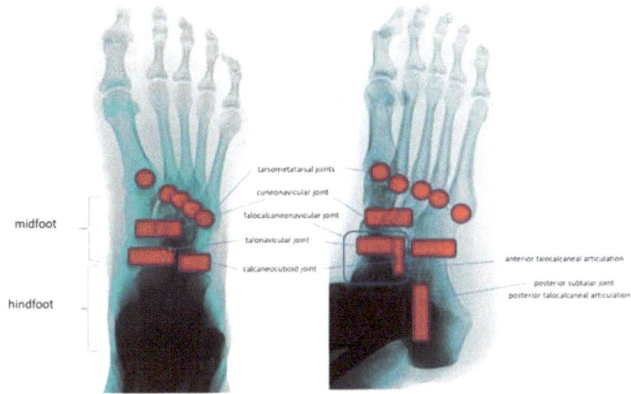

Fig. (34). The sites of the involvement with RA of the midfoot and the hindfoot.

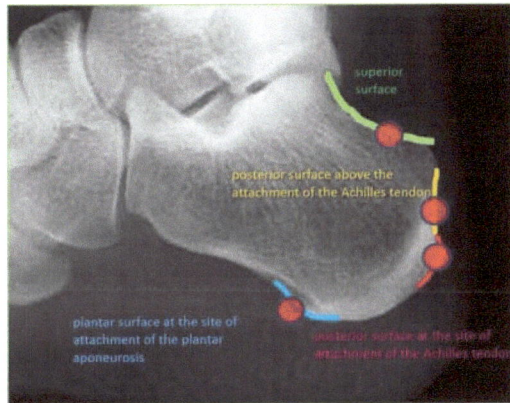

Fig. (35). The sites of the involvement with RA of the calcaneus.

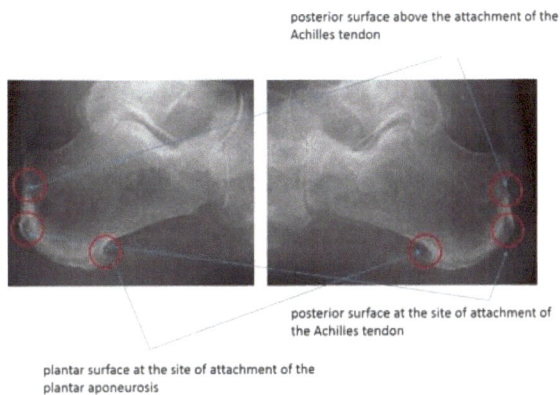

Fig. (36). The sites of the involvement of the calcaneus in a patient with RA.

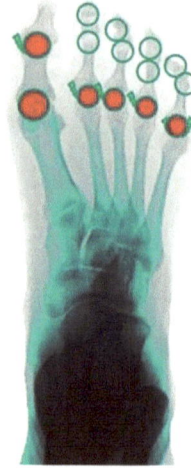

Fig. (37). The sites of arthritis and erosions of the forefoot in RA.

DISTRIBUTION IN THE REGIONS OF OTHER RHEUMATIC DISEASES

To perform accurate diagnosis of RA, the information of the distribution of arthritis in the regions including the hands and the feet of other rheumatic diseases is important. Moreover, the complication of other rheumatic diseases may occur in patients with RA. In those cases, the distribution appears atypical.

OA

The sites of the involvement with OA of the hand (Fig. **38**), the wrist (Fig. **39**), and the forefoot (Fig. **40**).

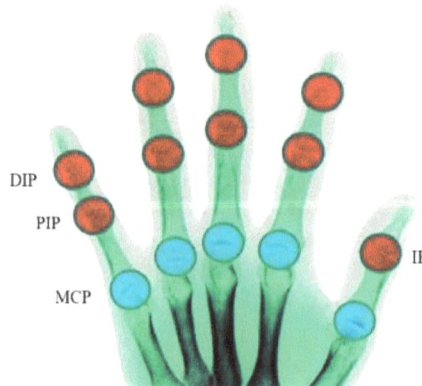

Fig. (38). The sites of the involvement with OA of the hand.

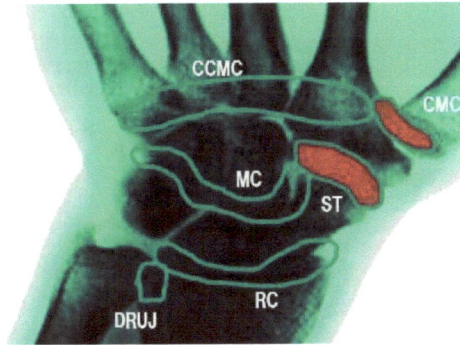

Fig. (39). The sites of the involvement with OA of the wrist.

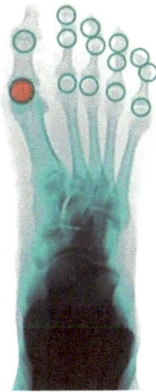

Fig. (40). The sites of the involvement with OA of the forefoot.

Erosive OA

The sites of the involvement with erosive OA of the hand (Fig. **41**) and the wrist (Fig. **42**).

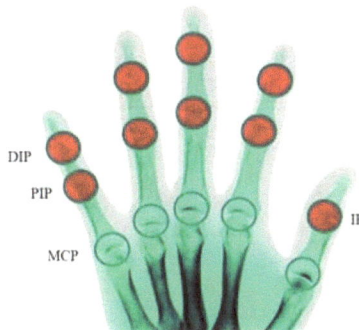

Fig. (41). The sites of the involvement with erosive OA of the hand.

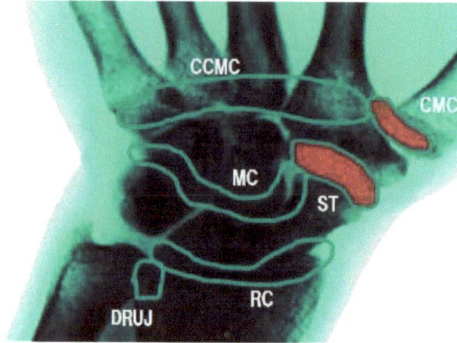

Fig. (42). The sites of the involvement with erosive OA of the wrist.

Gout

The sites of the involvement with gout of the hand (Fig. **43**), the wrist (Fig. **44**), and the forefoot (Fig. **45**).

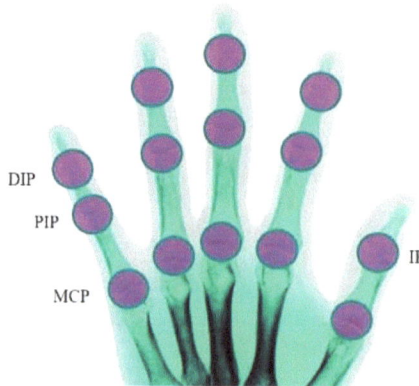

Fig. (43). The sites of the involvement with goat of the hand.

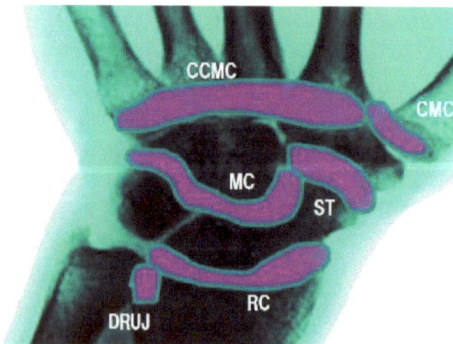

Fig. (44). The sites of the involvement with goat of the wrist.

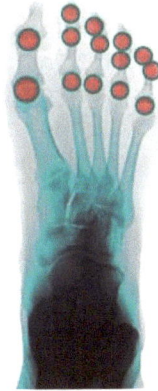

Fig. (45). The sites of the involvement with gout of the forefoot.

Calcium Pyrophosphate Dehydrate Deposition (CPPD) Crystal Deposition Disease

The sites of the involvement with CPPD crystal deposition disease of the hand (Fig. **46**) and the wrist (Fig. **47**).

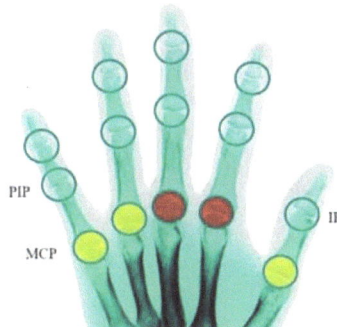

Fig. (46). The sites of the involvement with CPPD crystal deposition disease of the hand.

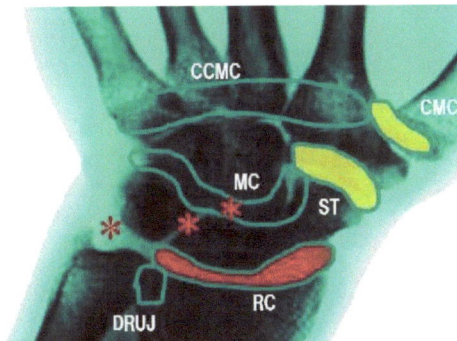

Fig. (47). The sites of the involvement with CPPD crystal deposition disease of the wrist.

Adult Onset Still's Disease (AOSD) and Juvenile Idiopathic Arthritis (JIA)

The sites of the involvement with AOSD and JIA of the hand (Fig. **48**) and the wrist (Fig. **49**).

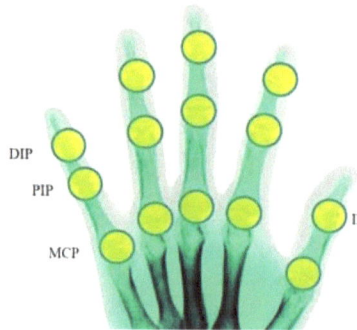

Fig. (48). The sites of the involvement with adult onset Still's disease (AOSD) and juvenile idiopathic arthritis (JIA) of the hand.

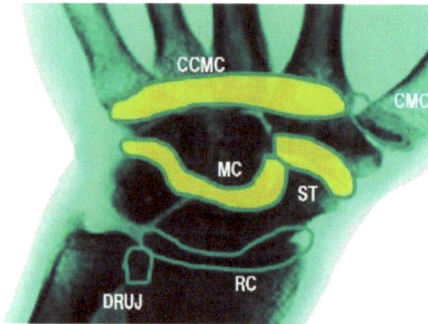

Fig. (49). The sites of the involvement with AOSD and JIA of the wrist, especially around the capitate.

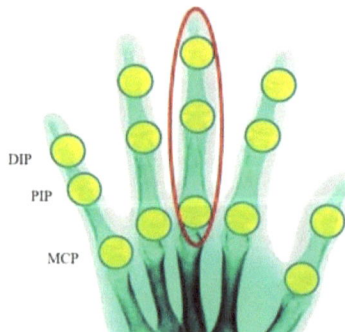

Fig. (50). The sites of the involvement with psoriatic arthritis (PsA) and dactylitis of the hand.

Psoriatic Arthritis (PsA)

The sites of the involvement with PsA of the hand (Figs. **50**, **52** and **53**), the wrist

(Figs. **51 - 53**), and the forefoot (Fig. **54**).

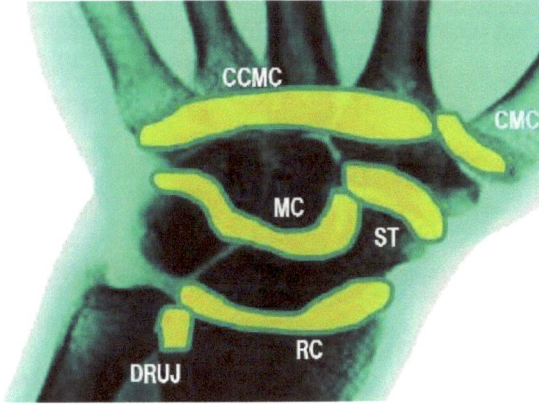

Fig. (51). The sites of the involvement with PsA of the wrist.

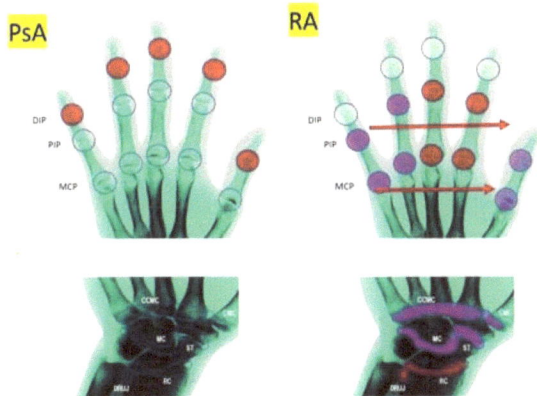

Fig. (52). The sites of the involvement with PsA and RA of the hand and the wrist.

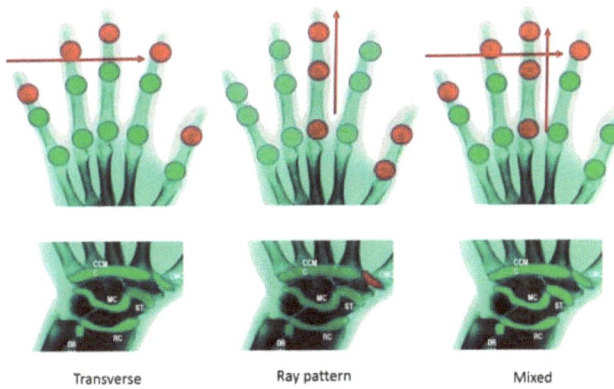

Fig. (53). The various patterns of the sites of the involvement with PsA of the hand and the wrist.

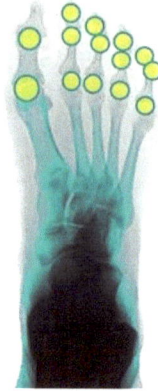

Fig. (54). The sites of the involvement with PsA of the forefoot.

Ankylosing Spondylitis (AS)

The sites of the involvement with AS of the hand (Fig. **55**) and the wrist (Fig. **56**).

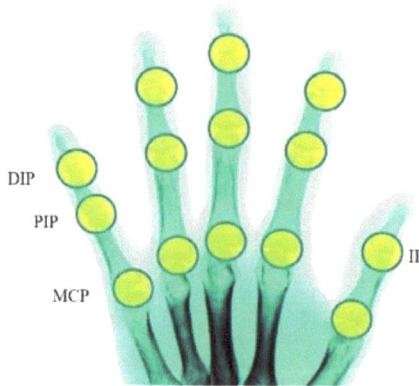

Fig. (55). The sites of the involvement with ankylosing spondylitis (AS) of the hand.

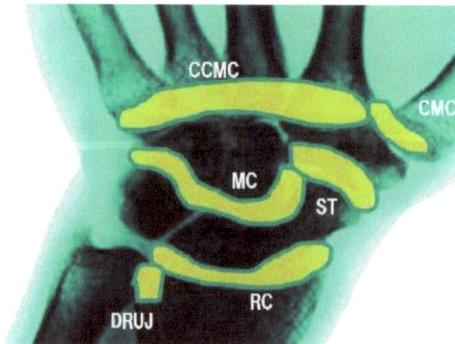

Fig. (56). The sites of the involvement with AS of the wrist.

Reactive Arthritis

The sites of the involvement with reactive arthritis of the hand (Fig. **57**), the wrist (Fig. **58**), and the forefoot (Fig. **59**).

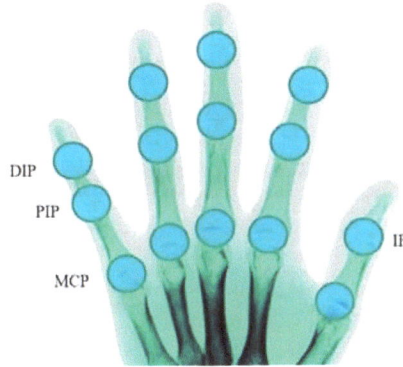

Fig. (57). The sites of the involvement with reactive arthritis of the hand.

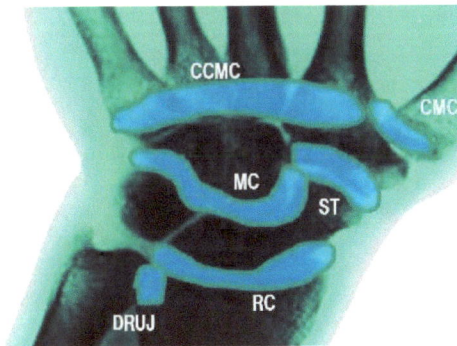

Fig. (58). The sites of the involvement with reactive arthritis of the wrist.

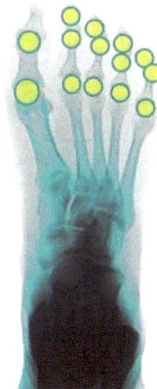

Fig. (59). The sites of the involvement with reactive arthritis of the forefoot.

Hemochromatosis

Hemochromatosis is inherited or caused by blood transfusions. The sites of the involvement with hemochromatosis of the hand (Fig. **60**) and the wrist (Fig. **61**).

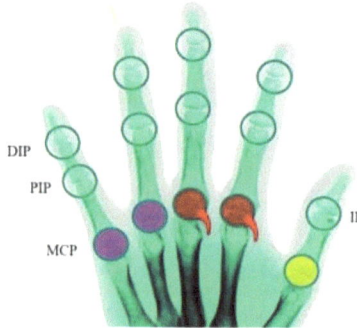

Fig. (60). The sites of the involvement with hemochromatosis of the hand.

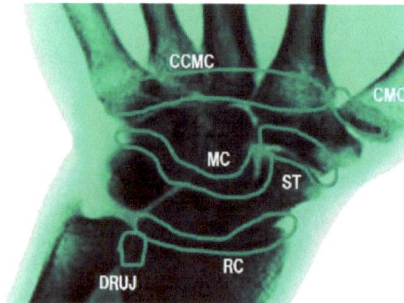

Fig. (61). The sites of the involvement with hemochromatosis of the wrist.

Sjögren's Syndrome (SS)

The sites of the involvement with SS of the hand and wirst (Figs. **62** - **64**).

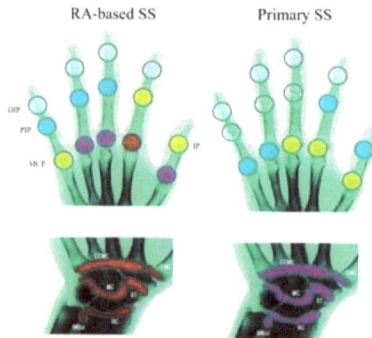

Fig. (62). The difference of the sites of the involvement with RA-based Sjögren's syndrome (SS) and primary SS of the hand and the wrist.

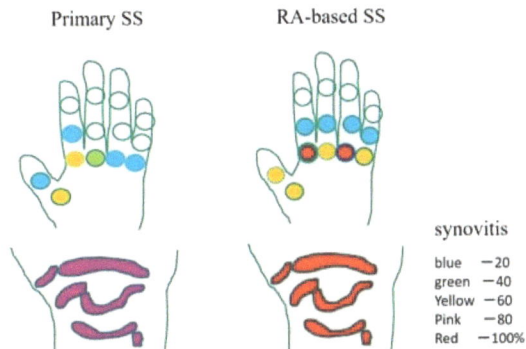

Fig. (63). The sites of synovitis in primary SS and secondary SS based on RA [4].

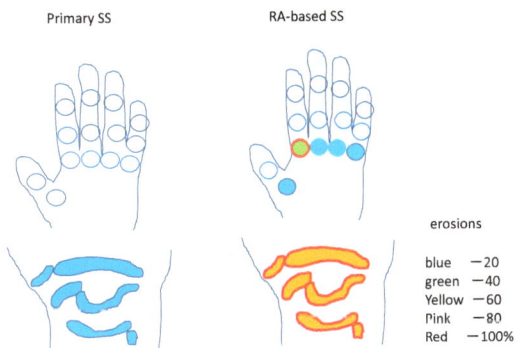

Fig. (64). The sites of erosions in primary SS and secondary SS based on RA [4].

Systemic Sclerosis (SSc)

The sites of the involvement with SSc of the hand (Figs. **65** and **67**), the wrist (Figs. **66** and **67**).

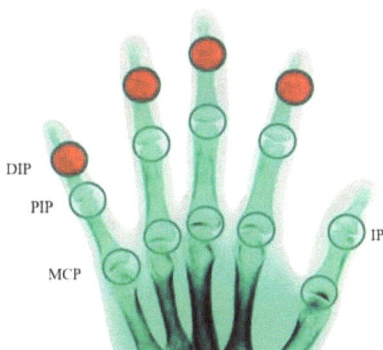

Fig. (65). The sites of the involvement with systemic sclerosis (SSc) of the hand.

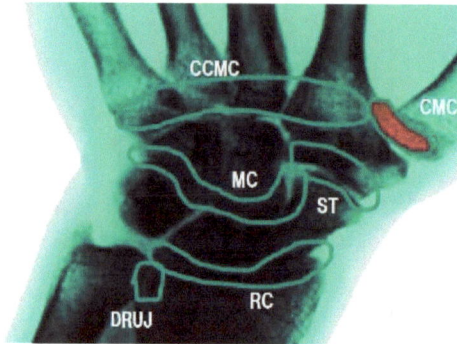

Fig. (66). The sites of the involvement with SSc of the wrist.

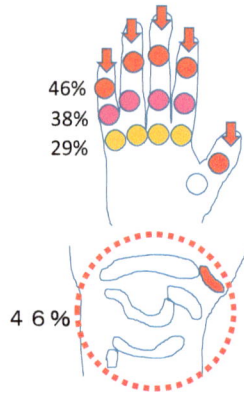

Fig. (67). Distribution of joint involvement in SSc [5].

Systemic Lupus Erythematosus (SLE)

The sites of the involvement with SLE of the hand and the wrist (Figs. **68** and **69**).

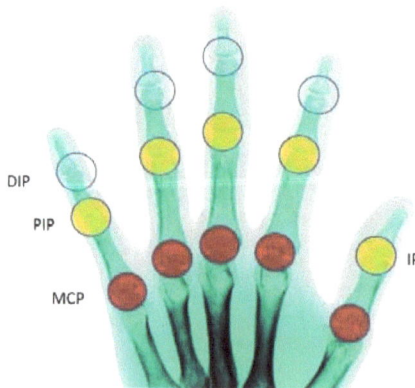

Fig. (68). The sites of the involvement with SLE of the hand.

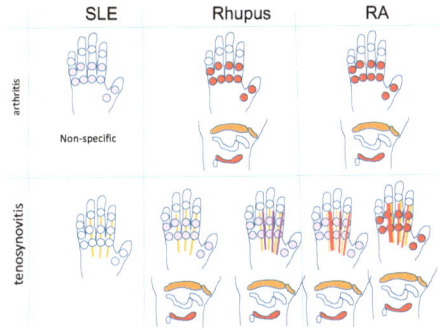

Fig. (69). The sites of the involvement with SLE, rhupus and RA of the hand.

Dermatomyositis (DM) and Polymyositis (PM)

The sites of the involvement with DM and PM of the hand and the wrist (Fig. **70**, **71**).

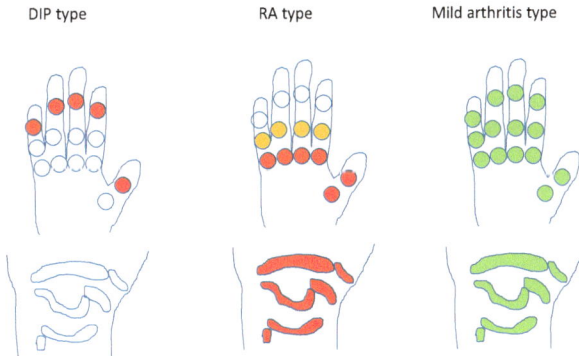

Fig. (70). The sites of the involvement with DM and PM of the hand.

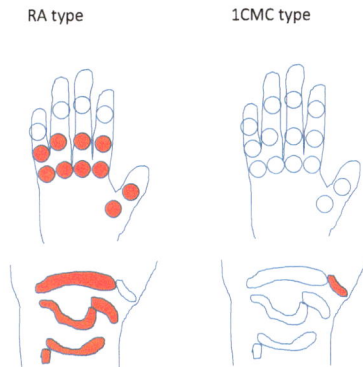

Fig. (71). The sites of the involvement with PM and DM having anti-aminoacyl tRNA synthetase (ARS) autoantibodies of the hand [6].

Hyperthyroidism

The sites of the involvement with hyperthyroidism of the hand and the wrist (Fig. **72**).

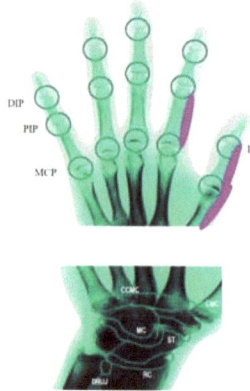

Fig. (72). The sites of the involvement with hyperthyroidism of the hand.

Hyperparathyroidism

The sites of the involvement with hyperparathyroidism of the hand and the wrist (Fig. **73**).

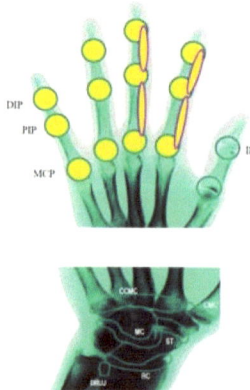

Fig. (73). The sites of the involvement with hyperparathyroidism of the hand. Subperiosteal bone resorption affects radial aspects of the proximal and the middle phalanges of the 2nd and the 3rd finger.

3. DISTRIBUTION IN JOINTS

The patterns of erosion in the joint in rheumatic diseases (Figs. **74 - 76**).

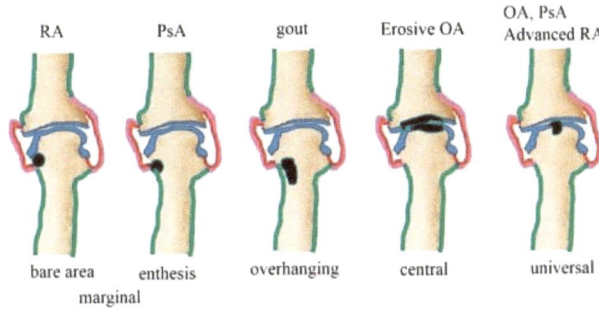

Fig. (74). The Patterns of Erosion in the Joint.

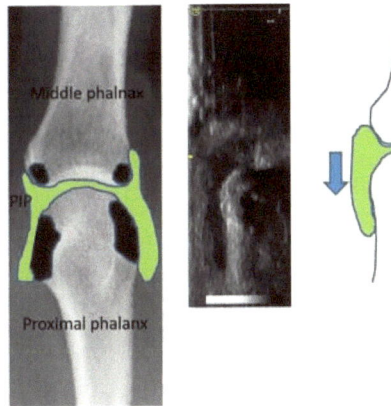

Fig. (75). The erosions are more extensive on the proximal phalanx than on the middle phalanx because the synovial surface of the head of the proximal phalanx is larger than the base of the middle phalanx. An ultrasound image illustrates that, in the PIP joint, the synovitis will extend proximally from the cleft between the articulations.

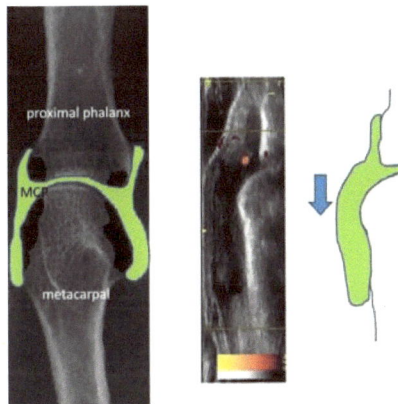

Fig. (76). The erosions are more extensive on the metacarpal than on the proximal phalanx because the synovial surface of the head of the metacarpal is much larger than the base of the proximal phalanx. An ultrasound image in a patient with RA shows the synovitis at the MCP joint. In the MCP joint, the synovitis will extend proximally from the cleft between the articulations.

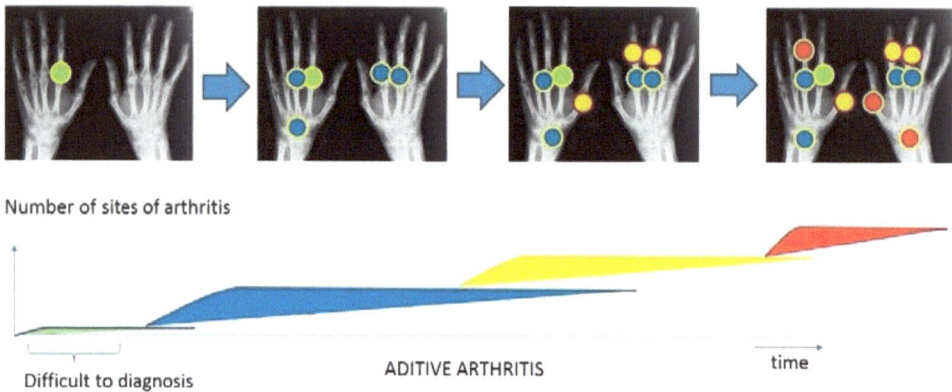

Fig. (77). RA is typical additive arthritis.

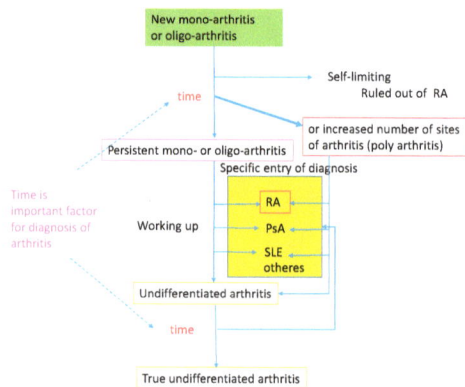

Fig. (78). In diagnosis of RA, time is a critical issue.

DISTRIBUTION IN THE TIME: DISEASE CHRONOLOGY

The pattern of arthritis in the time course is also important to diagnosis. Basically, RA is typical additive arthritis (Fig. **77**). However, it is difficult to diagnose RA in very early stage with mono- or oligo-arthritis (Fig. **78**).

CONSENT FOR PUBLICATION

Not applicable.

CONFLICT OF INTEREST

The author (editor) declares no conflict of interest, financial or otherwise.

ACKNOWLEDGEMENTS

The authors thank Ms. K. Eguchi and A. Ibe for secretarial assistance.

REFERENCES

[1]   Mies Richie A, Francis ML. Diagnostic approach to polyarticular joint pain. Am Fam Physician 2003; 68(6): 1151-60.
        [PMID: 14524403]

[2]   Rowbotham EL, Grainger AJ. Rheumatoid arthritis: ultrasound versus MRI. AJR Am J Roentgenol 2011; 197(3): 541-6.
        [http://dx.doi.org/10.2214/AJR.11.6798] [PMID: 21862794]

[3]   Villeneuve E, Emery P. Rheumatoid arthritis: what has changed? Skeletal Radiol 2009; 38(2): 109-12.
        [http://dx.doi.org/10.1007/s00256-008-0579-4] [PMID: 18773202]

[4]   Amezcua-Guerra LM, Hofmann F, Vargas A, *et al.* Joint involvement in primary Sjögren's syndrome: an ultrasound "target area approach to arthritis". BioMed Res Int 2013; 2013: 640265.
        [http://dx.doi.org/10.1155/2013/640265] [PMID: 23936829]

[5]   Avouac J, Clements PJ, Khanna D, Furst DE, Allanore Y. Articular involvement in systemic sclerosis. Rheumatology (Oxford) 2012; 51(8): 1347-56.
        [http://dx.doi.org/10.1093/rheumatology/kes041] [PMID: 22467084]

[6]   Kamo K, Nishino S, Matsuda Y, Kawashima A, Yoshimoto T. The normal thicknesses of entheseal insertions in the lower limbs of Japanese individuals. Japan Society of Ultrasonics in Medicine 2015; 46: 695-9.
        [http://dx.doi.org/10.3179/jjmu.JJMU.A.49]

CHAPTER 6

E: External Bone, Extra-Articular Manifestations

Syuichi Koarada* and **Akihito Maruyama**

Division of Rheumatology, Faculty of Medicine, Saga University, Saga, Japan

Abstract: Category "E" includes the eaternal bone, extra-articular manifestations. In this category, there are soft tissue swelling, dactylitis, rheumatoid nodules, bursitis, ganglions, tenosynovitis, enthesitis, tendonitis, and calcification in rheumatoid arthritis (RA).

Keywords: Bursitis, Dactylitis, Enthesitis, Ganglions, Rheumatoid arthritis, Rheumatoid nodules, Tenosynovitis, Tendonitis.

Rheumatoid arthritis (RA) has extra-articular or external bone musculoskeletal manifestations in soft tissues such as rheumatoid nodules, enthesopathy, bursitis, ganglions, tenosynovitis, and tendon ruptures.

SOFT TISSUES

Soft tissues consist of the tendons, the ligaments, the fascia, the skin, the fibrous tissues, the fat, the synovial membranes, the muscles, the nerves and the blood vessels. Soft tissue swelling is a common condition caused by various disorders. For example, swelling may occur suddenly following the bone fracture or gradually due to chronic tenosynovitis and arthritis. Especially, symmetrical soft tissue swelling due to synovitis and joint effusion with the shape of spindle is one of the characteristic features of RA. Bilateral osteophytes, hematoma, and bone fracture near the joint may also cause symmetrical soft tissue swelling.

The evaluation of soft tissue swelling at the PIP, the MCP and the wrist joints is usually performed by physical examination and plain radiographs of the hands. Ultrasound is helpful to evaluate the condition of the swelling.

* **Corresponding author Syuichi Koarada:** Division of Rheumatology, Faculty of Medicine, Saga University, Saga, Japan; Tel: 81-952-31-6511; E-mail: koarada@cc.saga-u.ac.jp

Soft Tissue Swelling Due to Arthritis

Soft tissue swelling of the hands and wrists (Figs. **1 - 8**), elbows (Fig. **9**), and knees (Figs. **10** and **11**) in RA.

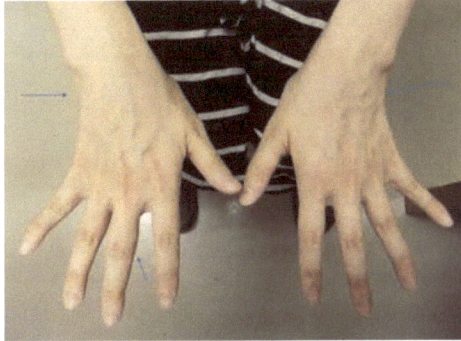

Fig. (1). Soft tissue swelling of the wrists and the right third PIP joint due to arthritis in a patient with RA.

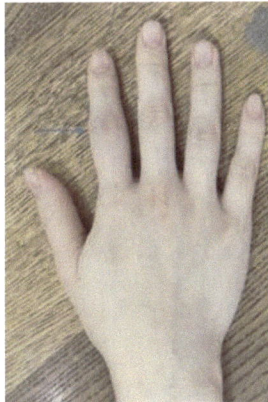

Fig. (2). Soft tissue swelling of the right second PIP joint due to arthritis in a patient with RA.

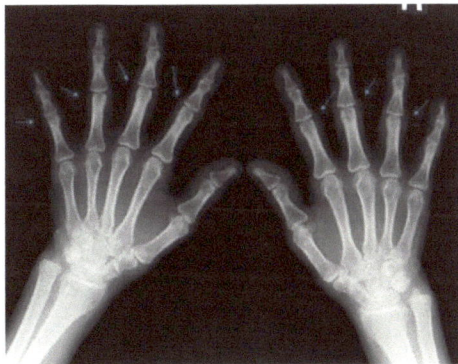

Fig. (3). Soft tissue swelling of most of the PIP joints in a patient with RA.

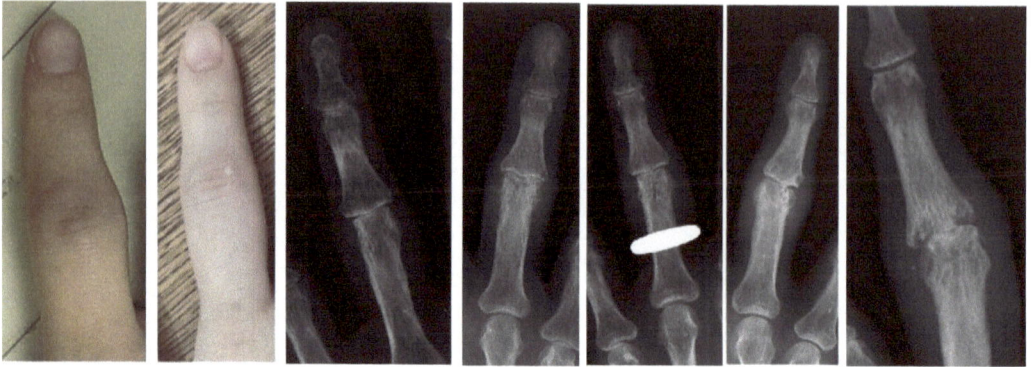

Fig. (4). Soft tissue welling of the PIP joints in RA.

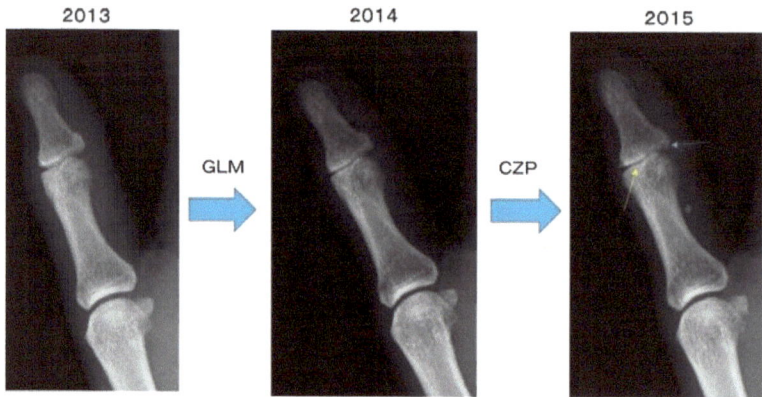

Fig. (5). Plain radiographs of the right first IP joint show improving of soft tissue swelling by the treatment with biological agents including golimumab (GLM) and certolizumab pegol (CZP) in a patient with RA. However, joint space narrowing (yellow arrow) and small erosion occur during the treatment.

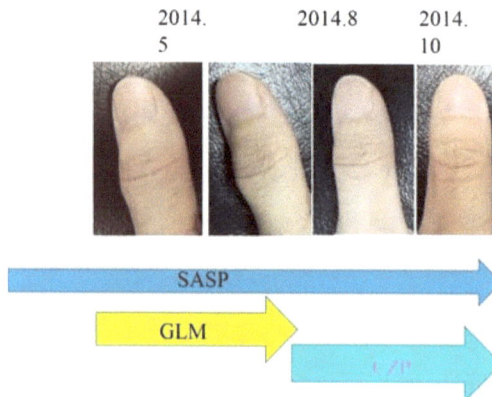

Fig. (6). Photographs of the first IP joint improved by the treatment in the same patient with RA (Fig. **5**).

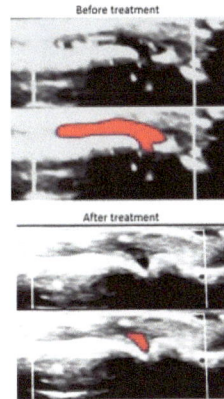

Fig. (7). Longitudinal power Doppler US images of dorsal aspect of the first IP joint before and after the treatment show improving of arthritis in the same patient with RA (Fig. **5**).

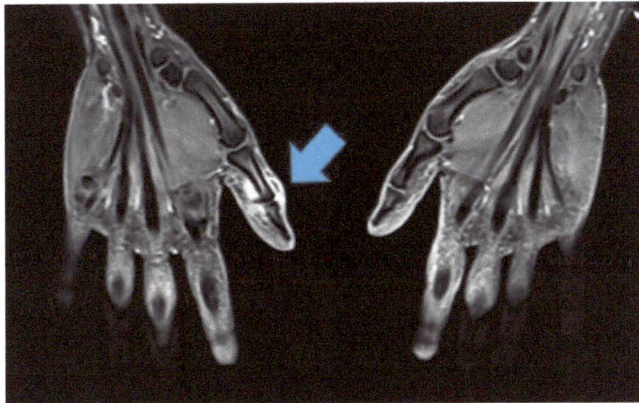

Fig. (8). Coronal gadolinium (Gd)-enhanced T1-weighted FS (fat-suppressed) scan shows enhancement of the inflammatory synovium in the right first IP joint in the same patient with RA as seen in Fig. (**6**). The synovitis induces soft tissue swelling of the first digit.

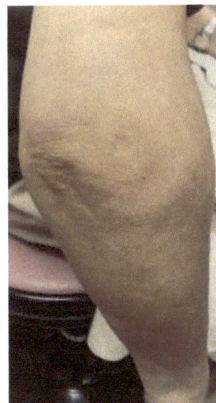

Fig. (9). Soft tissue welling of the right elbow in a patient with RA.

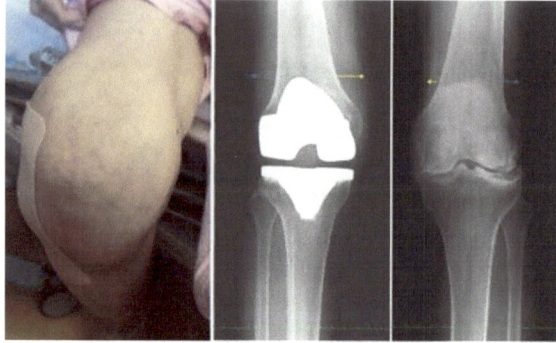

Fig. (10). Photograph and radiographs show soft tissue swelling of the right knee in a patient with RA.

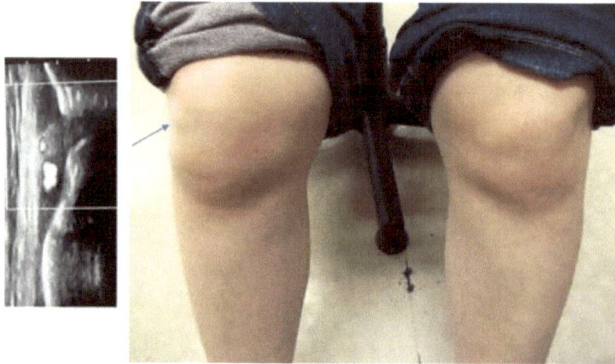

Fig. (11). Photograph and longitudinal US image show soft tissue swelling of the right knee in a patient with RA.

Ulnar deviation of the finger at the PIP joint resembles soft tissue swelling (Fig. 12).

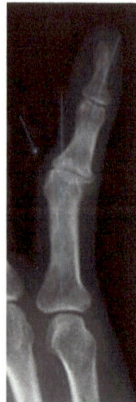

Fig. (12). Ulnar deviation of the finger at the PIP joint resembles soft tissue swelling. However, in radiograph, there is not soft tissue swelling.

Dactylitis

Sausage digit (hot dog digit, dactylitis) is soft tissue swelling of the entire digit (Figs. **13** and **14**).

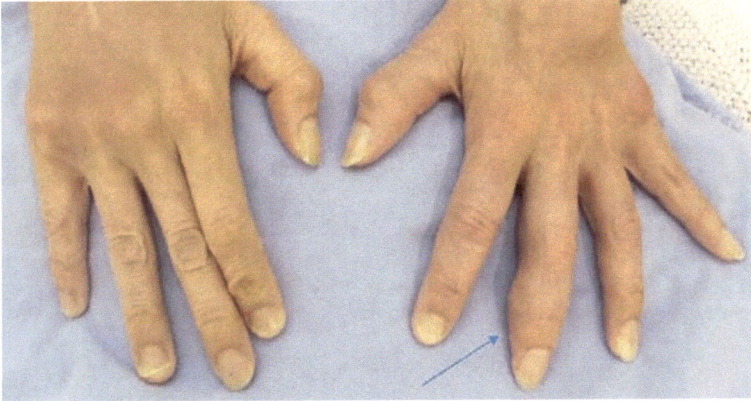

Fig. (13). Dactylitis in a patient with rhupus (RA and SLE).

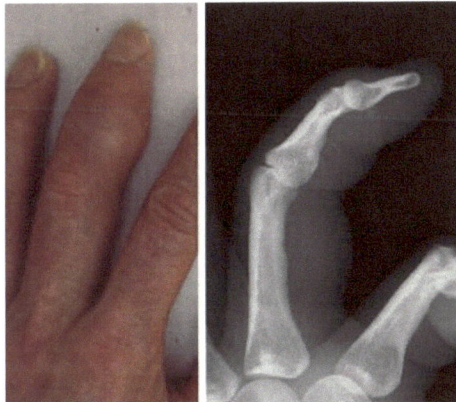

Fig. (14). Photograph and radiograph of the left third finger show soft tissue swelling of the entire digit, dactylitis in a patient with rhupus (RA and SLE).

Rheumatoid Nodules

Rheumatoid nodules are local swelling or tissue lumps in association with RA (Figs. **15 - 18**). Usually rheumatoid nodules are firm. They locate in subcutaneous tissues over bony prominences including the olecranon and the IP joints. The size of a rheumatoid node may fluctuate during the treatment of RA. It may enlarge in active disease, although the size can be changed by the treatment.

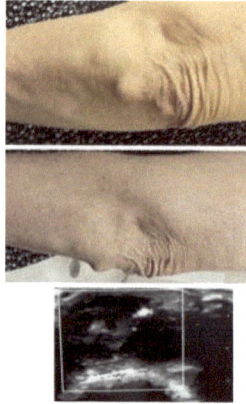

Fig. (15). The photographs show a rheumatoid nodule in a patient with RA. Longitudinal power Doppler US image of dorsal aspect of the olecranon at the elbow shows a heterogeneous hypoechoic nodular mass. This finding is consistent with a rheumatoid nodule.

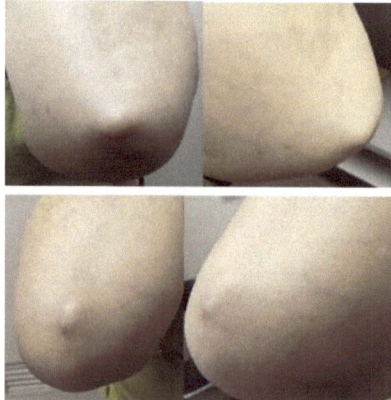

Fig. (16). Rheumatoid nodules are observed on the elbows in a patient with RA.

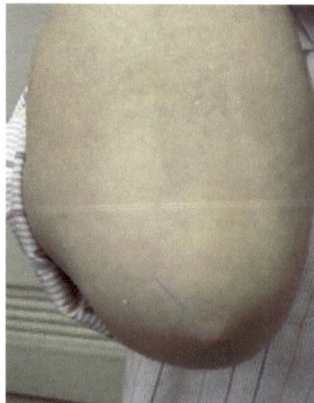

Fig. (17). Photograph shows a small-sized rheumatoid nodule in a patient with RA.

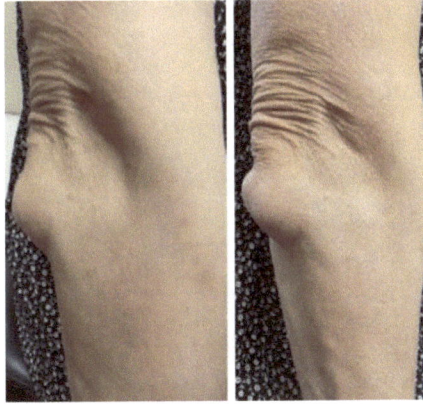

Fig. (18). A large-sized rheumatoid nodule at the elbow in a patient with RA.

BURSITIS

Bursae are normal potential spaces of thin, lubricated cushions with synovial membrane. Bursae are located at the points of friction between a bone and the surrounding soft tissues including the skin, the muscles, the ligaments and the tendons around the knee, the shoulder, the ankle, the elbow and so on. At least, there are 78 bursae in the body. Especially, 16 bursae are found around the knee. However, the precise numbers and the nomenclature are changeable by researchers. The most common location for bursae is in the knee. Bursitis and ganglion cysts are similar conditions, but not identical.

Elbows

Olecranon Bursitis

Olecranon bursitis is a small- to large-sized visible lump on the elbow with discomfort and elbow pain at rest and bending the arm (Figs. **19 - 21**). Moderate to severe elbow pain occurs by weight on the elbow.

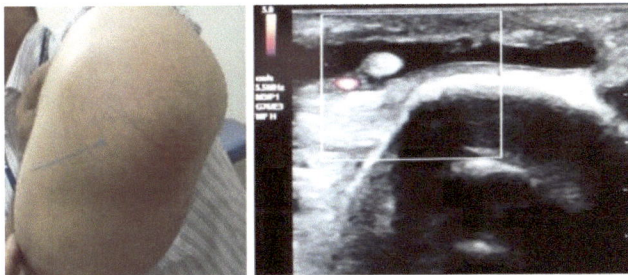

Fig. (19). Photograph and longitudinal power Doppler US image show olecranon bursitis in a patient with RA.

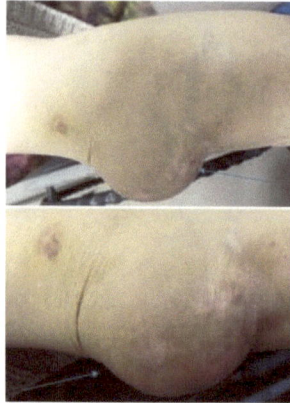

Fig. (20). Medium-sized chronic olecranon bursitis of the elbow.

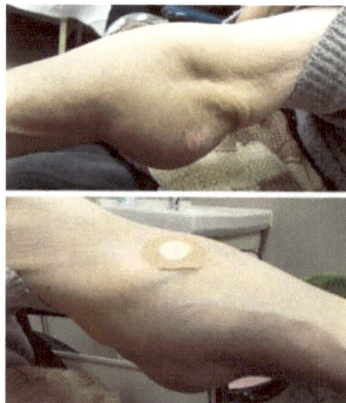

Fig. (21). Large-sized olecranon bursitis.

Shoulders

Bursae of the shoulder in RA (Figs. **22 - 25**).

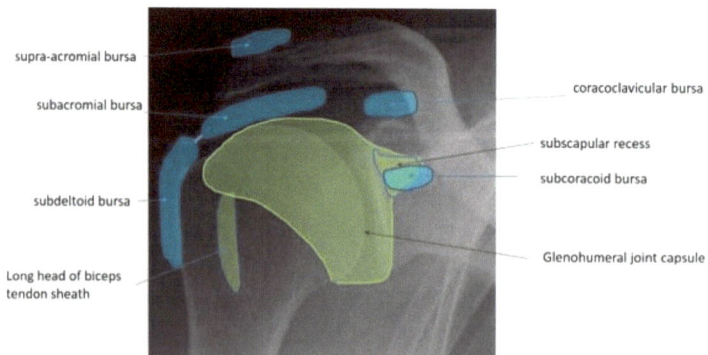

Fig. (22). Bursae of the shoulder.

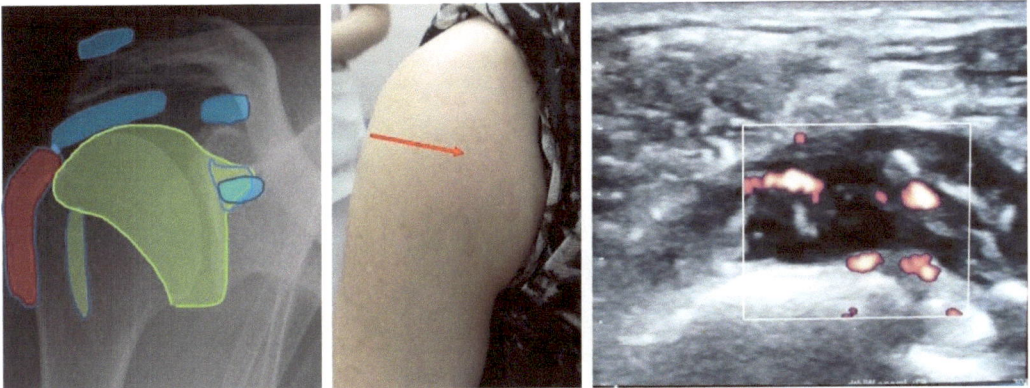

Fig. (23). Photograph and transverse power Doppler US image show subdeltoid bursitis in a patient with RA.

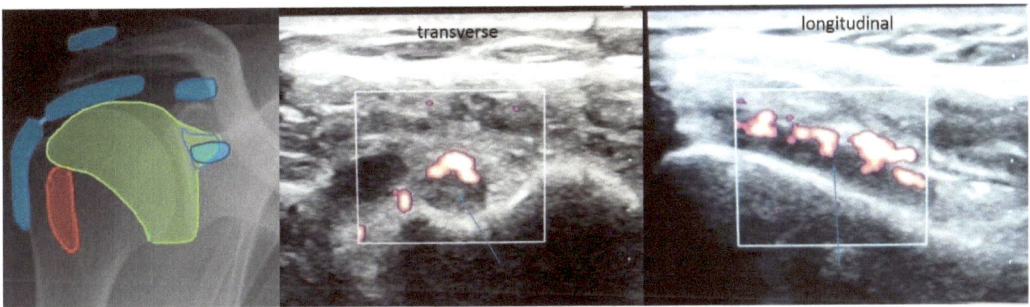

Fig. (24). US images of the shoulder are presented. Center panel; transverse image of the bicipital groove near the transverse humeral ligament. Right panel; longitudinal image of the bicipital groove. US images show tenosynovitis of the long head of biceps tendon sheath with remarked PD signals.

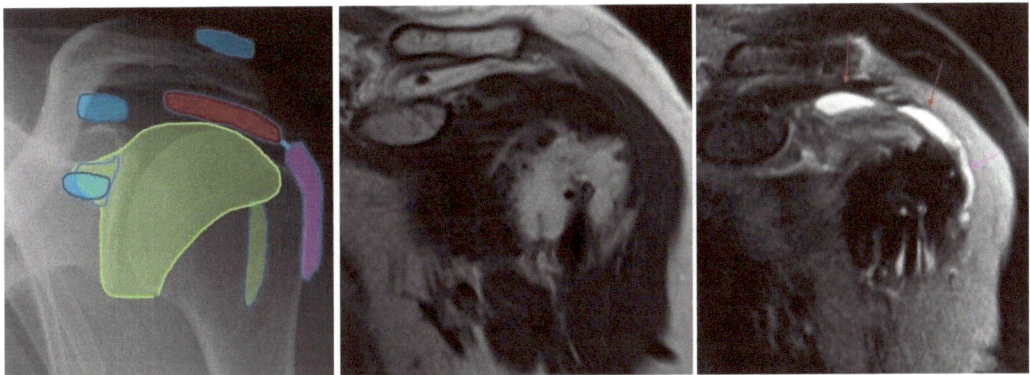

Fig. (25). MR images (T1 and T2 FS) of the left shoulder joint in a patient with RA show subacromial-subdeltoid bursitis with medial extension of subacromial-subdeltoid bursa.

Knees

Anterior

Five bursae (Fig. **26**)

Fig. (26). Anterior bursae of the knee.

1. The suprapatellar bursa or recess (K1) (Fig. **27**)

Between the anterior surface of the lower part of the femur and the deep surface of the quadriceps femoris for movement of the quadriceps tendon over the distal end of the femur.

Fig. (27). The suprapatellar bursa.

2. The subcutaneous prepatellar bursa (K2) (Fig. **28**)

The prepatellar bursa

The prepatellar bursa is a frontal bursa of the knee joint between the skin and the patella (Figs. **29 - 32**).

The bursa is one of the superficial bursae with a thin synovial lining

Bursitis is "housemaid's knee".

It allows movement of the skin over underlying patella.

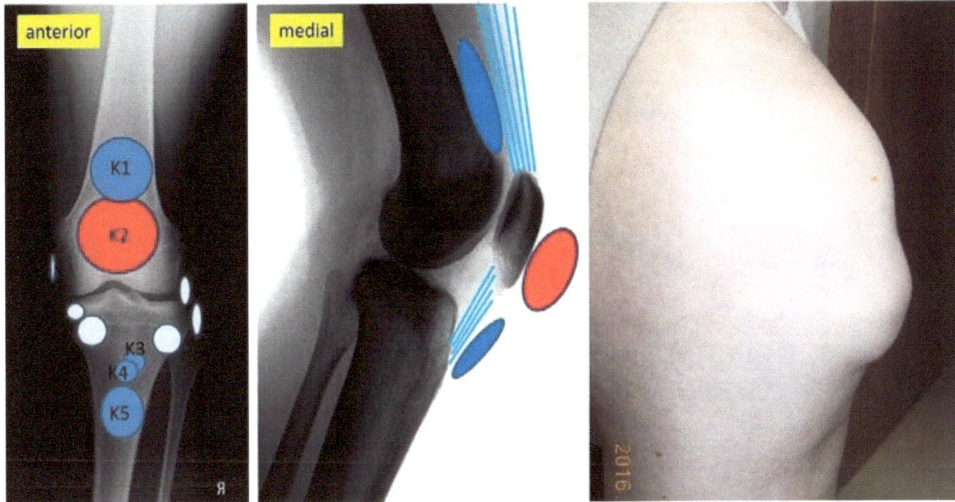

Fig. (28). The prepatellar bursa of the knee.

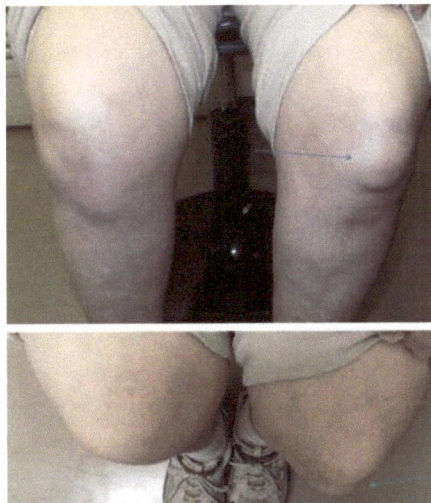

Fig. (29). Photographs of the prepatellar bursa.

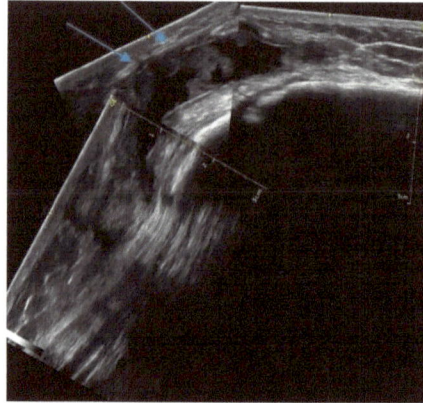

Fig. (30). Longitudinal gray-scale US image shows prepatellar bursitis of the knee in a patient with RA.

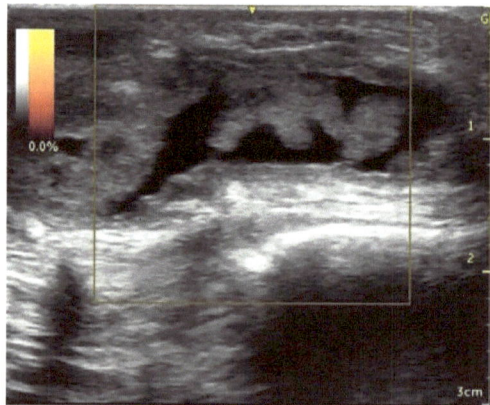

Fig. (31). Longitudinal power Doppler US image shows chronic prepatellar bursitis without PD signal.

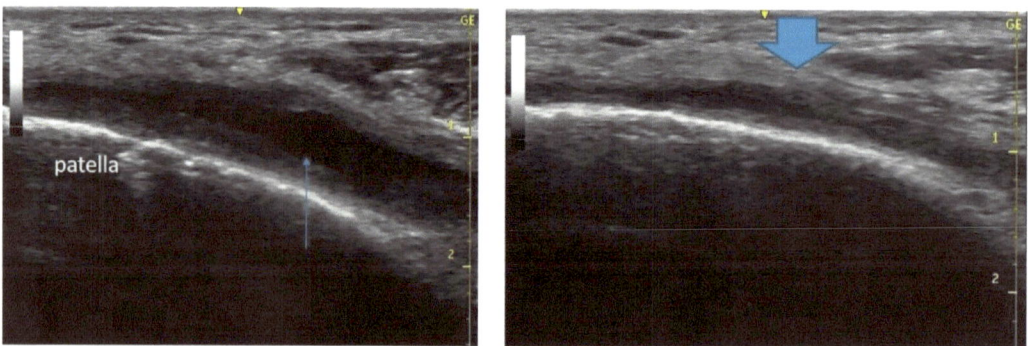

Fig. (32). Left panel; Prepatellar bursitis of the right knee in a patient with RA. Right panel: When the bursa is pressed, it will disappear.

3. The deep infrapatellar bursa (K3)

Between the upper part of the tibia and the patellar ligament.

For movement of the patellar ligament over the tibia.

4. The superficial infrapatellar bursa (K4)

The subcutaneous infrapatellar bursa

Between the patellar ligament and skin.

5. The pretibial bursa (K5) (Fig. **33**)

Between the tibial tuberosity and the skin.

For movement of the skin over the tibial tuberosity.

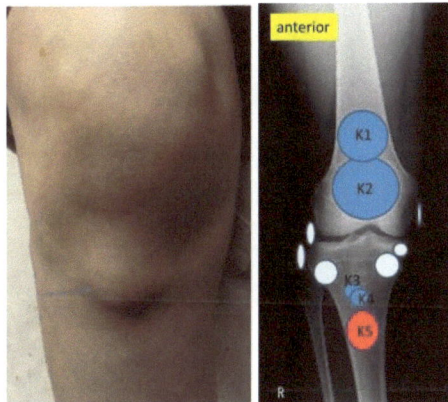

Fig. (33). Bursitis of the pretibial bursa in a patient with RA.

Medial

Six bursae (Figs. **34** and **35**)

6. The medial gastrocnemius [subtendinous] bursa (K6)

Between the medial head of the gastrocnemius and the joint capsule.

7. The anserine bursa (K7)

The subsartorial bursa

Pes anserinus bursa

Between the medial (tibial) collateral ligament and the tendons of the sartorius, gracilis, and semitendinosus.

8. The bursa semimembranosa between the medial collateral ligament and the

tendon of the semimembranosus (K8)

9. The bursa between the tendon of the semimembranosus and the head of the tibia (K9)

10. The bursa between the tendons of the semimembranosus and semitendinosus (K10)

11. The medial collateral ligament bursa (K11)

The bursa is located on the medial side of the knee between the superficial and deep layer of the medial collateral ligament.

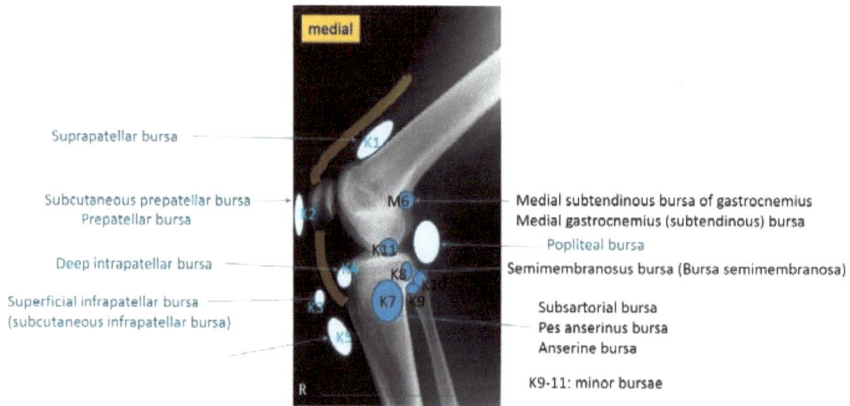

Fig. (34). Medial bursae of the knee.

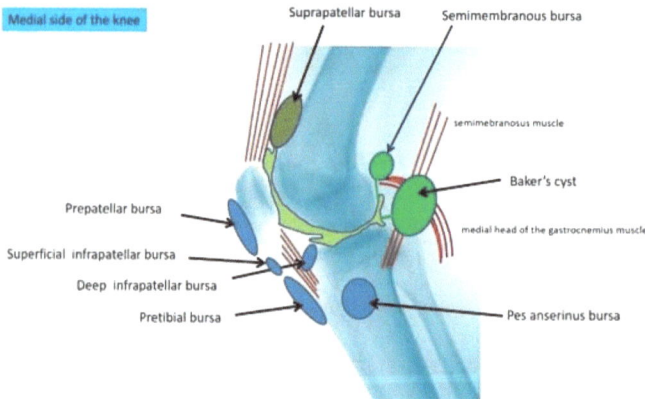

Fig. (35). A schema of the medial side bursae of the knee.

Lateral

Four (or five) bursae (Fig. 36)

12. The lateral gastrocnemius [subtendinous] bursa (K12)

Between the lateral head of the gastrocnemius and the joint capsule.

13. The fibular bursa (K13)

The subtendinous bursa of the biceps femoris muscle

The biceps femoris tendon inferior subtendinous bursa

Between the lateral (fibular) collateral ligament and the tendon of the biceps femoris.

14. The fibulopopliteal bursa (K14)

Between the fibular collateral ligament and the tendon of the popliteus.

15. The bursa deep to the iliotibial tract (K15)

The subpopliteal recess (or bursa)

Between the tendon of the popliteus and the lateral condyle of the femur.

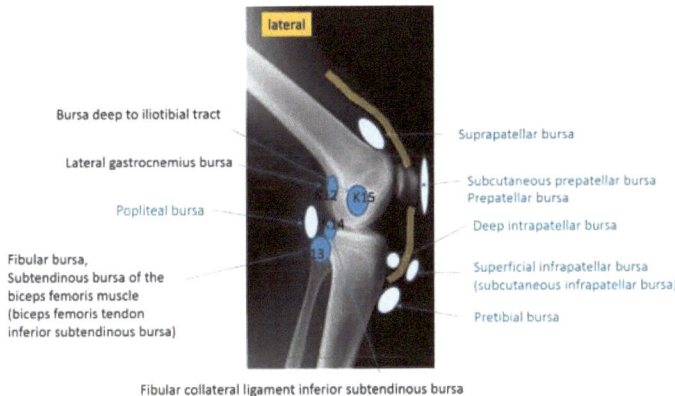

Fig. (36). Lateral bursae of the knee.

Posterior

16. The popliteal bursa (K16) (Fig. **37**)

Baker's Cyst

A Baker's cyst is a typical cyst in RA that extends into the soft tissues. The cyst at the back of the knee extends posteriorly, inferiorly or superiorly (Figs. **38 - 41**). Ultrasound imaging is helpful to diagnose the cystic lesion in the knee.

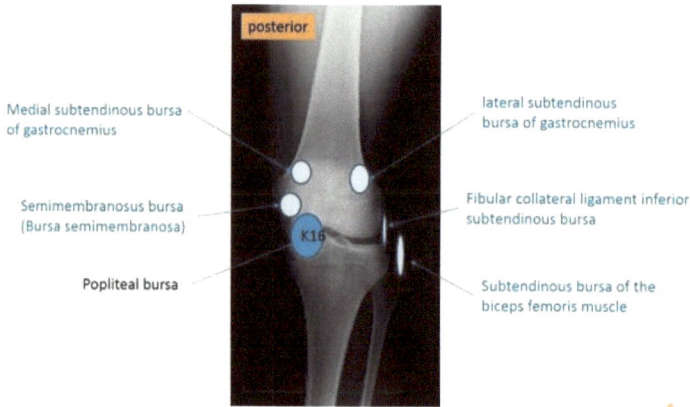

Fig. (37). Posterior bursae of the knee.

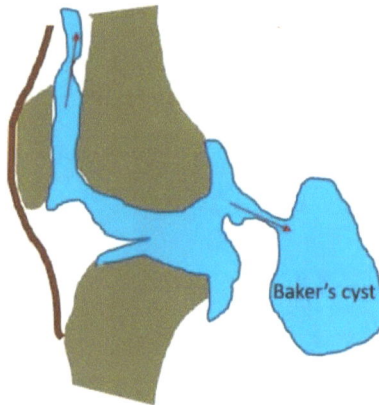

Fig. (38). A schema of a Baker's cyst.

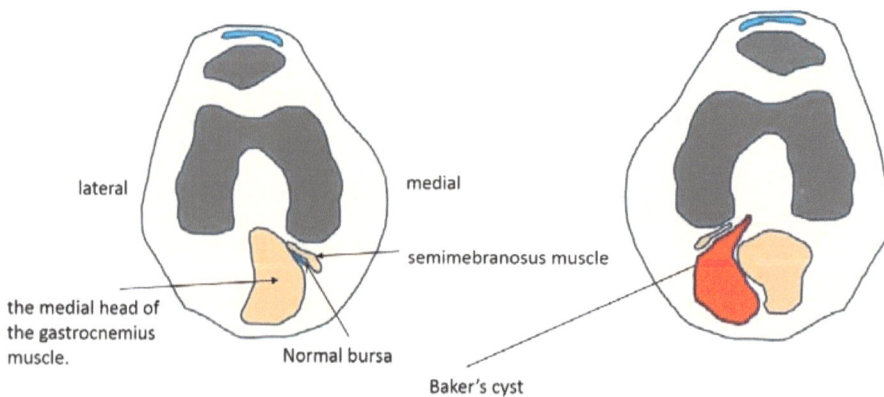

Fig. (39). A schema of a Baker's cyst. The cyst appears between the semimembranosus muscle and the medial head of the gastrocnemius muscle.

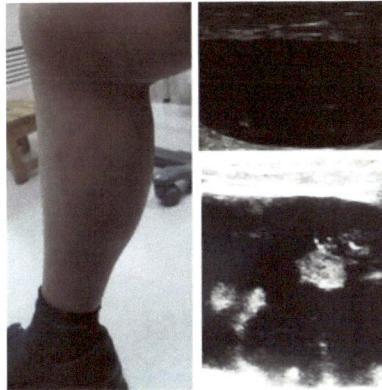

Fig. (40). A ruptured Baker's cyst in a patient with RA.

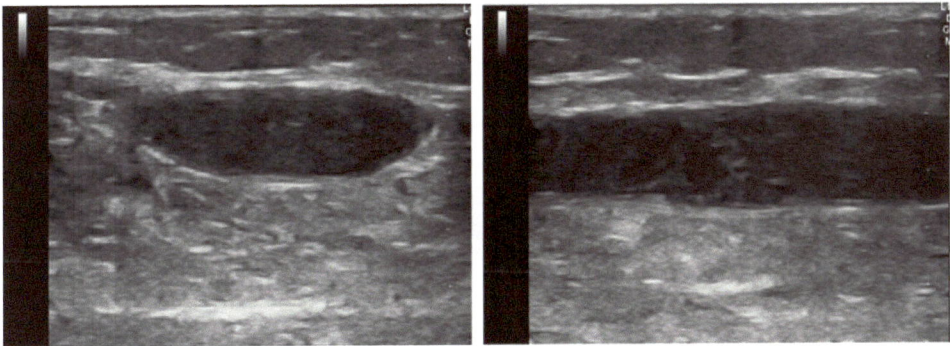

Fig. (41). Reduced size of the ruptured Baker's cyst of the same patient (Fig. **40**).

Ankles

Bursae of the ankle (Fig. **42**).

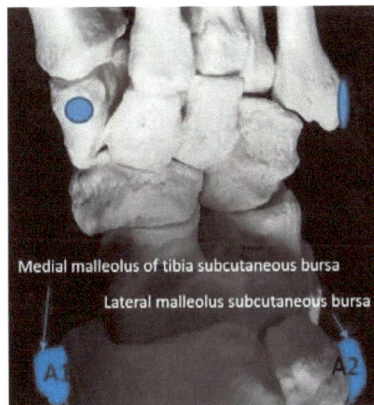

Fig. (42). Bursae of the ankle. The medial malleolus of the tibia subcutaneous bursa (A1) and the lateral malleolus subcutaneous bursa (A2).

Feet

Calcaneus

Bursae of the hindfoot (Figs. **43** and **44**).

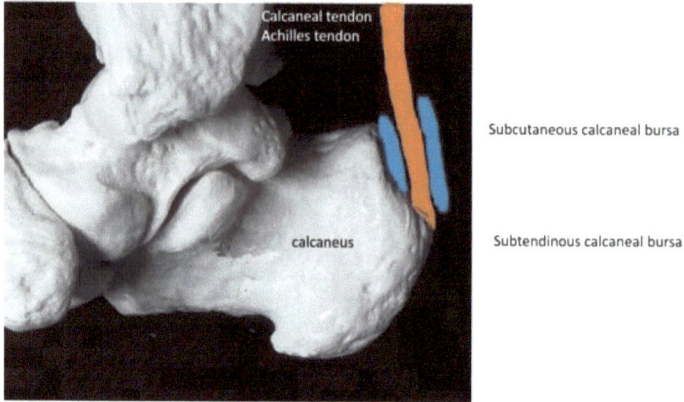

Fig. (43). Bursae of the hindfoot.

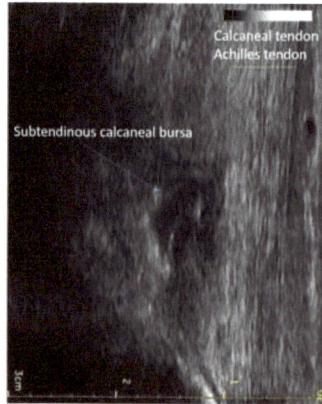

Fig. (44). Longitudinal gray-sacle US image of <u>the posterior surface of the distal Achillis tendon</u> shows the subtendinous calcaneal bursitis.

Bursae of the Foot

Bursae of the foot (Fig. **45**).

Interdigital bursitis (Figs. **46** and **47**) and subcutaneous bursitis at the tuberosity of the fifth metatarsal bone (Fig. **48**).

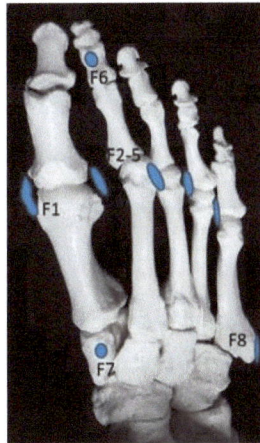

Fig. (45). Bursae of the foot.
Bunion (F1)
Intermetatarsophalangeal Bursae
The interdigital bursae (F2-F5)
Bursa of the toe (F6)
Subcutaneous bursa on the medial cuneiform (F7)
Subcutaneous bursa at the tuberosity of fifth metatarsal bone (F8)

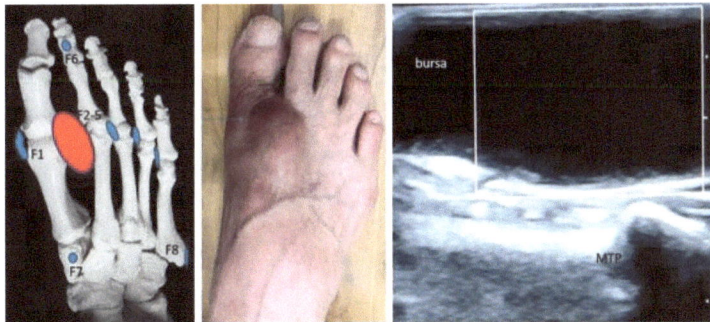

Fig. (46). Interdigital bursitis between the first and the second digit (F2).

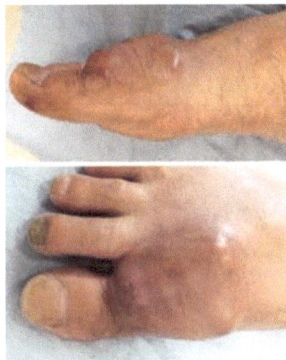

Fig. (47). Severe bursitis of the interdigital bursa between the first and the second digit (F2).

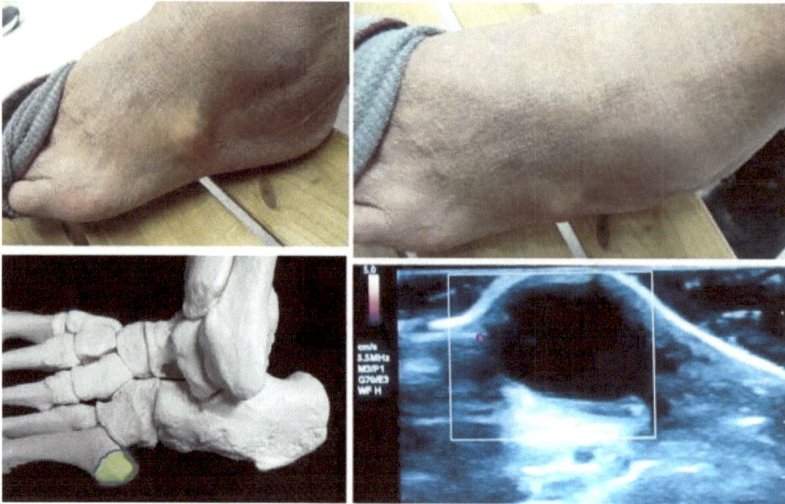

Fig. (48). Subcutaneous bursitis at the tuberosity of the fifth metatarsal bone (F8).

GANGLIONS

Ganglions are benign lumps filled with viscous synovial fluid. Ganglions occur mostly over the joints of the wrists, the hands, the ankles, and the feet. Also, ganglions appear around the tendons of the wrists, the hands and the feet. The size of the ganglions ranges from pea-size to an inch in diameter. They can arise from the joint spaces or the tendon sheaths.

Hands

Ganglion of the hands in patients with RA (Figs. **49 - 54**).

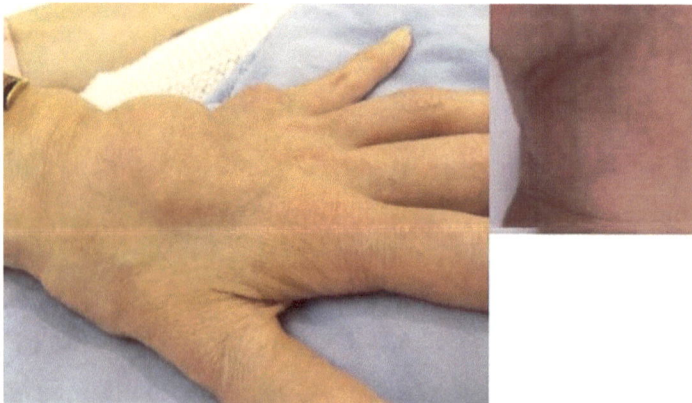

Fig. (49). A ganglion at the wrist in a patient with RA.

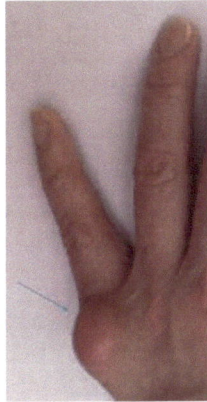

Fig. (50). A ganglion at the fifth MCP joint in a patient with RA.

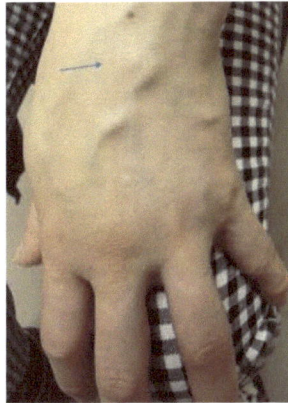

Fig. (51). A ganglion occurs at the dorsal side of the wrist joint of a patient with RA.

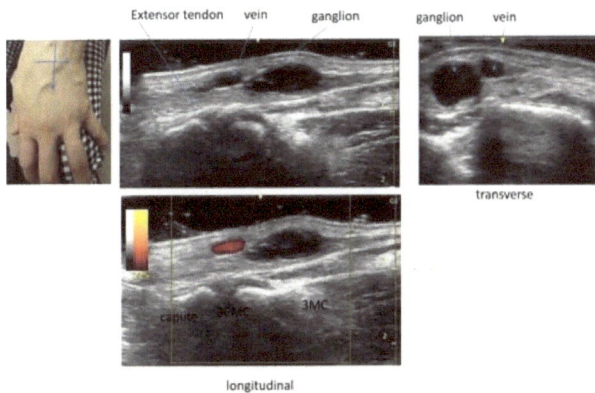

Fig. (52). Longitudinal and transverse US images show a ganglion over the extensor tendon at the third CMC joint. The vein can be observed near the ganglion.

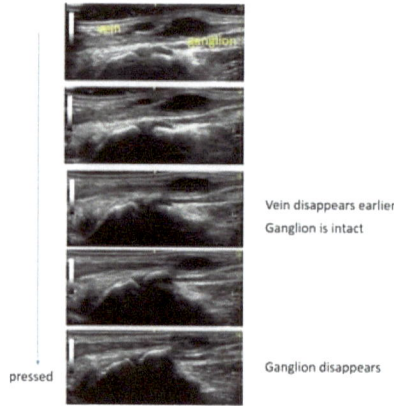

Fig. (53). The vein near the ganglion disappears much earlier than the ganglion by milder pressure. However, when the same ganglion is hardly pressed, it will disappear because the contents are liquid.

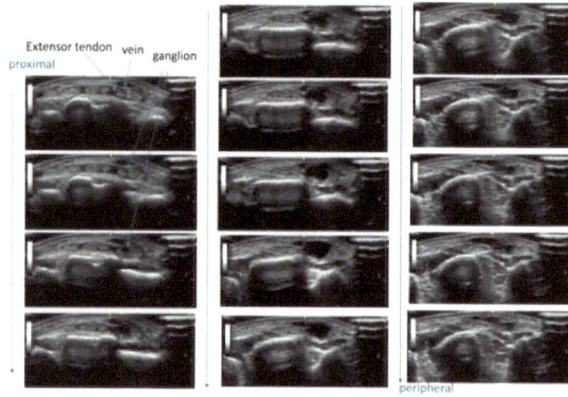

Fig. (54). Tansverse US images show that the ganglion starts in the extensor tendon at the proximal end, and then it extends to the peripheral direction.

Wrists

Ganglions of the wrists in patients with RA (Figs. **55** - **58**).

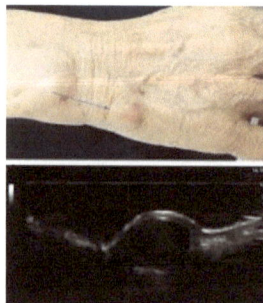

Fig. (55). A small ganglion of the wirst. Longitudinal gray-scale US image of the ganglion.

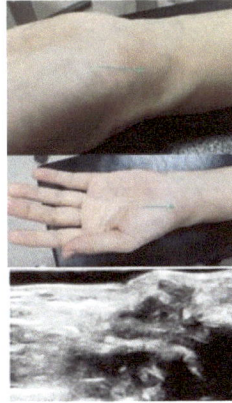

Fig. (56). A small-sized ganglion of the wrist in a patient with RA. The ganglion arises from the tendon sheath.

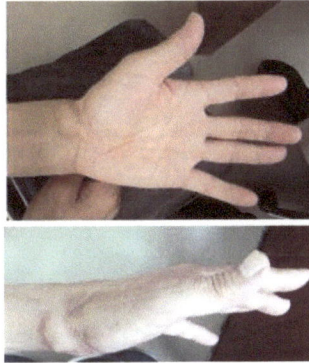

Fig. (57). A medium-sized ganglion of the wrist in a patient with RA.

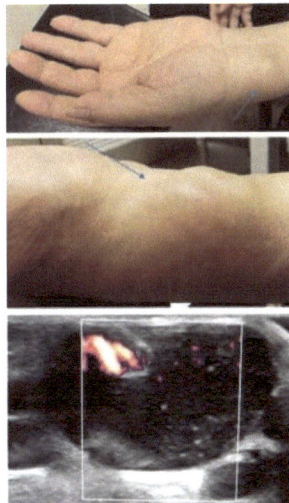

Fig. (58). A ganglion (or bursitis) of the wirst.

TENOSYNOVITIS

Tenosynovitis is common and inflammation of the synovium that surrounds a tendon in patients with RA. The patients with tenosynovitis present pain, swelling and restriction of moving at the affected joints.

Hands

Tenosynovitis of the hands in RA (Figs. **59 - 62**).

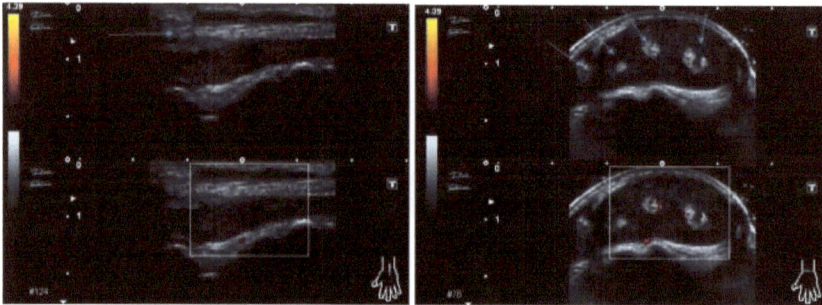

Fig. (59). Longitudinal and transverse gray-scale and power Doppler US images show severe tenosynovitis of the extensor digitorum (arrows) in a patient with RA and SLE.

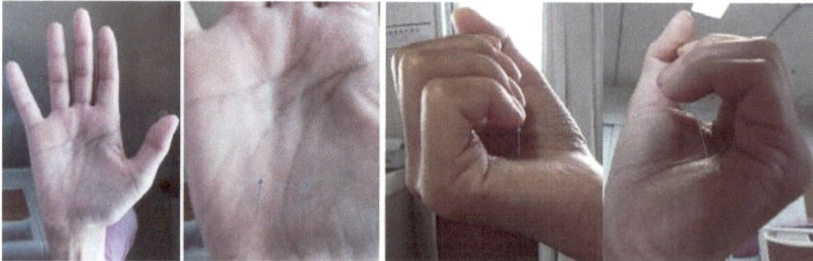

Fig. (60). Tenosynovitis of the flexor digitorum superficialis of the hands in a patient with RA and SLE (rhupus).

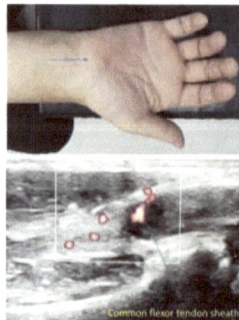

Fig. (61). Tenosynotitis of the common flexor tendon. Longitudinal US image shows swelling of the tendon sheath and positive PD signals.

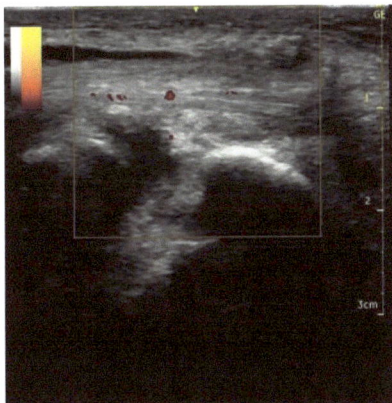

Fig. (62). Longitudinal power Doppler US image of the dorsal aspect of the foot shows a hypoechoic distended tendon sheath and increased PD signals of the extensor digitorum longus (EDL) consistent with tenosynovitis and tendonitis.

FINGERS

Extensor Tenosynovitis

Tenosynovitis of the extensor tendon in RA (Fig. **63**).

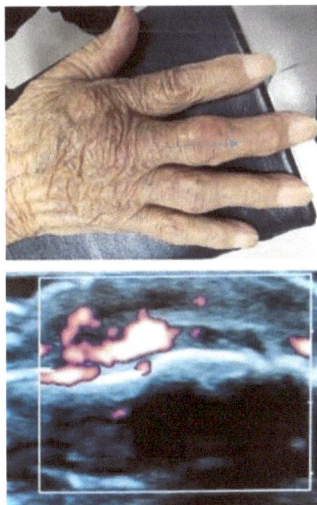

Fig. (63). Tenosynovitis of the extensor tendon and synovitis of the third PIP joint in a patient with RA.

Flexor Tenosynovitis

Flexor tenosynovitis (FT) causes disruption of normal flexor tendon function in the hand (Figs. **64 - 67**). Flexor tenosynovitis can be secondary to acute or chronic inflammation of the joints due to RA.

Dorsal aspect   Palmar aspect

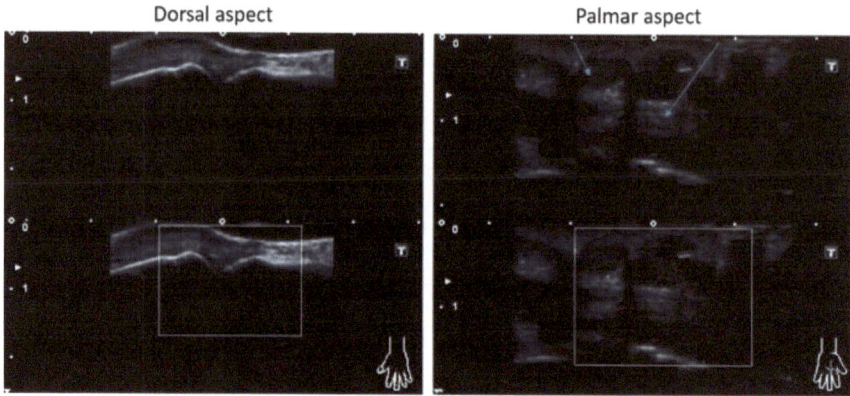

Fig. (64). Longitudinal gray-scale and power Doppler US images of the dorsal and the palmar aspect of the third PIP joint show the tenosynovitis of the flexten tendon in a patient with rhupus.

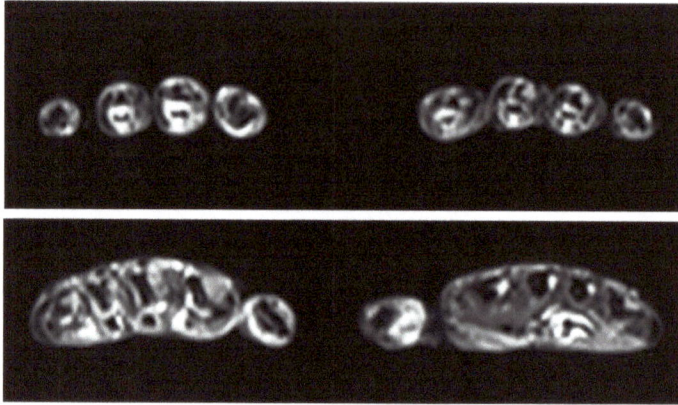

Fig. (65). T2-weighted STIR axial images at the level of the proximal phalanx and the metacarpal heads show synovitis of the digital flexor tendon sheaths of the fingers.

SLE   rhupus   RA

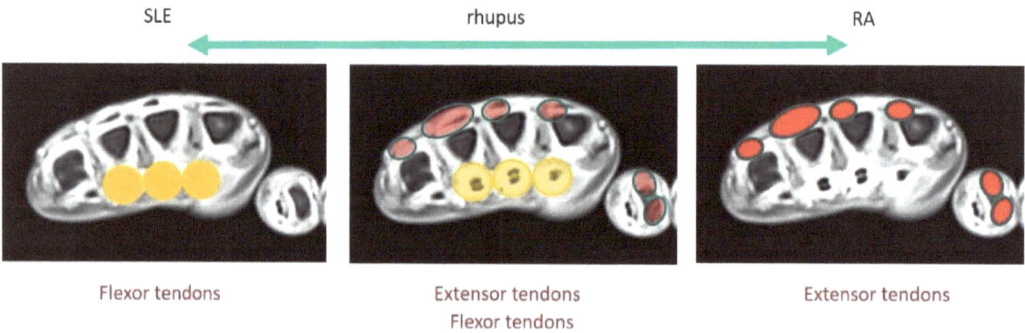

Flexor tendons   Extensor tendons   Extensor tendons
                        Flexor tendons

Fig. (66). The distribution of tenosynovitis in RA, SLE and rhupus syndrome (RA and SLE).

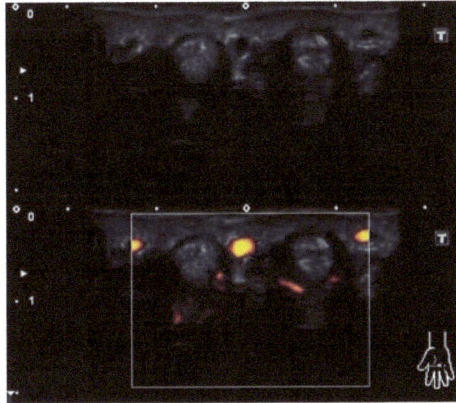

Fig. (67). Transverse gray-scale and power Doppler US images at the level of the metacarpals show tenosynovitis of the digital flexor tendon sheaths with PD signals.

Wrists

Extensor Tendon Compartments

The extensor tendons at the wrist run through the extensor retinaculum in six compartments with synovial sheaths (Figs. **68** and **69**).

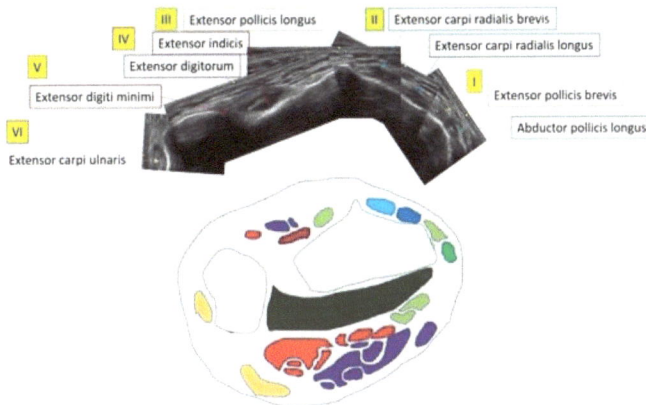

Fig. (68). The dorsal extensor tendons of the wrist in a normal person. There are six (1-6) separate compartments including I (APL, abductor pollicis longus; EPB, extensor pollicis brevis), II (ECRB, extensor carpi radialis brevis; ECRL, extensor carpi radialis longus), III (ECU, extensor carpi ulnaris), IV (EDC, extensor digitorum communis; EI, extensor indicis), V (EDM, extensor digiti minimi) and VI (extensor carpi ulnaris).

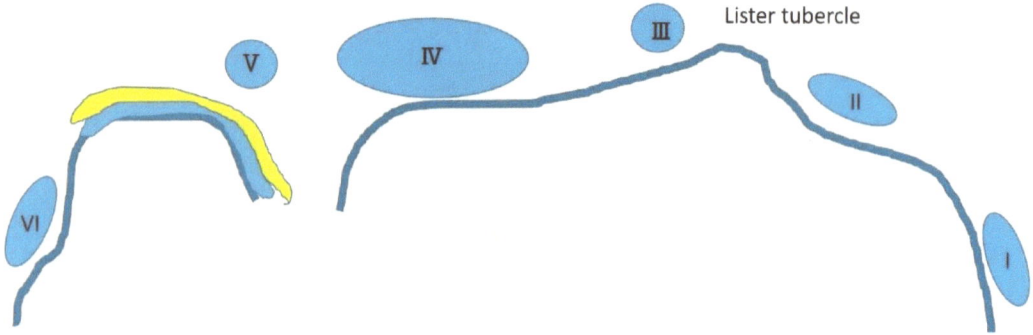

Fig. (69). A shame of the dorsal extensor tendons of the wrist.

The First Compartment

Locating the most radial side (Fig. **70**).

The extensor pollicis brevis and the abductor pollicis longus to insert to the thumb.

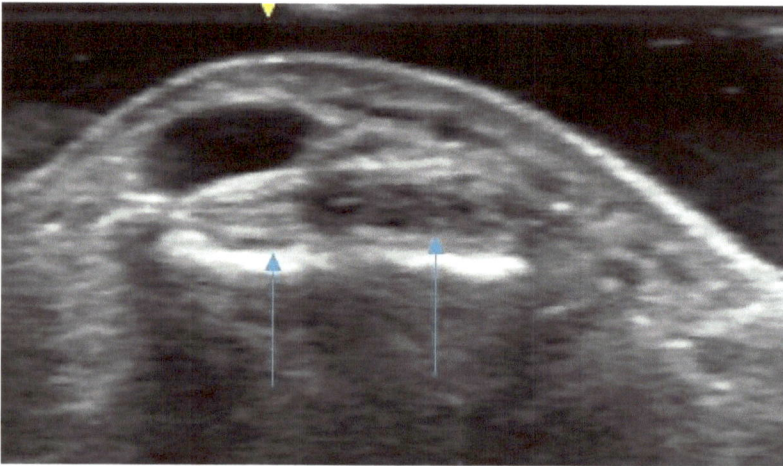

Fig. (70). Transverse gray-scale US image of the first compartment in a patient with RA.

The Second Compartment

Two radial wrist extensors (Fig. **71**)

The extensor carpi radialis longus

The extensor carpi radialis brevis

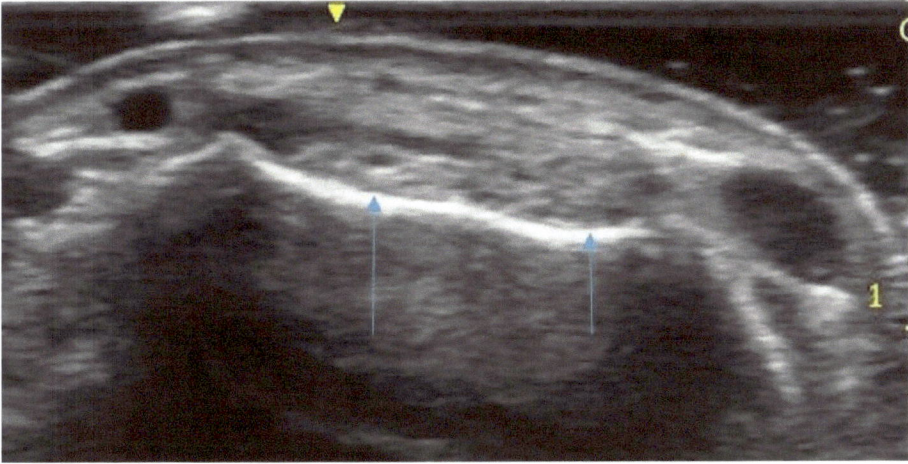

Fig. (71). Transverse gray-scale US image of the second compartment in a patient with RA.

The Third Compartment

The extensor pollicis longus (Fig. **72**)

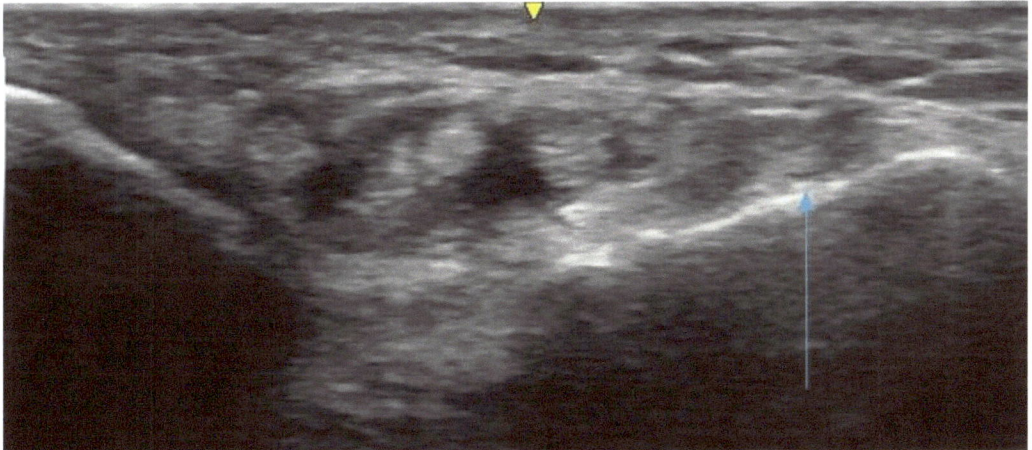

Fig. (72). Transverse gray-scale US image of the third compartment in a patient with RA.

The Fourth Compartment

The largest compartment (Figs. **73-76**)

The extensors of the digits

The extensor digitorum communis

The extensor indicis proprius

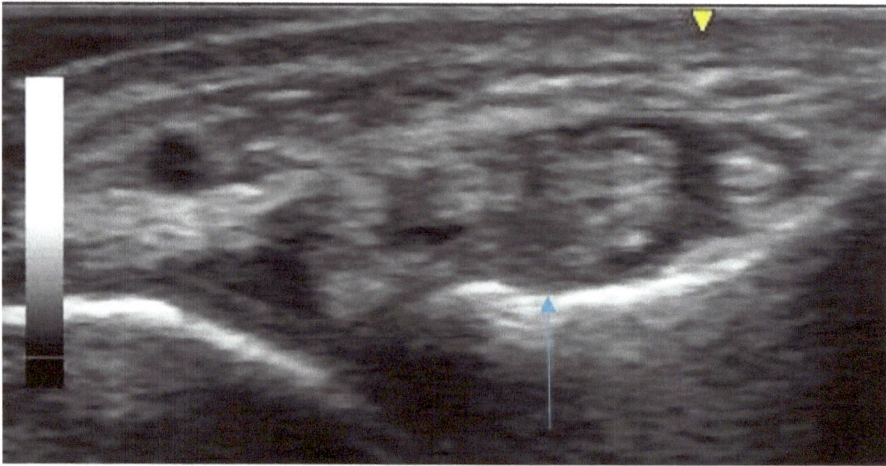

Fig. (73). Transverse gray-scale US image of the fourth compartment in a patient with RA.

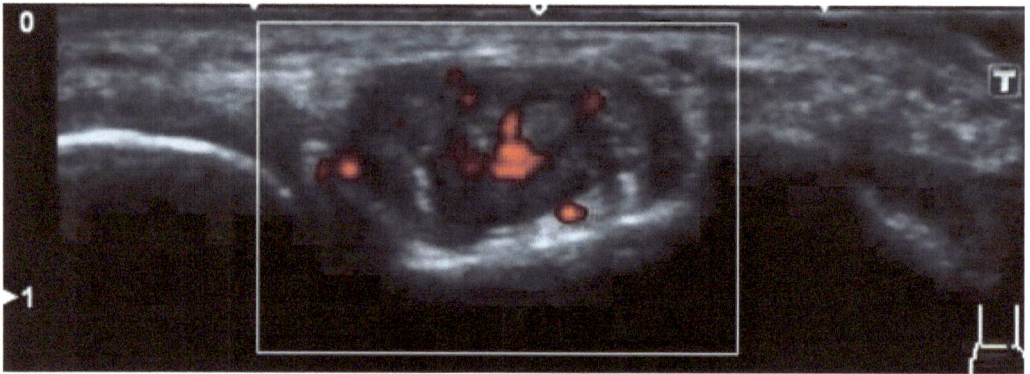

Fig. (74). Transverse power Doppler US image shows tenosynovitis of the extensor digitorum communis with PD signals.

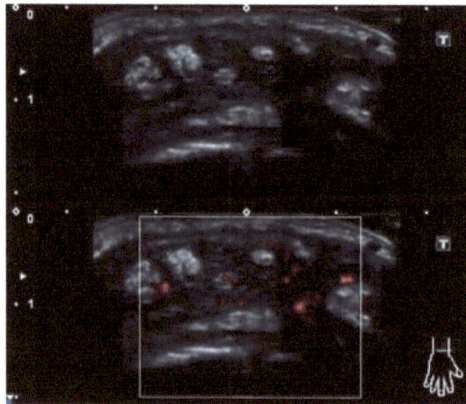

Fig. (75). Transverse gray-scale and power Doppler US images show the tenosynovitis of the fourth compartment in a patient with rhupus (RA and SLE).

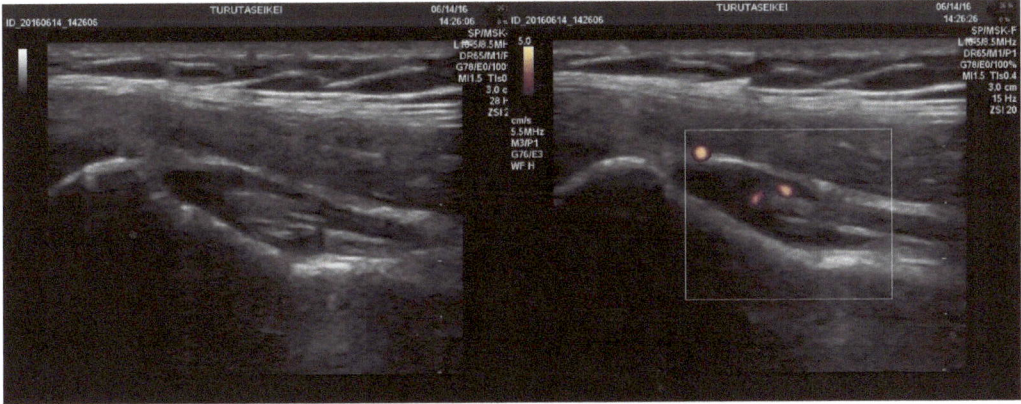

Fig. (76). Longitudinal power Doppler US images show tenosynovitis of the extensor digitorum communis (the fourth compartment).

The Fifth Compartment

The extensor digiti minimi (Fig. **77**)

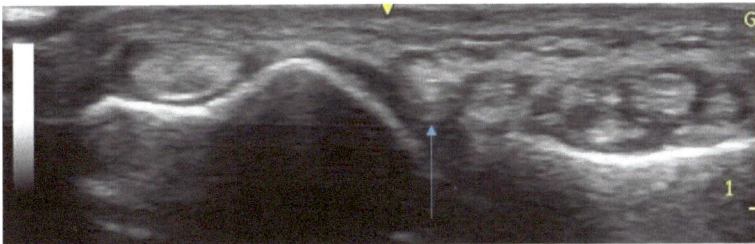

Fig. (77). Transverse gray-scale US image of the fifth compartment in a patient with RA.

The Sixth Compartment

The extensor carpi ulnaris (Figs. **78** and **79**)

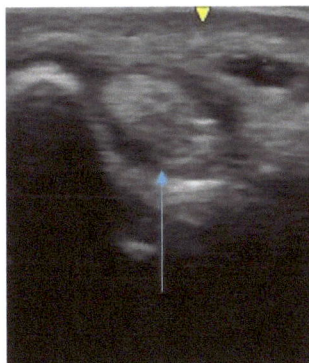

Fig. (78). Transverse gray-scale US image of the sixth compartment in a patient with RA.

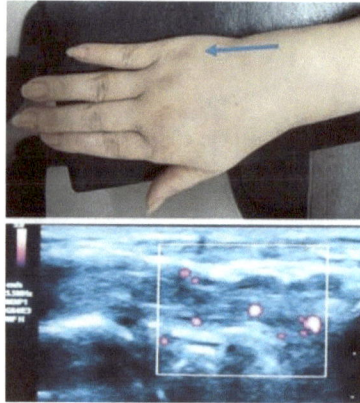

Fig. (79). Phtograph and longitudinal power Doppler US image show tenosynovitis of the compartment of VI (the extensor carpi ulnaris) in a patient with RA.

Flexor Tendons

Tenosynovitis of the flexor tendons in RA (Figs. **80** and **81**).

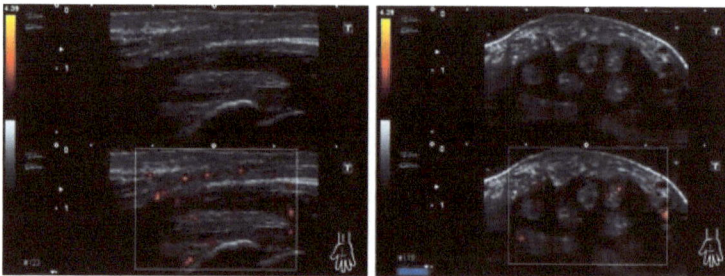

Fig. (80). Tenosynovitis of the flexor digitorum profundus and the flexor digitorum superficialis.

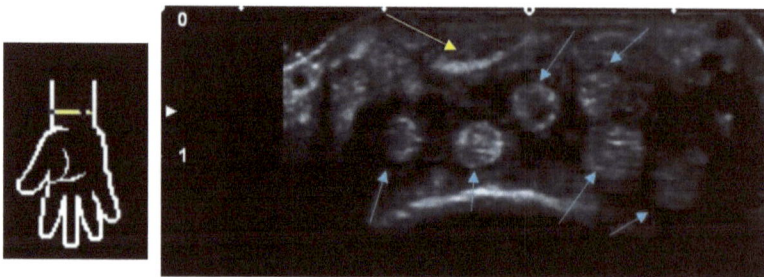

Fig. (81). Carpal tunnel synovitis in a patient with RA. Transverse gray-scale US image of the carpal tunnel shows increased PD signals around the flexor tendons (blue arrows) consistent with active tenosynovitis and bursitis. There is also compression of the median nerve within the carpal tunnel (yellow arrow).

Shoulders

Tenosytnovitis of the long head biceps in RA (Fig. **82**).

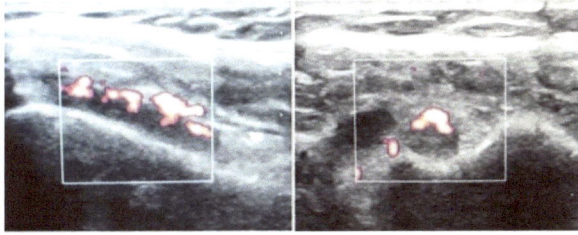

Fig. (82). Longitudinal and transverse power Doppler US images of the shoulder show long head biceps tenosytnovitis with PD signals.

Feet

Tenosynovitis of the tendon of extensor digitorum muscle in RA (Fig. **83**).

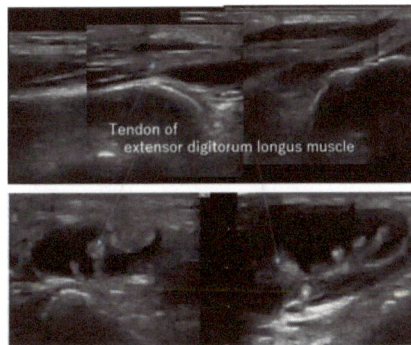

Fig. (83). Longitudinal (upper panel) and transverse (lower panels) gray-scale US images of the dorsal aspect of the foot show tenosynovitis of the tendon of extensor digitorum muscle.

ENTHESITIS AND TENDONITIS

Shoulders

Tendinitis of the supraspinatus tendon in RA (Fig. **84**).

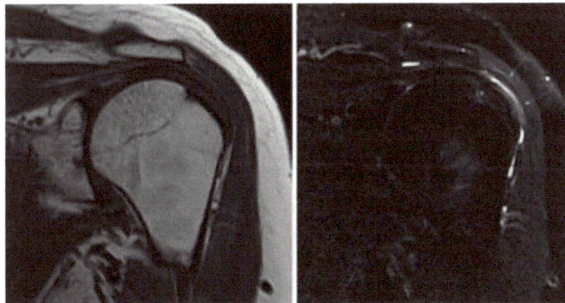

Fig. (84). MR images (left panel, T1 ; right panel, T2 FS) of the left shoulder show tendinitis of the supraspinatus tendon in a patient with RA.

Knees

Nomal Images of US of the knees (Figs. **85 - 89**).

Tendinitis and enthesitis of the knees in RA (Figs. **90-92**).

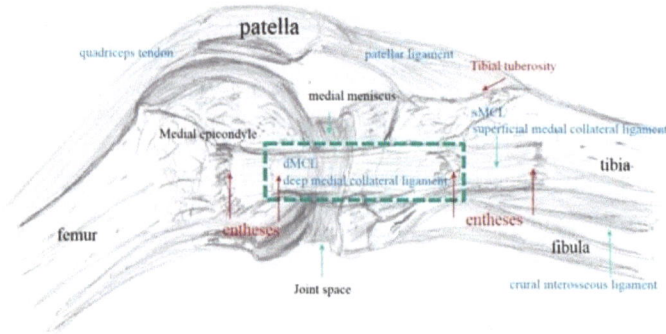

Fig. (85). A schema of the ligaments of the knees.

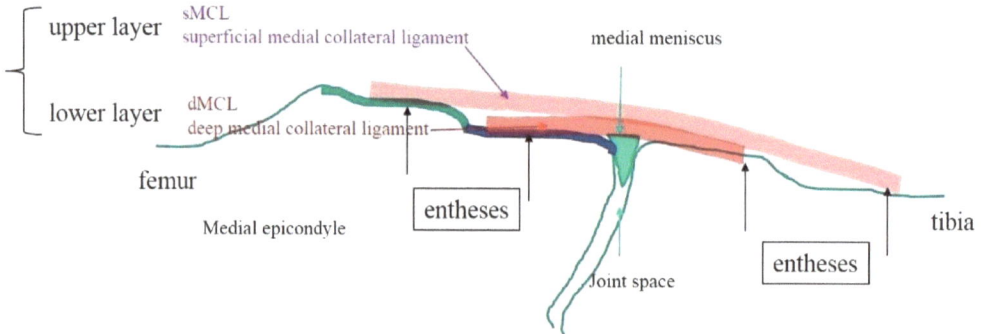

Fig. (86). A simplified schema of the ligaments of the medial aspect of the knee.

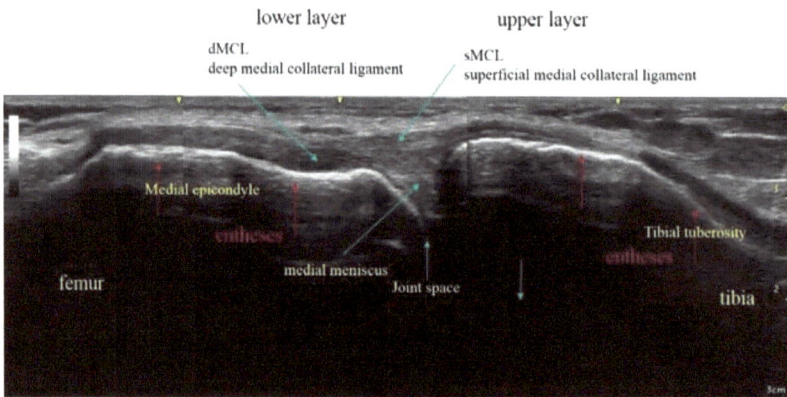

Fig. (87). Longitudinal gray-scale US image of medial aspect of the knee.

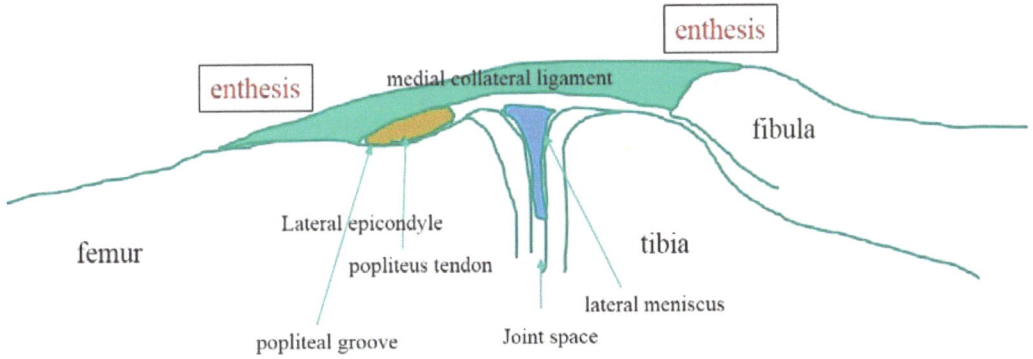

Fig. (88). A simplified schema of the ligaments of the lateral aspect of the knee.

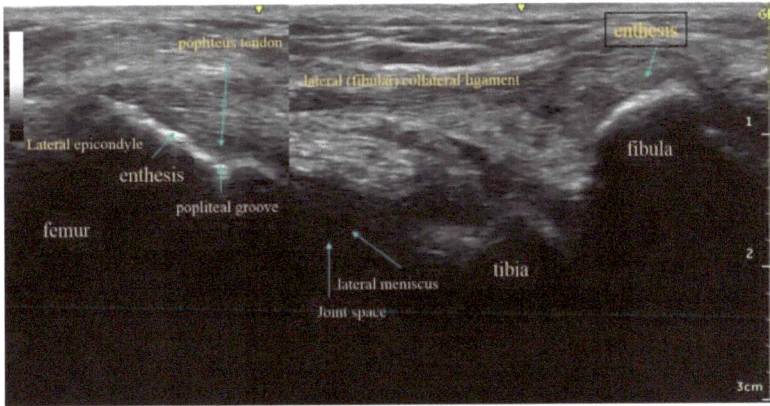

Fig. (89). Longitudinal gray-scale US image of the lateral aspect of the knee.

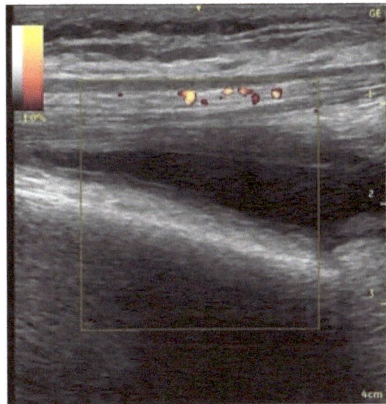

Fig. (90). US image of the tendon of the quadriceps shows PD signals that suggest tendonitis.

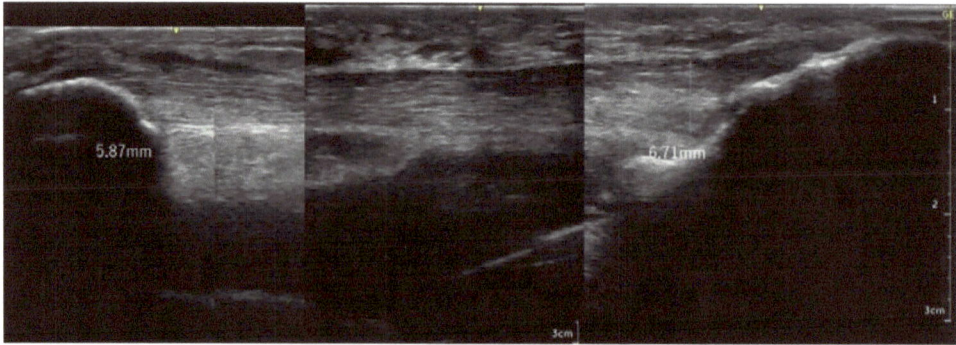

Fig. (91). Patella tendinitis. Longitudinal gray-scale US image shows thicknesses of the patella tendon and the entheseal insertions. In normal Japanese persons, the mean thickness of the proximal patellar tendon insertions is 3.25 (3.08-3.43) mm and that of the distal patellar tendon insertions is 3.84 mm (3.64-4.05) [1].

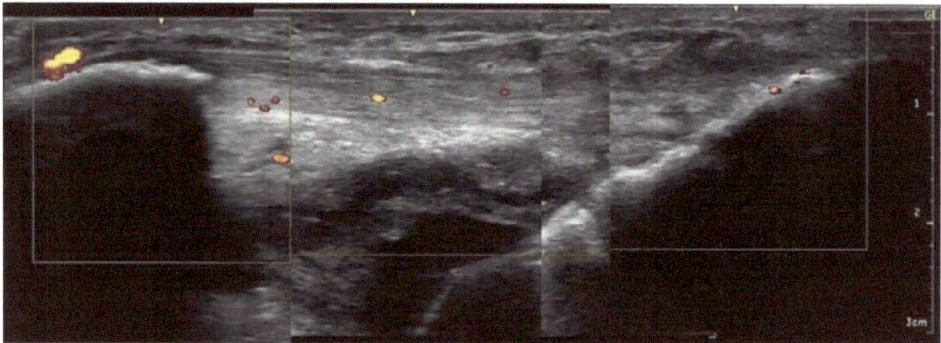

Fig. (92). Longitudinal power Doppler US image shows patella tendinitis and enthesitis in a patient with RA.

Feet

Tendinitis and enthesitis of the Achilles' tendon in RA (Figs. **93** and **94**).

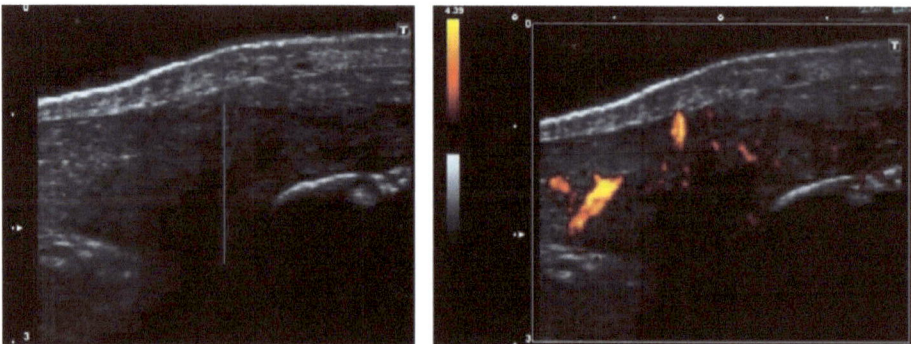

Fig. (93). Longitudinal gray-scale and power Doppler US images show tendinitis and enthesitis of the Achilles' tendon in a patient with RA. Thickness of the tendon and PD signals are observed.

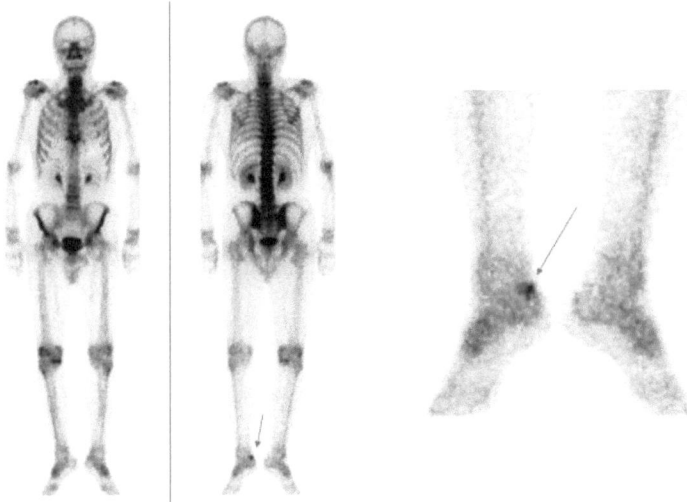

Fig. (94). Bone scan suggests enthesitis of the Achilles' tendon in a patient with RA.

CALCIFICATION

Hands

Calcification in a rheumatoid nodule (Fig. **95**).

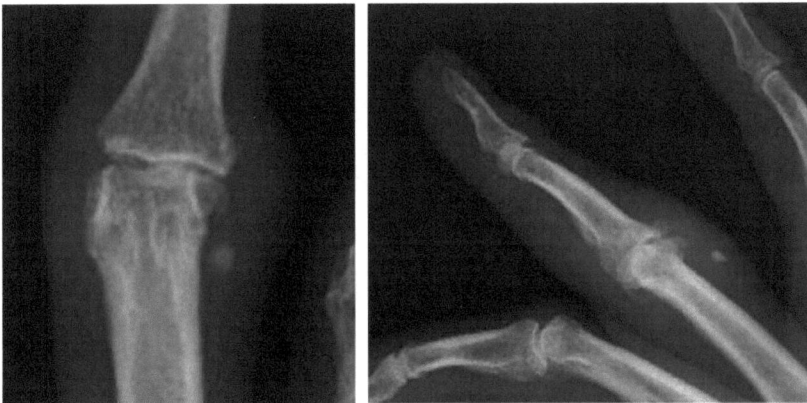

Fig. (95). Calcification in a rheumatoid nodule at the third PIP joint in a patient with RA.

Calcium hydroxyapatite can deposit in the soft tissues including the muscles, the capsules, the bursae and the tendon sheaths (Figs. **96** and **97**).

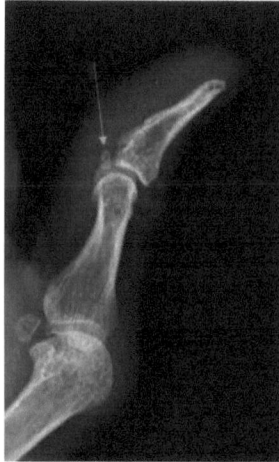

Fig. (96). Hydroxyapatite deposition at the first IP joint in a patient with RA.

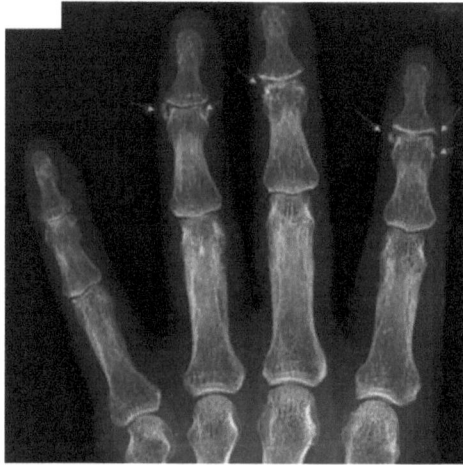

Fig. (97). Hydroxyapatite deposition at the DIP joints.

Elbows

Calcification of the elbows (Figs. **98 - 100**).

Shoulders

Calcification of the shoulders (Figs. **101 - 104**).

Legs

Calcification of the legs in RA (Figs. **105 - 107**).

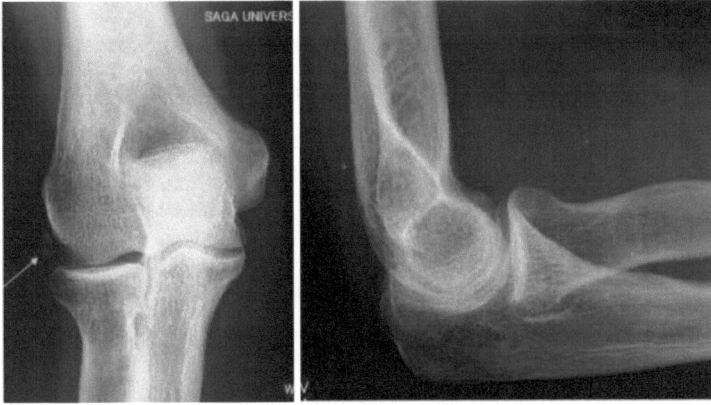

Fig. (98). Calcificartion of the extensor carpi radialis brevis (ECRB) and external humeral epicondylitis at the right elbow in a patient with RA.

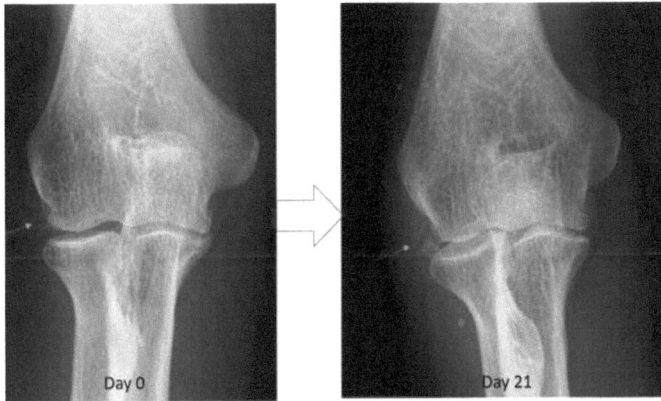

Fig. (99). Calcification at the right elbow eventually ruptures into the joint space and arthritis occurs.

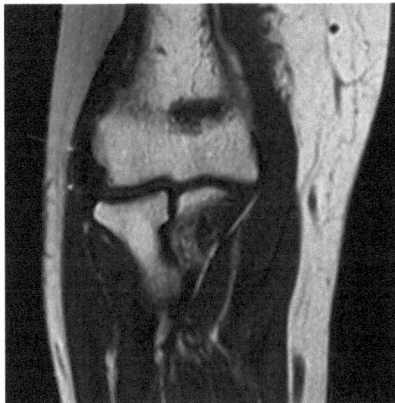

Fig. (100). T1-weighted MR image shows low signals in the tendon and the bursa of the elbow.

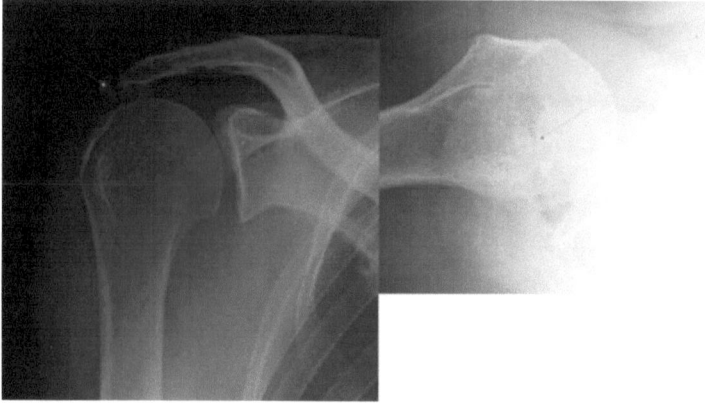

Fig. (101). Chronic calcifying tendonitis of the shoulder in a patient with RA. AP veiw of the right shoulder shows calcification of the tendons around the shoulder.

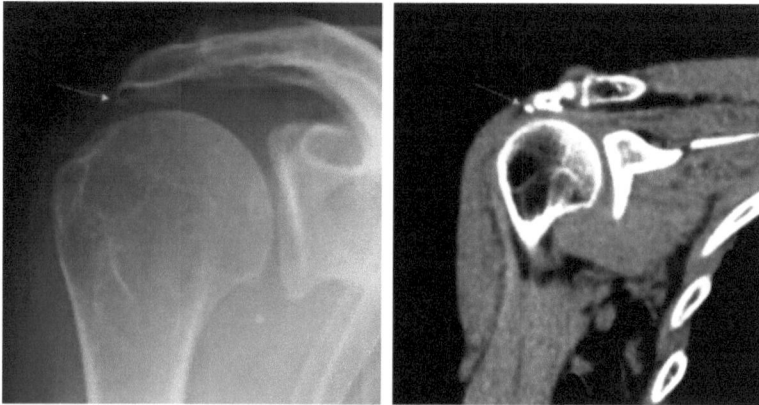

Fig. (102). Plain radiograph and CT image show calcification of the shoulder in a patient with RA.

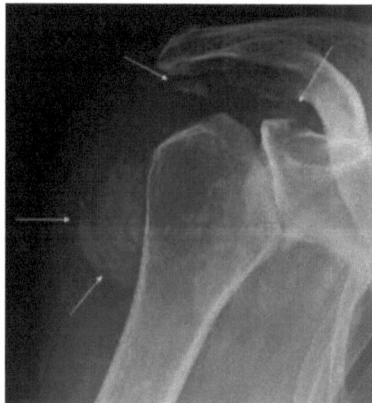

Fig. (103). Calcification of the shoulder due to hydroxyapatite deposition disease (HADD) ("Milwaukee shoulder"). Plain radiograph also shows a severely destructive arthropathy.

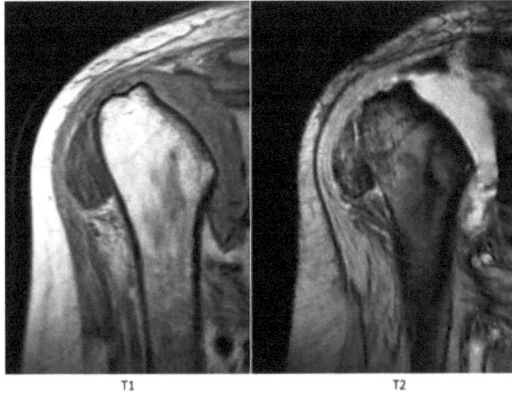

Fig. (104). T1- and T2-weighted MR images of the shoulder show <u>the features of HADD</u> in the same patient with RA (Fig. **103**).

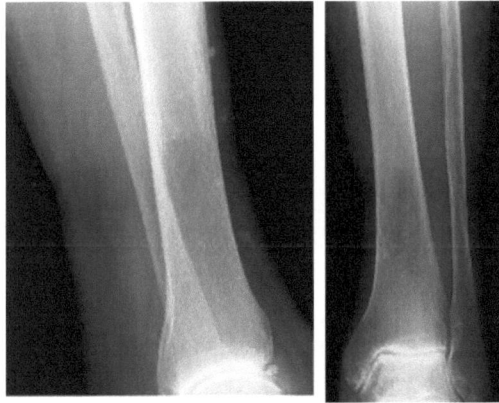

Fig. (105). Subcutaneous calcification in a patient with RA.

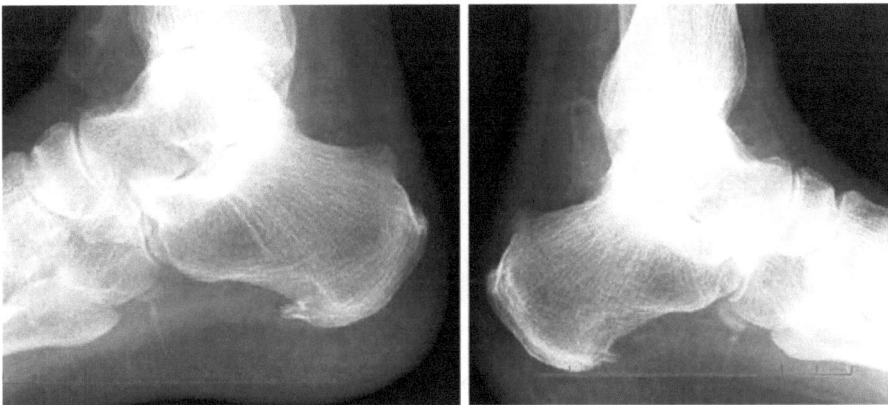

Fig. (106). Calcification of the feet in a patient with RA and HADD.

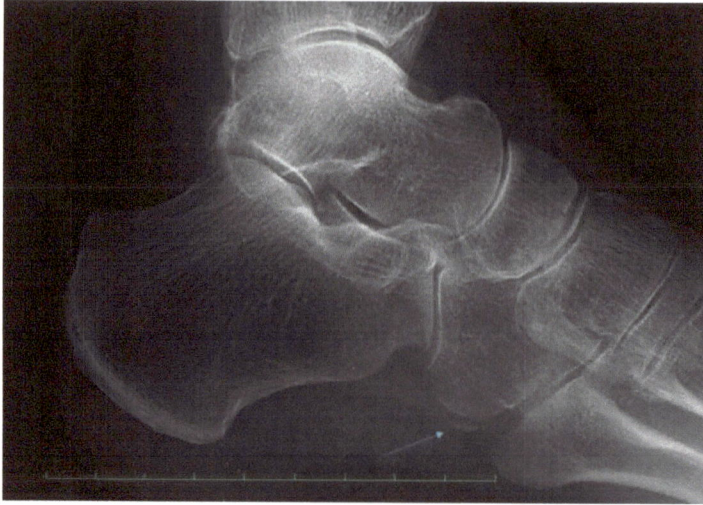

Fig. (107). Calcification of the feet in a patient with RA and HADD.

NERVES

Median Nerve

US image of the median nerve (Fig. **108**).

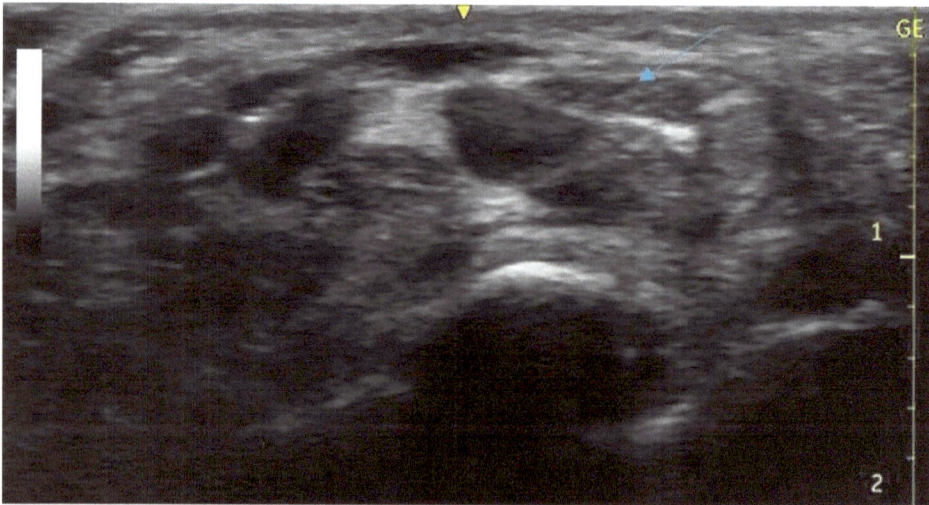

Fig. (108). Transverse gray-scale US image of the wrist shows the median nerve.

Carpal Tunnel Syndrome; Carpal Canal Syndrome; CTS

Carpal tunnel syndrome (CTS) (Fig. **109**).

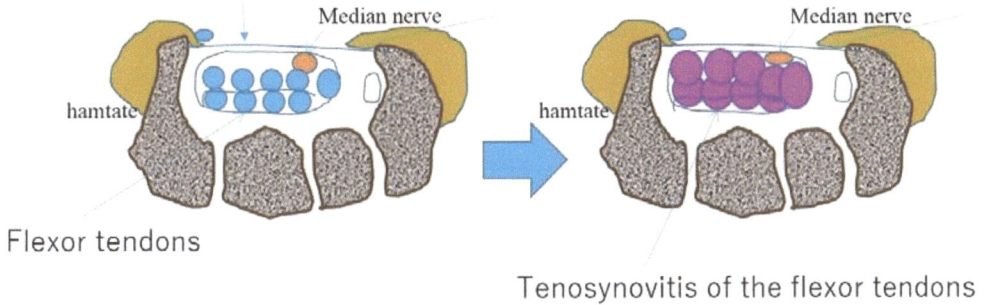

Fig. (109). Carpal tunnel syndrome (CTS) is caused by compression of the median nerve due to tenosynovitis of the flexor tendons in RA as it runs through the carpal tunnel at the wrist.

Vessels

Thrombophlebitis

The thrombophlebitis in RA is important because the symptoms are like the rupture of a Baker's cyst. Sometimes, the rupture of a Baker's cyst and thrombophlebitis coexist due to high pressure on the deep venous system by the cyst (Fig. **110**).

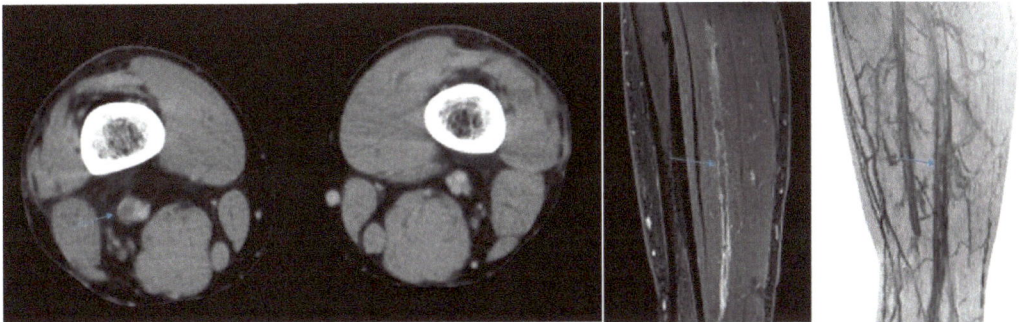

Fig. (110). Thrombophlebitis in a patient with RA.

CONSENT FOR PUBLICATION

Not applicable.

CONFLICT OF INTEREST

The author (editor) declares no conflict of interest, financial or otherwise.

ACKNOWLEDGEMENTS

The authors thank Ms. K. Eguchi and A. Ibe for secretarial assistance.

REFERENCES

[1]   Kamo K, Nishino S, Matsuda Y, Kawashima A, Yoshimoto T. The normal thicknesses of entheseal insertions in the lower limbs of Japanese individuals. Japan Society of Ultrasonics in Medicine 2015; 46: 695-9.
[http://dx.doi.org/10.3179/jjmu.JJMU.A.49]

[2]   Guerra I, Algaba A, Pérez-Calle JL, *et al.* Induction of psoriasis with anti-TNF agents in patients with inflammatory bowel disease: a report of 21 cases. J Crohn's Colitis 2012; 6(5): 518-23.
[http://dx.doi.org/10.1016/j.crohns.2011.10.007] [PMID: 22398059]

Appendixes

Normal Radiographs and Images of US and MRI.

HANDS AND WRISTS

Normal Radiographs and Images of US and MRI of the hands and wrists (Figs. **1-16**).

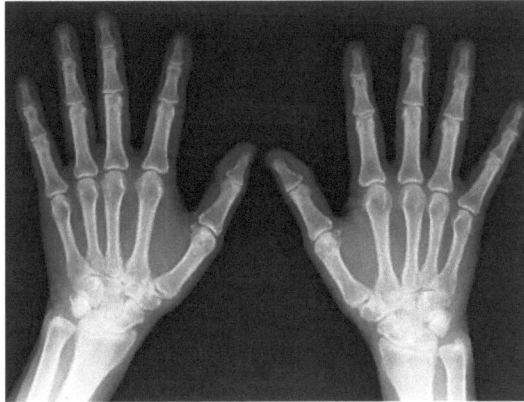

Fig. (1). PA view of the hands in a normal person.

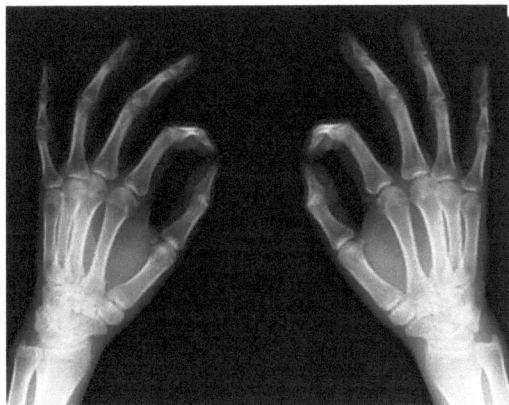

Fig. (2). Oblique view of the hands in a normal person.

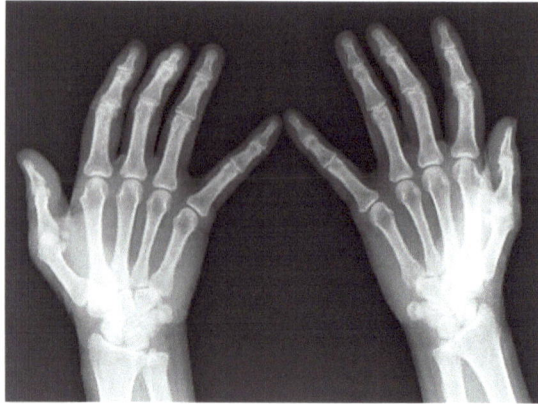

Fig. (3). Nørgaard view of the hands in a normal person.

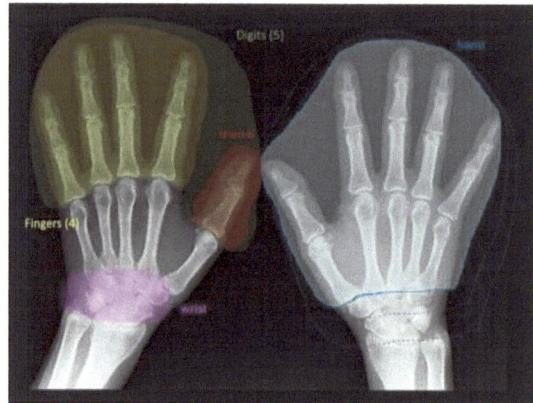

Fig. (4). Radiographic anatomy of the skeleton of the hands and wrists: PA view.

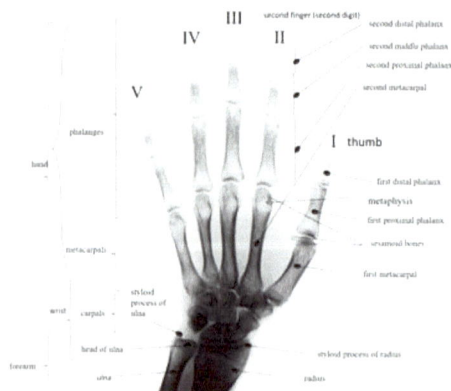

Fig. (5). Radiographic anatomy of the skeleton of the hand and the wrist: PA view.

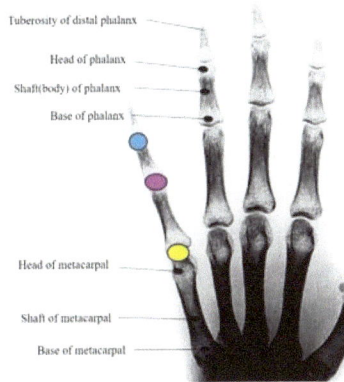

Fig. (6). The bones of the phalanges and metacarpals.

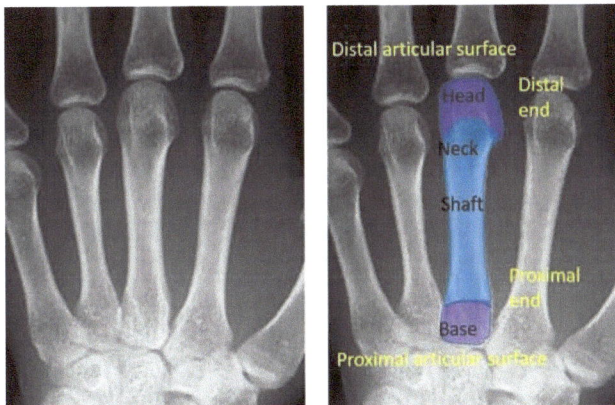

Fig. (7). Radiographic anatomy of the skeleton of the finger: PA view.

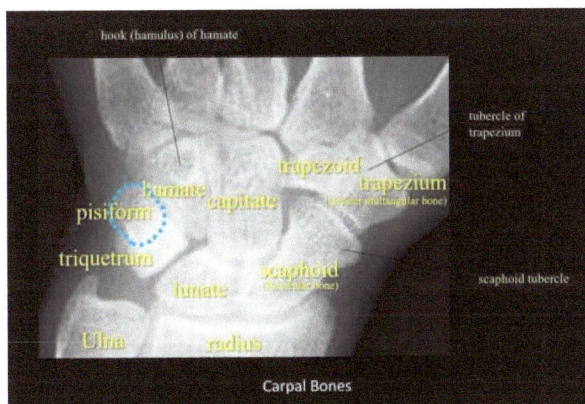

Fig. (8). Radiographic anatomy of the skeleton of carpal bones.

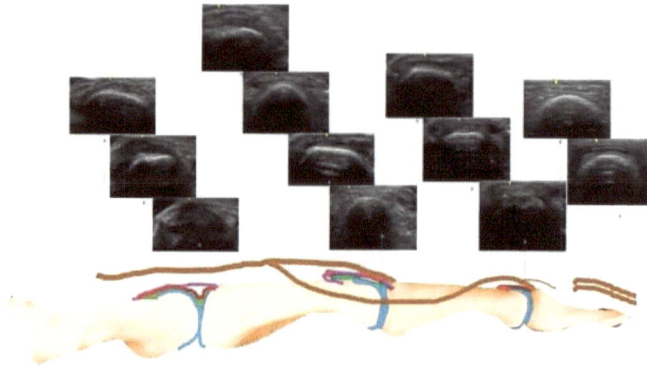

Fig. (9). The transverse gray-scale US images show normal bone shapes of the finger. Surface shapes of bones tell the position in the finger. Note the lack of bone at the joints.

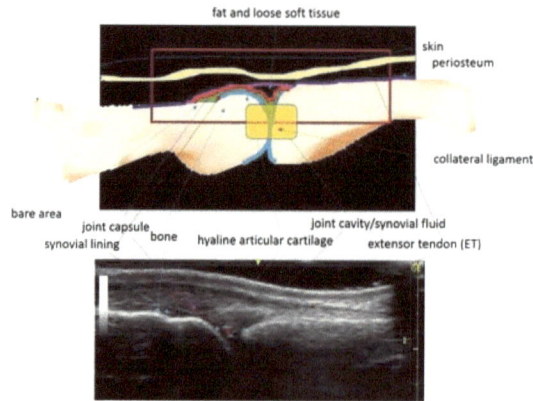

Fig. (10). US image of the MCP joint in a normal person.

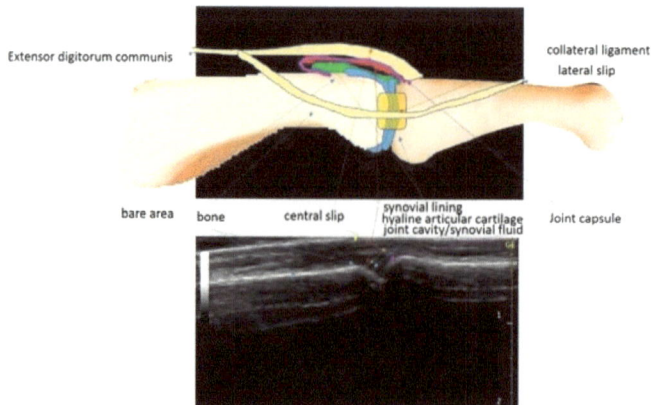

Fig. (11). US image of the PIP joint in a normal person.

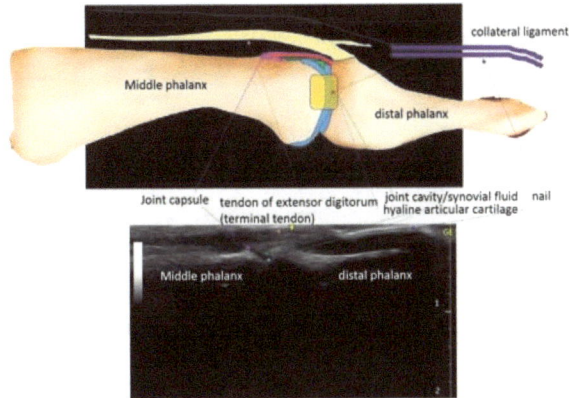

Fig. (12). US image of the DIP joint in a normal person.

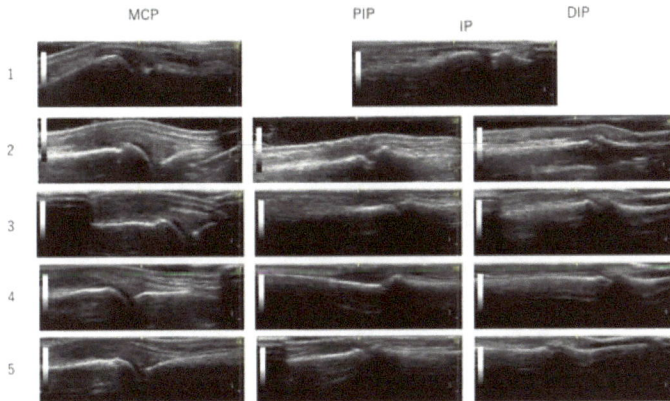

Fig. (13). Longitudinal gray-scale US images show normal joints of the hand.

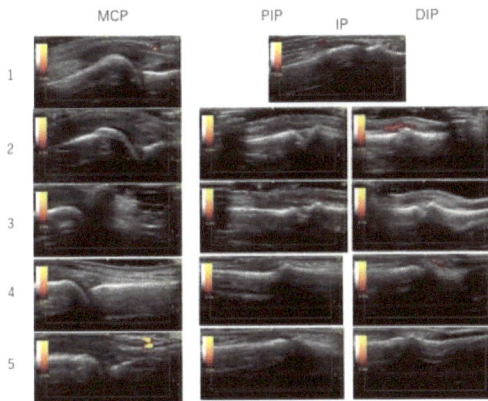

Fig. (14). Longitudinal power Doppler US images show normal joints of the hand.

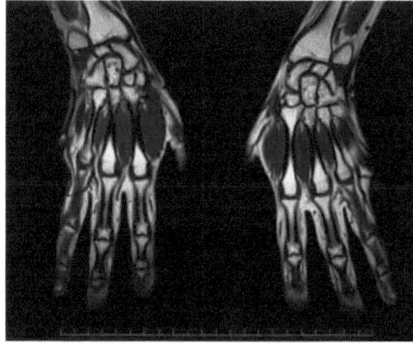

Fig. (15). Coronal T1 image (MRI) of the hands in a normal person.

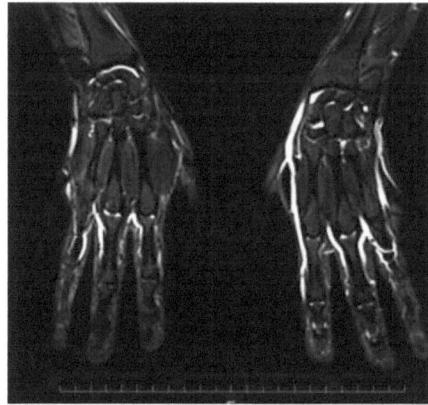

Fig. (16). Coronal T2-STIR (MRI) of the hands in a normal person.

ELBOWS

Normal Radiographs of the elbows (Figs. **17-21**).

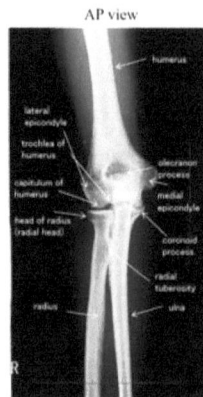

Fig. (17). Radiographic anatomy of the skeleton of the elbow: AP view.

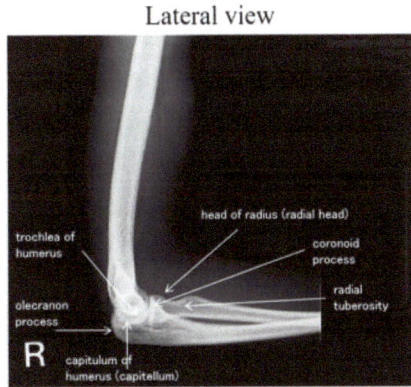

Fig. (18). Radiographic anatomy of the skeleton of the elbow: lateral view.

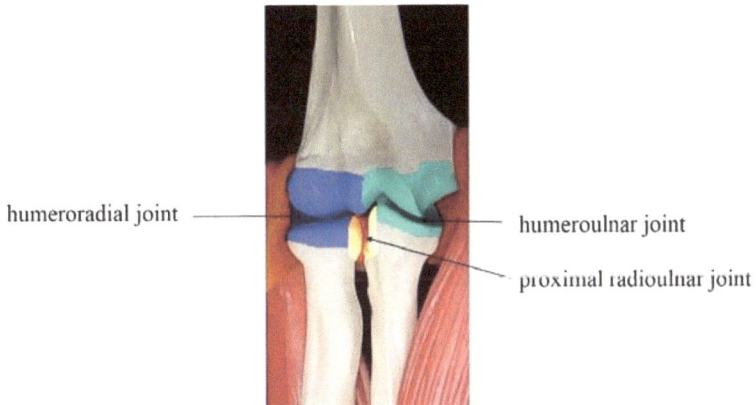

Fig. (19). Joints of the elbow. There are three joints in the elbow, the humeroradial joint, the humeroulnar joint and the proximal radioulnar joint.

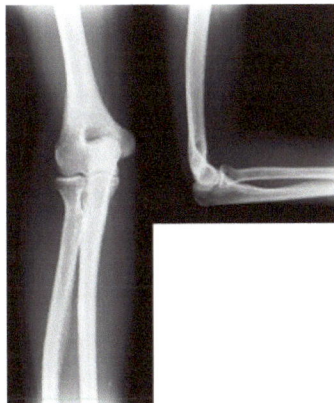

Fig. (20). PA and lateral views of the right elbow in a normal person.

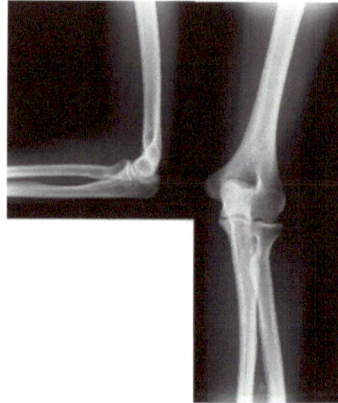

Fig. (21). PA and lateral views of the left elbow in a normal person.

SHOULDERS

Normal Radiographs of the shoulders (Figs. **22-25**).

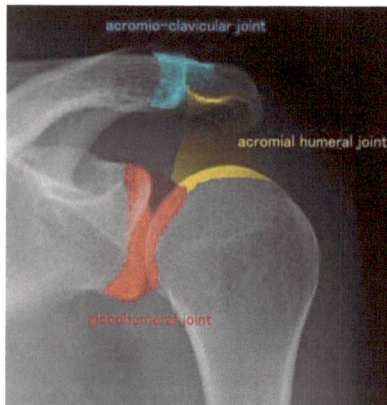

Fig. (22). There are three joints in the shoulder, the glenohumeral, the acromial humeral, and the acromioclavicular (AC) joint.

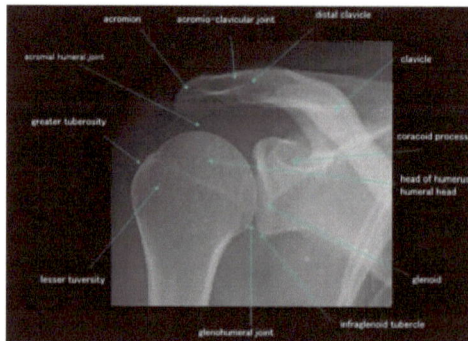

Fig. (23). Radiographic anatomy of the skeleton of the shoulder: AP view.

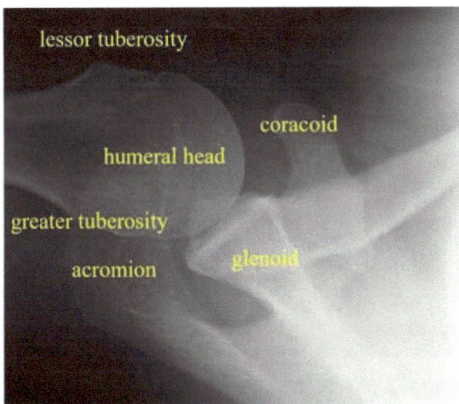

Fig. (24). Radiographic anatomy of the skeleton of the shoulder: axillary view.

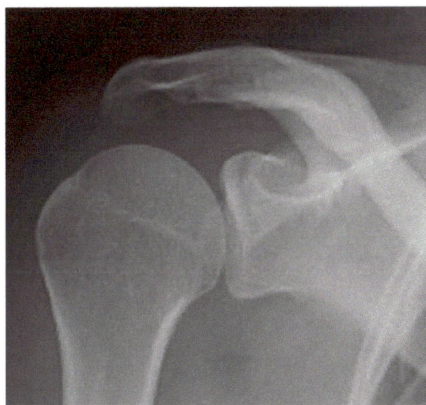

Fig. (25). AP views (with external and internal rotation) of the right shoulder in a normal person.

HIPS

Normal Radiographs of the hips (Figs. **26-28**).

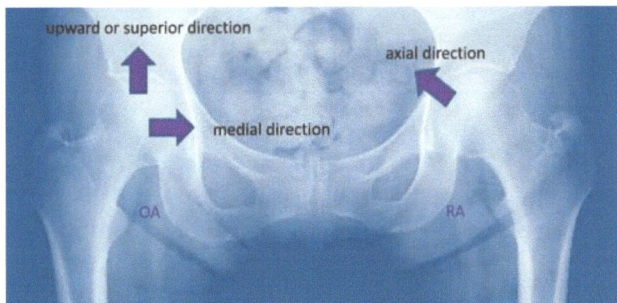

Fig. (26). In OA, the cartilage at the hip joint is not uniformaly lost and the femoral head migrates in an upward or a medial direction. However, in RA, the cartilage is uniformaly lost and then the femoral head migrates in an axial (superior medial) direction.

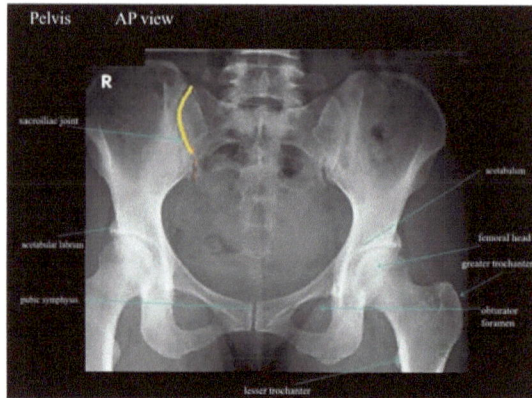

Fig. (27). Radiographic anatomy of the skeleton of the hip: AP view.

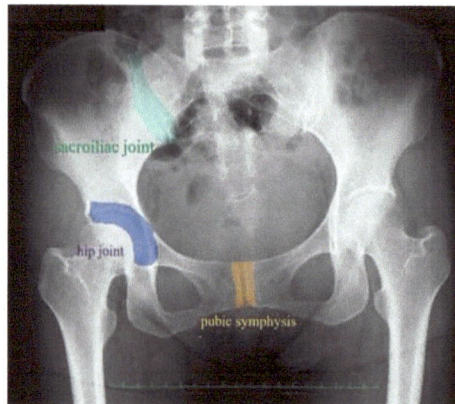

Fig. (28). There are three joints in the pelvis, the hip joint, the pubic symphysis, and the sacroiliac joint.

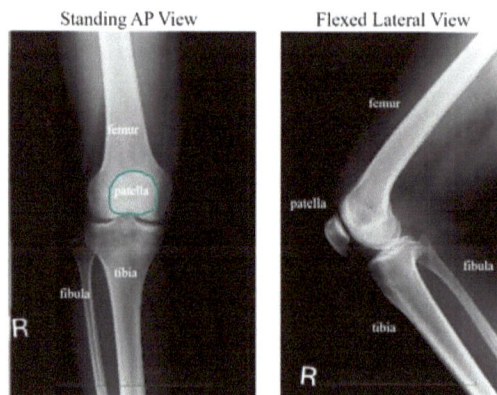

Fig. (29). Radiographic anatomy of the skeleton of the right knee: AP view and lateral view.

KNEES

Normal Radiographs and Images of US of the knees (Figs. **29-36**).

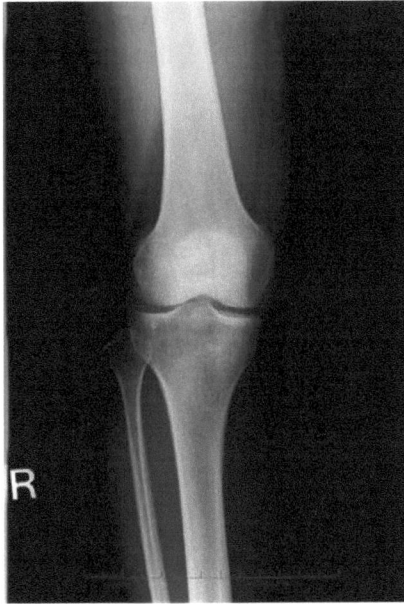

Fig. (30). AP view (with standing semiflexed position) of the right knee in a normal person.

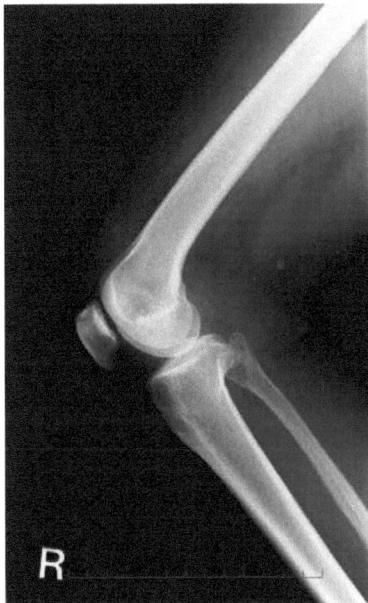

Fig. (31). Flexed lateral view (non-standing) of the right knee in a normal person.

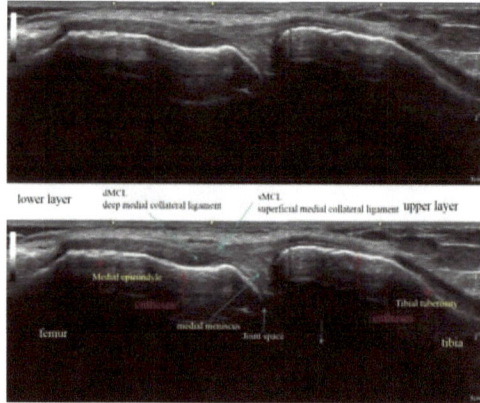

Fig. (32). Longitudinal gray-scale US image of medial aspect of the knee.

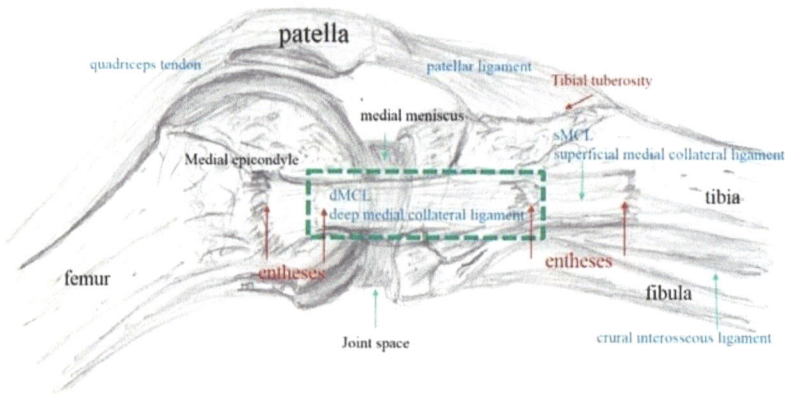

Fig. (33). A schema of the ligaments of the knees.

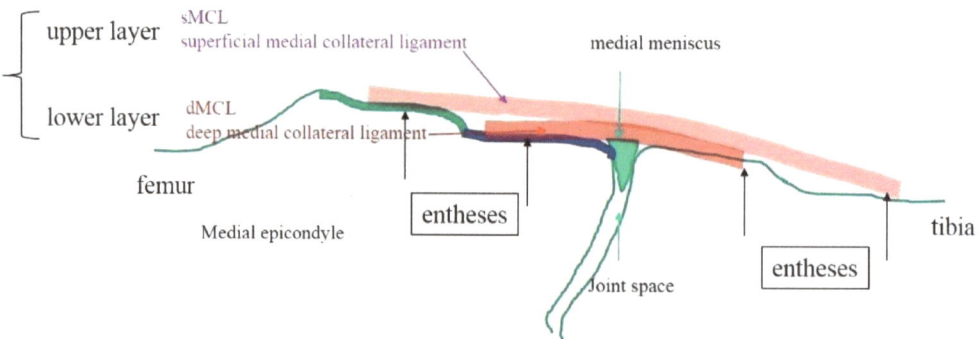

Fig. (34). A simplified schema of the ligaments of the medial aspect of the knee.

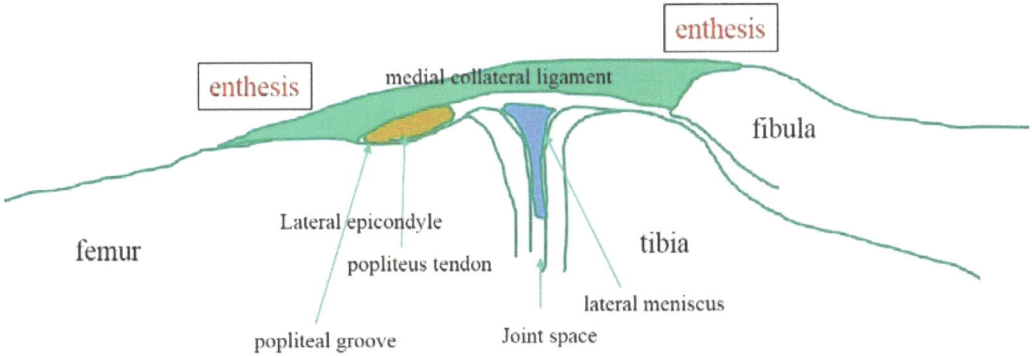

Fig. (35). A simplified schema of the ligaments of the lateral aspect of the knee.

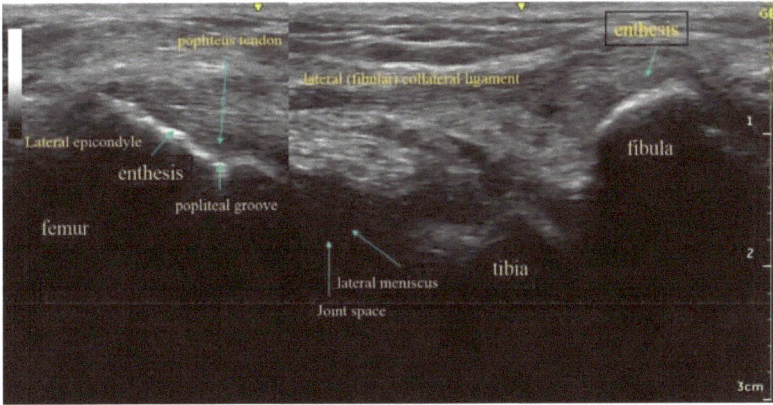

Fig. (36). Longitudinal gray-scale US image of the lateral aspect of the knee.

ANKLES

Normal Radiographs of the ankles (Figs. **37-39**).

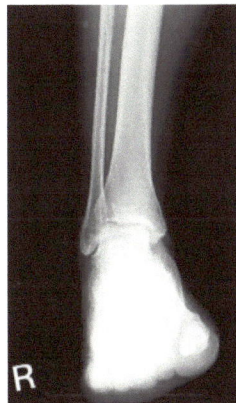

Fig. (37). AP view of the right ankle in a normal person.

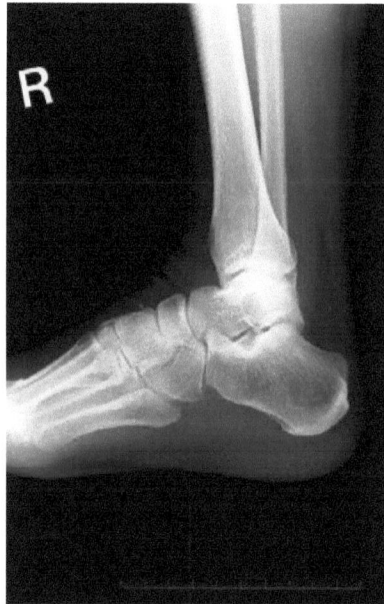

Fig. (38). AP view of the right ankle in a normal person.

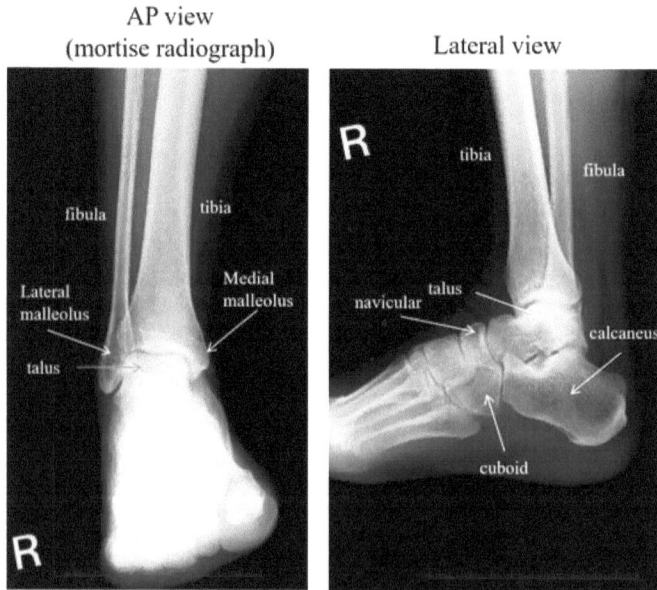

Fig. (39). Radiographic anatomy of the skeleton of the right ankle: AP view and lateral view.

FEET

Normal Radiographs of the feet (Figs. **40-44**).

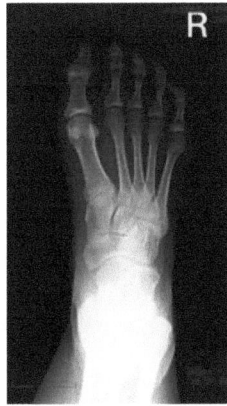

Fig. (40). AP view of the right foot in a normal person.

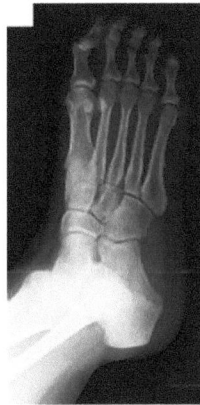

Fig. (41). Oblique view of the right foot in a normal person.

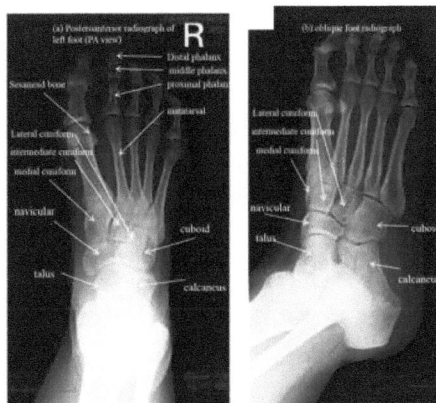

Fig. (42). Radiographic anatomy of the skeleton of the right foot: AP view and oblique view.

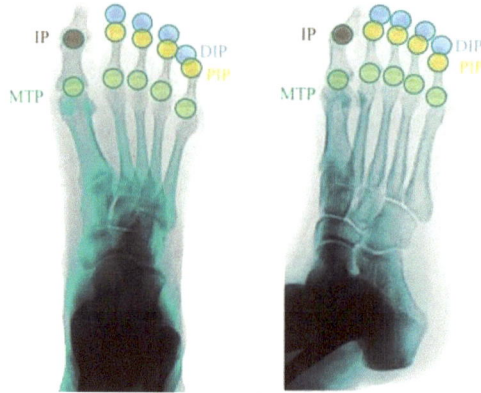

Fig. (43). Joints of the forefoot.

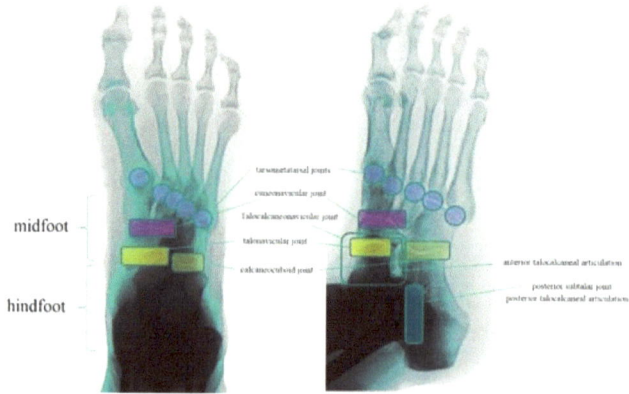

Fig. (44). Joints of the mid- and hindfoot.

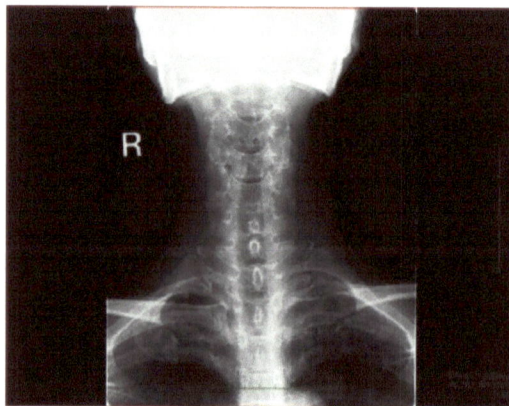

Fig. (45). AP view of the cervical spine in a normal person.

CERVICAL SPINE

Normal Radiographs of the cervical spine (Figs. **45-48**).

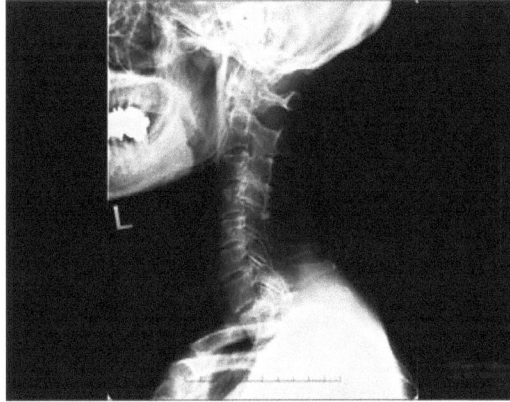

Fig. (46). Lateral view of the cervical spine in a normal person.

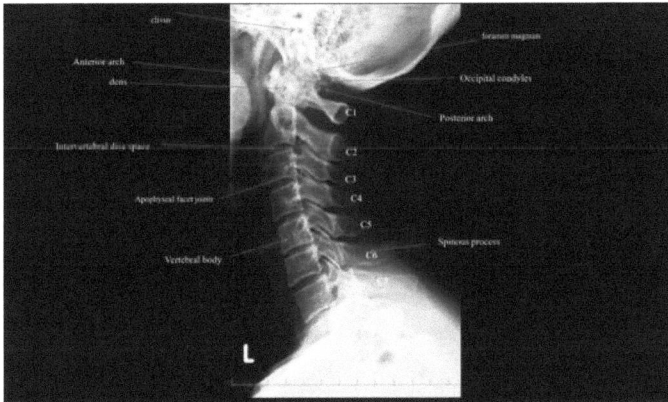

Fig. (47). Radiographic anatomy of the skeleton of the cervical spine: Lateral view.

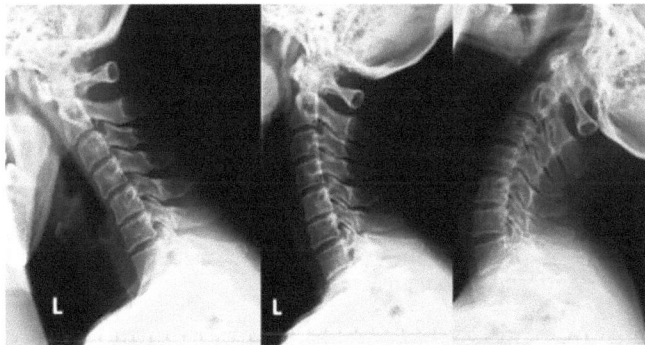

Fig. (48). Flexion and extension lateral radiographs of the cervical spine.

THORACIC SPINE

Normal Radiographs of the thoracic spine (Fig. **49**).

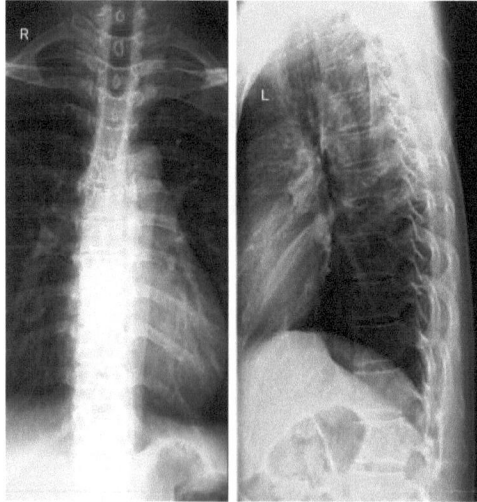

Fig. (49). Thoracic spine in a normal person.

LUMBAR SPINE

Normal Radiographs of the lumbar spine (Figs. **50-55**).

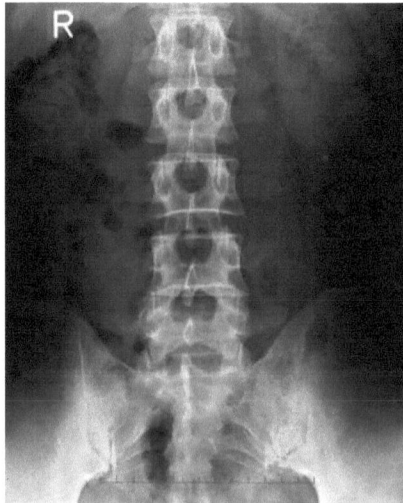

Fig. (50). AP view of the lumbar spine in a normal person.

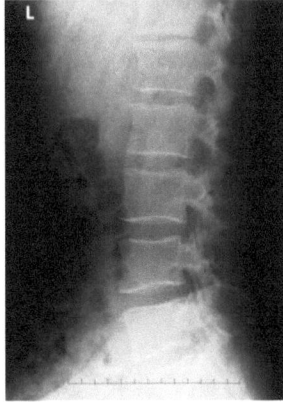

Fig. (51). Lateral view of the lumbar spine in a normal person.

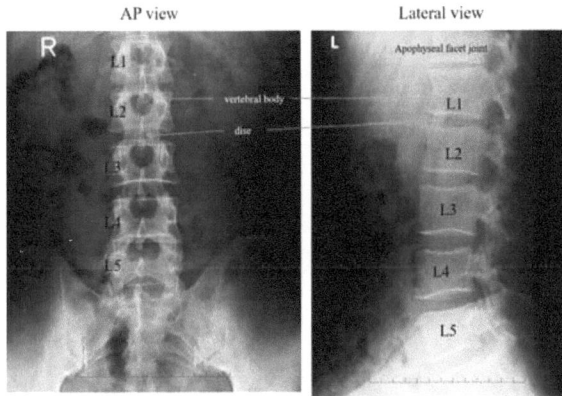

Fig. (52). Lumbar spine 2 views ; AP view and lateral view.

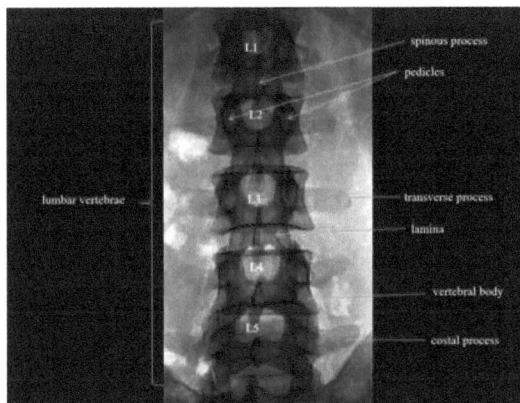

Fig. (53). Radiographic anatomy of the skeleton of the lumbar spine: AP view.

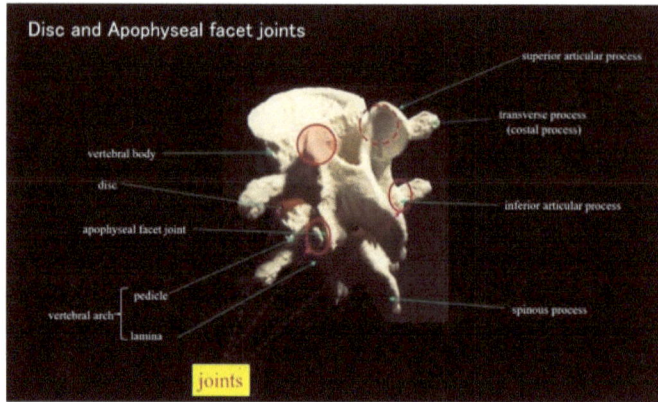

Fig. (54). Disc and apophyseal facet joints.

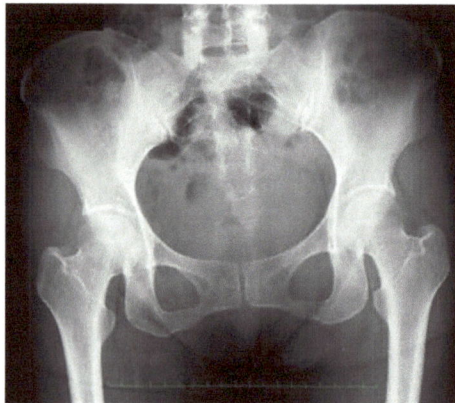

Fig. (55). AP view of the hips in a normal person.

MRI finding in RA (Fig. **56**).

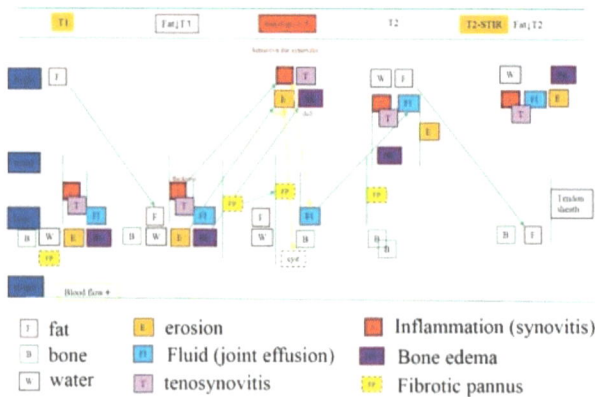

Fig. (56). MRI findings in RA.

SUBJECT INDEX

www.ingramcontent.com/pod-product-compliance
Lightning Source LLC
Chambersburg PA
CBHW050816220326
41598CB00006B/232

* 9 7 8 1 6 8 1 0 8 6 6 2 0 *